Statistics for Biology and Health

Series Editors
M. Gail, K. Krickeberg, J. Samet, A. Tsiatis, W. Wong

Statistics for Biology and Health

Borchers/Buckland/Zucchini: Estimating Animal Abundance: Closed Populations.

Burzykowski/Molenberghs/Buyse: The Evaluation of Surrogate Endpoints.

Everitt/Rabe-Hesketh: Analyzing Medical Data Using S-PLUS.

Evens/Grant: Statistical Methods in Bioinformatics: An Introduction.

Gentleman/Carey/Huber/Izirarry/Dudoit: Bioinformatics and Computational Biology Solutions Using R and Bioconductor.

Hougaard: Analysis of Multivariate Survival Data.

Keyfitz/Caswell: Applied Mathematical Demography 3rd ed.

Klein/Moeschberger: Survival Analysis: Techniques for Censored and Truncated Data, 2nd ed.

Kleinbaum: Survival Analysis: A Self-Learning Text, 2nd ed.

Kleinbaum/Klein: Logistic Regression: A Self-Learning Text, 2nd ed.

Lange: Mathematical and Statistical Methods for Genetic Analysis, 2nd ed.

Manton/Singer/Suzman: Forecasting the Health of Elderly Populations.

Martinussen/Scheike: Dynamic Regression Models for Survival Data.

Moyé: Multiple Analyses in Clinical Trials: Fundamentals for Investigators.

Nielsen: Statistical Methods in Molecular Evolution.

Parmigiani/Garrett/Irizarry/Zeger: The Analysis of Gene Expression Data: Methods and Software.

Proschan/Lan/Wittes: Statistical Monitoring of Clinical Trials: A Unified Approach.

Salsburg: The Use of Restricted Significance Tests in Clinical Trials.

Simon/Korn/McShane/Radmacher/Wright/Zhao: Design and Analysis of DNA Microarray Investigations.

Sorensen/Gianola: Likelihood, Bayesian, and MCMC Methods in Quantitative Genetics.

Stallard/Manton/Cohen: Forecasting Product Liability Claims: Epidemiology and Modeling in the Manville Asbestos Case.

Therneau/Grambsch: Modeling Survival Data: Extending the Cox Model.

Ting: Dose Finding in Drug Development.

Vittinghoff/Glidden/Shiboski/McCulloch: Regression Methods in Biostatistics: Linear, Logistic, Survival, and Repeated Measures Models.

Zhang/Singer: Recursive Partitioning in the Health Sciences.

Michael A. Proschan
K.K. Gordan Lan
Janet Turk Wittes

Statistical Monitoring
of Clinical Trials

A Unified Approach

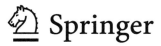 Springer

Michael A. Proschan
Biostatistics Research Branch, NIAID
Bethesda, MD 20892
USA
ProschaM@mail.nih.gov

K.K. Gordon Lan
Johnson & Johnson
Raritan, NJ 08869
glan@prdus.jnj.com

Janet Turk Wittes
Statistics Collaborative
Washington, DC 20036
USA

Series Editors

M. Gail
National Cancer Institute
Rockville, MD 20892
USA

K. Krickeberg
Le Chatelet
F-63270 Manglieu
France

J. Sarnet
Department of
  Epidemiology
School of Public Health
Johns Hopkins University
615 Wolfe Street
Baltimore,
      MD 21205-2103
USA

A. Tsiatis
Department of Statistics
North Carolina State University
Raleigh, NC 27695
USA

W. Wong
Department of Statistics
Stanford University
Stanford, CA 94305-4065
USA

ISBN-13: 978-0-387-30059-7

Library of Congress Control Number: 2005939187

Printed in the United States of America.

Printed on acid-free paper.

9 8 7 6 5 4 3 2 (corrected printing as of the 2nd printing, 2007)

springer.com

To the National Heart, Lung, and Blood Institute, which allowed biostatisticians to learn, to contribute, and to flourish.

Preface

We statisticians, especially those of us who work with randomized clinical trials within a regulatory environment, typically operate within the constraints of careful prespecification of analyses. We worry lest ad hoc response to data that we see affect the integrity of our inference. When we are involved in interim monitoring of clinical trials, however, we must have the latitude to respond with intellectual agility to unexpected findings. Perhaps that very mixture of careful prespecification—to protect the scientific integrity of the study—and data-driven modifications—to protect the interest of the participants in the trial—explains why so many of us enjoy the challenge of interim monitoring of clinical trials. Of course we must, even in that context, carefully describe the analyses we plan to conduct and the nature of the inference to which various outcomes will lead us; on the other hand, if our analyses lead to a premature—in contrast to an early—stopping of the clinical trial, there is no putting the train back on the track. The past half century has seen an explosion of methods for statistical monitoring of ongoing clinical trials with the view toward stopping the trial if the interim data show unequivocal evidence of benefit, worrisome evidence of harm, or a strong indication that the completed trial will likely show equivocal results. The methods appear to come from a variety of different underlying statistical frameworks. In this book we stress that a common mathematical unifying formulation—Brownian motion—underlies most of the basic methods. We aim to show when and how the statistician can use that framework and when the statistician must modify it to produce valid inference. We hope that our presentation will help the reader understand the relationships among commonly used methods of group-sequential analysis, conditional power, and futility analysis. The level of the book is appropriate to graduate students in biostatistics and to statisticians involved in clinical trials. One of our goals is to provide biostatisticians with tools not only to perform the necessary calculations but to be able to explain the methodology to our clinical colleagues. When the process of statistical decision-making becomes too opaque, the clinicians with whom we work tune out and leave important parts of the discussion to the statisticians.

We believe the stark separation of clinical and biostatistical thinking cannot be healthy to intelligent, thoughtful decision-making, especially when it occurs in the middle of a trial. The book represents our distillation of years of collaboration with many colleagues, both from the clinical and biostatistical worlds. All three of us spent formative years at the National Heart, Lung, and Blood Institute where Claude Lenfant, Director, encouraged the growth of biostatistics. We learned much from the many lively discussions we had there with coworkers as we grappled collectively with issues related to ongoing monitoring of clinical trials. Especially useful was the opportunity we had to attend as many Data Safety Monitoring Board meetings as we desired; those experiences formed the basis for our view of data monitoring. We hope that the next generation of biostatisticians will find themselves in an organization that recognizes the value of training by apprenticeship. We particularly want to acknowledge the insights we gained from other members of the biostatistics group—Kent Bailey, Erica Brittain, Dave DeMets, Dean Follmann, Max Halperin, Marian Fisher, Nancy Geller, Ed Lakatos, Joel Verter, Margaret Wu, and David Zucker. Physician colleagues who, while they were at NHBLI and in later years, have been especially influential have been the two Bills (William Friedewald and William Harlan), as well as Larry Friedman, Curt Furberg (who pointed out to us the distinction between premature and early stopping of trials), Gene Passamani, and Salim Yusuf. One of us (it is not hard to guess which one) is especially indebted to insights gained from Robert Wittes, who for four decades has provided thoughtful balanced judgment to a variety of issues related to clinical trials (and many other topics). And then there have been so many others with whom we have had fruitful discussions about monitoring trials over the years. Of particular note are Jonas Ellenberg, Susan Ellenberg, Tom Fleming, Genell Knatterud, and Scott Emerson. Dave DeMets has kindly agreed to maintain a constant free version of his software so that readers of this book would have access to it. We thank Mary Foulkes, Tony Lachenbruch, Jon Turk, and Joe Shih for their helpful comments on earlier versions of the book. Their suggestions helped strengthen the presentations. It goes without saying that any errors or lapses of clarity remaining are our fault. Without further ado, we stop this preface early.

Michael A. Proschan
K.K. Gordon Lan
Janet Turk Wittes
Washington D.C.
3/2006

Contents

1

Introduction

Advancement of clinical medicine depends on accurate assessment of the safety and efficacy of new therapeutic interventions. Relevant data come from a variety of sources—theoretical biology, *in vitro* experimentation, animal studies, epidemiologic data—but the ultimate test of the effect of an intervention derives from randomized clinical trials. In the simplest case, a new treatment is compared to a control in an experiment designed so that some participants receive the new treatment and others receive the control. A random mechanism governs allocation to the two groups. Well-designed, carefully conducted randomized clinical trials are generally considered the most valid tests of the effect of medical interventions for reasons both related and unrelated to randomization. Randomization produces comparable treatment groups and eliminates selection bias that could occur if the investigator subjectively decided which patients received the experimental treatment. Clinical trials often use double blinding whereby neither the patient nor the investigator/physician knows which treatment the patient is receiving. Blinding the patient equalizes the placebo effect—feeling better because one thinks one is receiving a beneficial treatment—across arms. Blinding the investigator/physician protects against the possibility of differential background treatment across arms that might result from "feeling sorry" for the patient who received what was perceived, rightly or wrongly, as the inferior treatment. Determination of whether a patient had an event is based on unambiguous criteria prespecified in the trial's protocol and applied blinded to the patient's treatment assignment whenever possible. Because the experimental units are humans, and because randomization and blinding are used, these trials require a formal process of informed consent as well as assurance that the safety of the participants is monitored during the course of the study.

Ethical principles mandate that such a clinical trial begin with uncertainty about which treatment under study is better. Uncertainty must obtain even during the study, for if interim data were sufficiently compelling, ethics would demand that the trial stop and the results be made public. But who decides whether the interim data have erased uncertainty and what are the criteria for deciding? As George Eliot said in *Daniel Deronda*, "We can do nothing safely without some judgment as to where we are to stop."

Evaluating ongoing data is often the job of the Data and Safety Monitoring Board (DSMB), a committee composed of experts not otherwise affiliated with the trial, who advise the sponsor—typically a government body such as the National Institutes of Health or a pharmaceutical company—whether to stop the trial and declare that the experimental treatment is beneficial or harmful. Such boards often struggle between two sometimes conflicting considerations: the welfare of patients in the trial (so-called "individualethics") and the welfare of future patients whose care will be impacted by the results of the trial (so-called "collective ethics"). Stopping a trial too late means needlessly delaying the study participant from receiving the better treatment. On the other hand, stopping before the evidence is sufficiently strong may fail to convince the medical community to change its practice or to persuade regulatory bodies to approve the product, thus depriving future patients of the better treatment.

The Cardiac Arrhythmia Suppression Trial (CAST) [CAST89] provides a classic example of the conflict between individual and collective ethics. CAST aimed to see whether suppression of cardiac arrhythmias in patients with a prior heart attack would prevent cardiac arrest and sudden death. Arrhythmias are known to predispose such patients to cardiac arrest and sudden death, so it seemed biologically reasonable that suppressing arrhythmias should prevent these events. Each prospective participant in CAST received antiarrhythmic drugs in a predetermined order until a drug was found that suppressed at least 80 percent of the person's arrhythmias. If such a drug was found, the patient was randomized to receive either that drug or its matching placebo. If none was found, the patient was not enrolled in the study. When the study was designed, many in the medical community believed that arrhythmia suppression would help prevent cardiac arrest and sudden death; few believed that suppression could be harmful. Indeed, some experts in the field felt strongly that the trial was unethical because half of the patients with suppressible arrhythmias were being denied medication that would suppress their arrhythmias (Moore, 1995 [M95], page 217). The trial was originally designed using a one-tailed statistical test of benefit. In other words, the possibility of harm was not even entertained statistically. Before they examined any data, however, the members of the DSMB recommended including a symmetric lower boundary for harm.

The DSMB chose to remain blinded to treatment arm when they reviewed outcome data for the first time on September 16, 1988; that is, they saw the data separated by arm (antiarrhythmic drug or placebo), but they did not know which arm was which. All they knew was that three sudden deaths or cardiac arrests occurred in arm A and 19 in arm B (Table 1.1); they did not know whether arm A represented the antiarrhythmic drugs or the placebo.

The board reviewed the data and concluded that regardless of the direction of the results, the board would not stop the trial. If arm A were the

Table 1.1. Number of arrhythmic deaths/cardiac arrests in CAST as of 9/16/88

	Event		
	Yes	No	
Arm A	3	573	576
Arm B	19	552	571
	22	1125	1147

antiarrhythmic arm, which the board believed, the data were not sufficiently compelling to conclude benefit. They argued that even if arm A were the placebo, it was still so early in the life of the trial that the results might not be convincing enough to change medical practice. Over time, the difference between arms A and B grew larger. In April 1989, the DSMB unblinded itself at the request of the unblinded coordinating center. The board discovered to its surprise and alarm that arm A was indeed the placebo. That is, these early data indicated that using a drug to suppress arrhythmias was harmful. The decision to recommend stopping was still difficult. Many in the medical community "knew" that antiarrhythmic therapy was beneficial (although the fact that many physicians were willing to randomize patients suggested that the evidence of benefit was not strong). Some members of the board argued that the problem was not that too many people were dying on the drugs, but that too few people were dying on placebo! But the board worried that the number of events seen thus far, about 5 percent of the number expected by trial's end, was unlikely to sway physicians who had been convinced of the benefit of suppressing arrhythmias. The lower than expected placebo mortality rate, a common phenomenon in clinical trials, highlights the folly of relying on historical controls in lieu of conducting a clinical trial like CAST. Though the DSMB considered the impact on medical practice of stopping the trial, its primary responsibility was the welfare of the patients in the trial. In April 1989, the board recommended discontinuing encainide and flecainide, the two drugs that appeared to be associated with the excess events. Two years later, they recommended stopping the third drug, moricizine [CAST92]. A detailed account of the DSMB's deliberations may be found in Friedman et al. (1993) [FBH93].

Should the CAST DSMB have recommended stopping the trial earlier? Did they stop too early? In 1989 the board was accused of both errors, but virtually everyone now agrees that both the decision to stop and the time of stopping were appropriate.

A second example comes from the Multicenter Unsustained Tachycardia Trial (MUSTT) (Buxton et al., 1999 [BLF99]), another trial using antiarrhythmic drugs to treat patients with cardiac arrhythmias. The major difference between CAST and MUSTT was that MUSTT used electrophysiologic (EP) testing to guide antiarrhythmic treatment. Patients for whom drug therapy was not successful received an implantable cardiac defibrillator (ICD). Figure

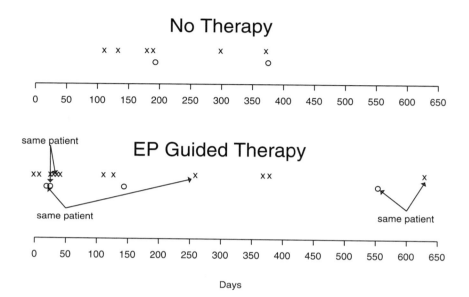

Fig. 1.1. Early results of the Multicenter Unsustained Tachycardia Trial (MUSTT). Xs represent deaths and circles represent cardiac arrests.

1.1 shows the early results of MUSTT. Nine of the first 12 events occurred in the EP-guided arm. The specter of CAST loomed over the DSMB's deliberations. There were tense discussions, but the DSMB decided the trial should continue. Ultimately, the DSMB's decision was vindicated; despite the early negative trend, by trial's end the data showed a statistically significant treatment benefit. Had the trial stopped early, both the participants in the trial and future patients would have received the less beneficial treatment.

Our third example is from the estrogen/progesterone replacement therapy (PERT) trial of the Women's Health Initiative (WHI) [WHI02], which compared PERT to placebo in post-menopausal women who still had their uterus (i.e., women without a hysterectomy). The study was designed as a 12-year trial. A DSMB charged with monitoring the trial met twice yearly to review the safety and efficacy of PERT. The trial had a number of endpoints and hypotheses—the most important being that PERT would decrease the rate of heart attack, hip fracture, and colorectal cancer while it would increase the rate of pulmonary embolism, invasive breast cancer, and endometrial cancer.

The DSMB made no prior hypothesis about the effect of PERT on stroke, although it monitored its occurrence. During the course of the trial, the DSMB noted that most interim findings were consistent with the hypotheses; however, the rates of heart attack and stroke in the PERT arm were higher than in the placebo arm. The DSMB recommended stopping the study 3 years before the planned end when it judged that the overall risks of therapy outweighed the overall benefits.

How does one determine whether emerging trends are real or merely reflect the play of chance? Repeated examination of accumulating data increases the probability of declaring a treatment difference even if there is none. Just as our confidence in a dart thrower who hits the bull's-eye is eroded if we learn he had many attempts, so too is our confidence about a true treatment effect when the test statistic has had many "attempts." How to take this into account through the construction of statistical boundaries is the topic of this book.

All three of the introductory examples have dealt with harm—in the case of CAST and WHI, the treatments led to worse outcomes than did the placebo. In the MUSTT trial, the early interim data suggested harm, but the DSMB—not convinced by the apparent trend—allowed the trial to continue and ultimately the treatment showed benefit. In designing a trial, we hope and expect that the treatment under study provides benefit, but we must be alert to the possibility of harm. This asymmetrical tension between harm and benefit underlies much of the discussion in the subsequent chapters. We will be describing methods for creating statistical boundaries that correct for the multiple looks at the data. In considering these methods, the reader needs to recognize intellectually and emotionally that emerging data differ from data at the end of a trial. Emerging data form the basis of decisions about whether to continue a trial; data at the end of a trial form the basis of inference about the effect of the treatment. The considerations about emerging data for safety and efficacy differ fundamentally. For efficacy, a clinical trial needs to show, to a degree consistent with the prespecified type 1 error rate, that the treatment under study is beneficial. In other words, the trial aims to "prove" efficacy. On the other hand, trials do not aim to "prove" harm; few people would agree to enter a trial if they knew its purpose was to demonstrate that a new therapy was harmful.

This difference between benefit and harm has direct bearing on the way to regard the "upper" and "lower" monitoring boundaries. Crossing the upper boundary demonstrates benefit while crossing the lower boundary suggests, but does not usually demonstrate, harm. The difference also bears on whether to perform one-sided or two-sided tests. Consider for a moment the typical nonsequential scientific experiment. Sound scientific principles dictate two-sided statistical testing in such cases, for the experimenter would be embarrassed to produce data showing the experimental arm worse than the control but being forced by a one-sided test to conclude that the two treatments do not differ from each other. Thus, the typical nonsequential experiment uses a symmetrical two-sided test of the null hypothesis that the two treatments are the same against the alternative that they differ.

In a prototypical sequential randomized clinical trial, on the other hand, the DSMB looks at the data several times during the course of the study. The trial compares a new treatment to placebo (or often, a new treatment plus standard of care to placebo plus standard of care). The participant, before enrolling in the trial, signs an informed consent document that describes the risks and potential benefits of the new therapy. The document states that while physicians do not know whether the experimental treatment is beneficial, data from previous studies provide hope that it may be. The document lists the known risks the participant might incur by virtue of entering the study. In a trial with a DSMB, the informed consent document states that if data during the course of the trial emerge that change the balance of risk to benefit, the study leadership will so inform the participants.

The informed consent document represents an agreement between the participant and the trial management whereby the participant volunteers to show whether the treatment under study is beneficial. For statisticians, this informed consent document provides the basis for the development of our technical approaches to monitoring the emerging data. Therefore, the upper boundary of our sequential plans must be consistent with demonstrating benefit. Throughout this book, we stress the need for statistical rigor in creating this upper boundary. Note that the fact of interim monitoring forces the boundary to be one-sided; we stop if we show benefit, not merely if we show a difference.

The lower boundary dealing with harm is also one-sided, but its shape will often differ considerably from that of its upper partner's. It is designed not to *prove* harm, but to prevent participants in the trial from incurring unacceptable risk. In fact, a given trial may have many lower boundaries, some explicit but some undefined. One can regard a clinical trial that compares a new treatment to placebo or to an old treatment as having one clearly defined upper one-sided boundary—the one whose crossing demonstrates benefit— and a number of less well defined one-sided lower boundaries, the ones whose crossing worries the DSMB.

Most of this book deals with the upper boundary, for it reflects the statistical goals of the study and allows formal statistical inference. But the reader needs to recognize that considerations for building the lower boundary (or for monitoring safety in a study without a boundary) differ importantly from the approaches to the upper boundary. The preceding discussion has assumed that the trial under consideration is comparing a new therapy to an old, or to a standard, therapy. Some trials are designed for other purposes where symmetric monitoring boundaries are appropriate. A trial may be comparing two or more therapies, all of which are known to be effective, to determine which is best. Equivalence or non-inferiority trials aim to show that a new treatment is not very different from an old (the "equivalence trial") or not unacceptably worse than the old (the "noninferiority trial").

The sequential techniques discussed in subsequent chapters have sprung from a long history of a methodology originally developed with no thought to clinical trials. The underlying theoretical basis of sequential analysis rests on Brownian motion, a phenomenon discovered in 1827 by the English botanist Robert Brown, who saw under the microscope that pollen grains suspended in water jiggled in a zigzag path. In 1905 Albert Einstein developed the first mathematical theory of Brownian motion, a contribution for which he received the Nobel prize. As the reader will see, Brownian motion is the unifying mathematical theme of this book.

The methods of sequential analysis in statistics date from World War II when the United States military was looking for methods to reduce the sample size of tests of munitions. Wald's classic text on sequential analysis led to the application of sequential methods to many fields (Wald, 1947 [W47]). Sequential methods moved to clinical trials in the 1960s. The early methods, introduced by Armitage in 1960 and in a later edition in 1975 (Armitage, 1975 [A75]), required monitoring results on a patient-by-patient basis. These methods were, in many cases, cumbersome to apply. In 1977, Pocock [P77] proposed looking at data from clinical trials not one observation at a time, but rather in groups. This so-called group-sequential approach spawned many techniques for clinical trials. This book presents a unified treatment of group-sequential methods.

2

A General Framework

A randomized clinical trial asks questions about the effect of an intervention on an outcome defined by a continuous, dichotomous, or time-to-failure variable. While the test statistics associated with these outcomes may appear quite disparate, they share a common thread—all behave like standardized sums of independent random variables. In fact, they all have the same asymptotic joint distribution over time, provided that we define the time parameter appropriately. Understanding the distribution of the test statistic over time is essential because typically we monitor data several times throughout the course of a trial, with an eye toward stopping if data show convincing evidence of benefit or harm. In clinical trials, the term "monitoring" often refers to a procedure for visiting clinical sites and checking that the investigators are carrying out the protocol faithfully and recording the data accurately. In statistics, and in this book, "monitoring" refers to the statistical process of assessing the strength of emerging data for making inferences or for estimating the treatment effect.

This chapter distinguishes between hypothesis testing (Section 2.1) and parameter estimation (Section 2.2). We begin with simple settings in which the test statistic and treatment effect estimator are a sum and mean, respectively, of independent and identically distributed (i.i.d.) random variables. We show that in less simple settings, the test statistic and treatment effect estimator behave *as if* they were a sum and mean, respectively, of i.i.d. random variables. This leads naturally to the concept of a sum process (S-process) behaving like a sum and an estimation process (E-process) behaving like a sample mean. Following the approach of Lan and Zucker (1993) [LZ93] and Lan and Wittes (1988) [LW88], we show the connection between S-processes, E-processes, and Brownian motion. We use Brownian motion to approximate the joint distribution of repeatedly computed test statistics over time for many different trial settings, including comparisons of means, proportions, and survival times, with or without adjustment for covariates. Because of our extensive use of Brownian motion, we were tempted to subtitle this chapter "Brown v. the Board of Data Monitoring."

This chapter, which presents the general framework for the rest of the book, is necessarily long. The reader may prefer to read the first three sections containing the essential ideas applied to tests of means, proportions, and survival, and then proceed to the next chapter showing how to apply Brownian motion to compute conditional power. The reader may then return to this chapter to see how to use the same ideas in more complicated settings such as maximum likelihood or minimum variance estimation, or even mixed models. While digesting the next sections, the reader should keep in mind the essential idea throughout this chapter—test statistics and estimators behave like sums and sample means, respectively, of i.i.d. random variables.

Lest the reader get the wrong impression that Brownian motion, like gravity, always works, we close the chapter with an example in which Brownian motion fails to provide a good approximation to the joint distribution of a test statistic over time.

2.1 Hypothesis Testing: The Null Distribution of Test Statistics Over Time

This section focuses on the null distribution of test statistics over time, while the next section deals with the distribution under an alternative hypothesis. We begin with paired data assuming the paired differences are independent and identically distributed normals with known variance. Because this ideal setting rarely holds in clinical trials, we then back away from these assumptions, one by one, to see which are really necessary.

2.1.1 Continuous Outcomes

Imagine a trial with a continuous outcome, and suppose first that the data are paired. For example, the data might come from a crossover trial studying the effects of two diets on blood pressure, or from a trial comparing two different treatments applied directly to the eyes, one to the left eye and the other to the right. Let X_i and Y_i be the control and treatment observations, respectively, for patient i and let $D_i = Y_i - X_i$. Assume that the D_i are normally distributed with mean δ and known variance σ^2. We wish to test whether $\delta = 0$.

At the end of the trial the z-score is

$$Z_N = v_N^{-1/2} \sum_{i=1}^{N} D_i, \qquad (2.1)$$

where $S_N = \sum_{i=1}^{N} D_i$ and $v_N = \text{var}(S_N) = N\text{var}(D_1)$. Treatment is declared beneficial if $Z_N > z_{\alpha/2}$, where z_a, for $0 < a < 1$, denotes the $100(1-a)$th percentile of a standard normal distribution.

Now imagine an interim analysis after n of the planned N observations in each arm have been evaluated. Note that

$$Z_N = \{S_n + S_N - S_n\}/\sqrt{v_N}$$

$$= S_n/\sqrt{v_N} + (S_N - S_n)/\sqrt{v_N} \tag{2.2}$$

is the sum of two independent components. We call the first term of (2.2) the *B-value* because of its connection to Brownian motion established later in this chapter. We term the ratio

$$t = v_n/v_N = \mathrm{var}(S_n)/\mathrm{var}(S_N) \tag{2.3}$$

the *trial fraction* because it measures how far through the trial we are. In this simple case, t simplifies to n/N, the fraction of participants evaluated thus far; $t = 0$ and $t = 1$ correspond to the beginning and end of the trial, respectively.

Denote the interim z-score $S_n/v_n^{1/2}$ at trial fraction t by $Z(t)$. Define the B-value $B(t)$ at trial fraction t by

$$B(t) = \frac{S_n}{\sqrt{v_N}} \tag{2.4}$$

$$= \sqrt{t}\, Z(t). \tag{2.5}$$

We could monitor using either the z-score or the B-value; in this book we use both. We use z-scores for setting boundaries (i.e., calculations assuming the null hypothesis is true), whereas for deciding whether observed results follow the expected trend (i.e., calculations assuming the alternative hypothesis is true), we find it advantageous to think in terms of B-values.

At the end of the trial, $B(1) = Z(1) = S_N/v_N^{1/2}$, so (2.2) becomes

$$B(1) = B(t) + \{B(1) - B(t)\}. \tag{2.6}$$

The decomposition (2.2) leading to (2.6) clearly implies that $B(t)$ and $B(1) - B(t)$ are independent (note, however, that the forthcoming derivation of the covariance structure of $B(t)$ is valid even when $B(t)$ and $B(1) - B(t)$ are uncorrelated, but not independent). At trial fraction t, $B(t)$ reflects the past while $B(1) - B(t)$ lies in the future.

More generally, let $t_0 = 0, t_1 = n_1/N, \ldots, t_k = n_k/N$ and let $B(t_0) = 0, B(t_1) = S_{n_1}/v_N^{1/2}, \ldots, B(t_k) = S_{n_k}/v_N^{1/2}$ be interim B-values at trial fractions $t_0 = 0, t_1, \ldots, t_k$. Then the successive increments $B(t_1) - B(t_0) = S_{n_1}/v_N^{1/2}, B(t_2) - B(t_1) = (S_{n_2} - S_{n_1})/v_N^{1/2}, \ldots, B(t_k) - B(t_{k-1}) = (S_{n_k} - S_{n_{k-1}})/v_N^{1/2}$ are independent because they involve nonoverlapping sums. Further, (2.5) implies that

$$\mathrm{var}\{B(t)\} = t\, \mathrm{var}\{Z(t)\} = t.$$

For $t_i \le t_j$,

$$\begin{aligned}
\mathrm{cov}\{B(t_i), B(t_j)\} &= \mathrm{cov}\{S_{n_i}/v_N^{1/2}, S_{n_j}/v_N^{1/2}\} \\
&= v_N^{-1}\mathrm{cov}\{S_{n_i}, S_{n_i} + S_{n_j} - S_{n_i}\} \\
&= v_N^{-1}\{\mathrm{cov}(S_{n_i}, S_{n_i}) + \mathrm{cov}(S_{n_i}, S_{n_j} - S_{n_i})\} \\
&= v_N^{-1}\{\mathrm{var}(S_{n_i}) + 0\} = v_{n_i}/v_N = t_i.
\end{aligned} \tag{2.7}$$

Thus, the distribution of $B(t)$ has the following structure:

- B1: $B(t_1), B(t_2), \ldots, B(t_k)$ have a multivariate normal distribution.
- B2: $\mathrm{E}\{B(t)\} = 0$.
- B3: $\mathrm{cov}\{B(t_i), B(t_j)\} = t_i$ for $t_i \leq t_j$.

Properties B1-B3 and relationship (2.5) confer the following properties to z-scores:

- Z1: $Z(t_1), Z(t_2), \ldots, Z(t_k)$ have a multivariate normal distribution.
- Z2: $\mathrm{E}\{Z(t)\} = 0$.
- Z3: $\mathrm{cov}\{Z(t_i), Z(t_j)\} = (t_i/t_j)^{1/2}$ for $t_i \leq t_j$.

We have been somewhat loose in that we have defined $B(t)$ only at trial fraction values $t = 0, 1/N, \ldots, N/N = 1$. That the set of points at which we defined the B-value depends on N suggests that we really should use the notation $B_N(t)$. The natural way to extend the definition of $B_N(t)$ to the entire unit interval is by linear interpolation: if $t = \lambda(i/N) + (1 - \lambda)\{(i + 1)/N\}$, we define $B_N(t)$ to be $\lambda B_N(i/N) + (1 - \lambda)B_N\{(i + 1)/N\}$. This makes $B_N(t)$ continuous on $t \in (0, 1)$ but nondifferentiable at the "sharp" points $t = 0, 1/N, \ldots, N/N = 1$. As $N \to \infty$, the set of t at which $B_N(t)$ is nondifferentiable becomes more and more dense. In the limit, we get *standard Brownian motion*, a random, continuous, but nondifferentiable, function $B(t)$ satisfying B1-B3 (Figure 2.1).

The approach we take throughout the book is first to transform a probability involving z-scores $Z_N(t)$ to one involving B-values $B_N(t) = t^{1/2}Z_N(t)$, and then to approximate that probability by one involving the limiting Brownian motion process, $B(t) = \lim_{N\to\infty} B_N(t)$. A major advantage to this approach is that properties and formulas involving Brownian motion are well known, having been studied extensively by mathematicians and physicists. The following example demonstrates in detail the process of using Brownian motion to approximate probabilities of interest. In the future, we jump right to $B(t)$, eliminating the intermediate step of arguing that probabilities involving $B_N(t)$ can be approximated by those of $B(t)$.

Example 2.1. Consider a trial comparing two different treatments for the eye. Each volunteer receives treatment 1 in one randomly selected eye and treatment 2 in the other. The outcome for each volunteer is the difference between the results from the eye treated with treatment 1 and the eye treated with treatment 2. Suppose we take an interim analysis after 50 of the 100 planned patients are evaluated, and the paired t-statistic is 1.44. The sample size is sufficiently large to regard the t-statistic as a z-score.

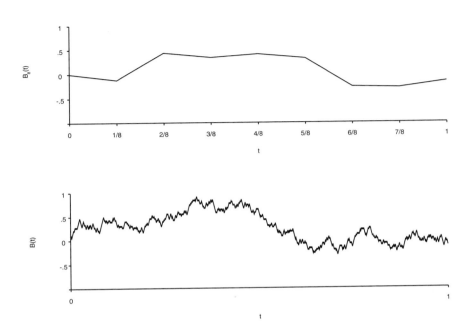

Fig. 2.1. Top panel: The B-value $B_N(t)$ for a trial with $N = 8$ pairs; $B_8(t)$ is defined by linear interpolation for t other than $i/8$, $i = 0, \ldots, 8$. The resulting random function is continuous everywhere but not differentiable at the "sharp" points $t = i/8$, $i = 0, \ldots, 8$. Bottom panel: As the sample size N increases, the set of points at which $B_N(t)$ is not differentiable becomes denser. The limiting case of $B_N(t)$ as $N \to \infty$ is Brownian motion, a random function continuous everywhere but differentiable nowhere, satisfying B1-B3. This nondifferentiability reflects the zigzagging Brown noted when he looked at pollen through his microscope (see the end of Chapter 1).

The trial fraction is $t = 50/100 = 0.50$, so $Z(0.50) = 1.44$. The B-value is $B(0.50) = (0.50)^{1/2}(1.44) = 1.018$. We can approximate the joint distribution of the interim and final B-values, $B_{100}(0.50)$ and $B_{100}(1)$, by those of $B(0.50)$ and $B(1)$, where $B(t)$ is Brownian motion. For example, we could compute boundaries a_1 and a_2 such that $\Pr(B(0.50) \geq a_1) = 0.01$ and $\Pr(B(0.50) \geq a_1 \cup B(1) \geq a_2) = 0.05$ (equivalently, z-score boundaries c_1 and c_2 such that $\Pr(Z(0.50) \geq c_1) = 0.01$ and $\Pr(Z(0.50) \geq c_1 \cup Z(1) \geq c_2) = 0.05$). We can also use Brownian motion to compute more complicated probabilities such as the effect on type 1 error rate of monitoring continuously from now to the end of the trial without adjusting for multiple looks (i.e., using critical value 1.96). The actual type 1 error rate, $\Pr(Z_{100}(i/N) \geq 1.96$ for some $i = 50, 51, \ldots, 100)$, can be approximated by $\Pr(B(t)/t^{1/2} \geq 1.96$ for some $1/2 \leq t \leq 1)$.

Our next step is to show that Brownian motion approximates the null distribution over t for many other testing scenarios. We reexamine the assumptions in Section 2.1.1 to see which ones we can relax.

First, the differences need not be normally distributed. Even if D is not normally distributed, the increments are independent and, by the central limit theorem (CLT), each increment is approximately normally distributed. Consequently, the joint distribution of partial sums is approximately multivariate normal even if the individual observations are not normally distributed.

Second, the sample variance need not be known. As we argued in the example above, Brownian motion holds approximately even if v_n is a consistent estimate of $\mathrm{var}(S_n)$ (that is, $\mathrm{var}(S_n)/v_n$ tends to 1 in probability—see Section 2.9.1 for a formal proof).

Third, we do not need paired observations, as we illustrate in the next section.

2.1.2 Dichotomous Outcomes

Consider a parallel arm trial with a dichotomous outcome such as 28-day mortality. Denote by $I(A)$ the indicator function taking the value 1 if the event A occurs and 0 otherwise. Although the data are not paired differences, we can view the difference in proportions after n patients per arm as S_n/n, where S_n is the sum of n paired differences (we get the same difference in proportions irrespective of how we pair treatment and control observations). The observations $D_i = I(\text{patient } i \text{ of treatment arm has an event}) - I(\text{patient } i \text{ of control arm has an event})$, $i = 1, \ldots, N$ are i.i.d. with null mean 0 and variance $2p(1 - p)$, where p is the null probability that a randomly selected patient has an event. The z-statistic at the end of the trial is given by (2.1), where $v_N = \mathrm{var}(S_N) = 2Np(1 - p)$ is the null variance of S_N. As the true p is unknown, to compute the z-score one replaces p by the sample proportion of all patients with events. The result is the usual (unpaired) z-statistic for a test of proportions. Decomposition (2.2) still holds. Define t by (2.3), which again simplifies to n/N. Brownian motion is again a good approximation for $B(t)$ defined by (2.4). Also, the joint distribution of z-scores is asymptotically the same for a dichotomous outcome trial as for a continuous outcome trial. We can use the same boundaries to monitor either type of trial.

Of course, we do not actually pair the data from a parallel arm trial. In fact, it is unusual for the control and treatment sample sizes to be exactly the same even at the end of a trial, let alone at all interim analyses. Later we will see how to use Brownian motion even in the unequal sample size setting.

Example 2.2. Suppose we design a trial of 200 breast cancer patients randomly assigned in a 1:1 ratio to the standard treatment plus a new treatment or to the standard treatment plus placebo. We want to compare the proportion of patients whose tumor regresses by 3 months after randomization. Interim analyses occur after 50, 75, and 100 patients per arm have been evaluated. The corresponding trial fractions are $t_1 = 50/100 = 0.50$, $t_2 = 75/100 = 0.75$, and $t_3 = 100/100 = 1$. If the z-scores for the usual test of proportions are $Z(0.50) = 0.55$, $Z(0.75) = -0.20$, and $Z(1) = 0.23$, the B-values are $B(0.50) = (0.50)^{1/2}(0.55) = 0.389$, $B(0.75) = (0.75)^{1/2}(-0.20) = -0.173$, and $B(1) = (1)^{1/2}(0.23) = 0.230$. The joint distribution of $B(0.50)$, $B(0.75)$, and $B(1)$, and therefore the joint distribution of $Z(0.50)$, $Z(0.75)$, and $Z(1)$, is the same as for a trial with a continuous outcome monitored at those trial fractions. Any boundary developed for continuous outcome trials would be valid for this dichotomous outcome trial as well. For any z-score boundary c_1, c_2, and c_3 we could compute the probability of crossing at various times. For example, suppose the upper boundary is $c_1 = 2.963$, $c_2 = 2.359$, and $c_3 = 2.014$. The probability of crossing the boundary at $t = 0.50$ is $\Pr(Z(0.50) \geq 2.963) = 1 - \Phi(2.963) = 0.0015$. The cumulative probability of crossing by the second look depends on the joint distribution of $Z(0.50)$ and $Z(0.75)$, which by properties Z1-Z3 is bivariate normal with zero means, unit variances, and covariance $(0.50/0.75)^{1/2} = 0.816$. We can use numerical integration (described in Section 4.7) to show that the cumulative crossing probability by $t = 0.75$ is $\Pr[\{Z(0.50) \geq 2.963\} \cup \{Z(0.75) \geq 2.359\}] = 0.0097$. Similarly, for the cumulative crossing probability by $t = 1$, we use the fact that

$$\mathrm{cov}\{Z(0.50), Z(0.75)\} = 0.816$$
$$\mathrm{cov}\{Z(0.50), Z(1)\} = (0.50/1)^{1/2} = 0.707$$
$$\mathrm{cov}\{Z(0.75), Z(1)\} = (0.75/1)^{1/2} = 0.866.$$

The cumulative crossing probability by $t = 1$ is $\Pr[\{Z(0.50) \geq 2.963\} \cup \{Z(0.75) \geq 2.359\} \cup \{Z(1) \geq 2.014\}] = 0.025$.

We next relax the assumption of independent observations. Notice that the steps leading to (2.7) remain valid even if the D_is are merely uncorrelated. Thus, even when the observations are uncorrelated but not independent, the B-values have the same correlation structure as Brownian motion. If we are willing to accept that the joint distribution of the B-values is asymptotically multivariate normal, then it must be that of Brownian motion. In the next section, we apply this idea to comparison of survival curves using the logrank statistic.

2.1.3 Survival Outcomes

In many clinical trials, the outcome is the time to some event. For simplicity, assume the event is death so that each person can only have one event; the same ideas apply for events that can recur, but in those cases we restrict attention to the first event for each patient. We use the logrank statistic to compare the treatment and control arms. Assume for now that all patients are randomized simultaneously. We show that the logrank statistic is also of the form (2.1) for uncorrelated, mean 0 random variables D_i. Brownian motion can approximate its null joint distribution at different analysis times. See Chapter 13 for further discussion of the logrank and related tests.

Let N be the total number of deaths at the end of the trial instead of the per-arm sample size. The numerator of the logrank statistic at the end of the trial is $\sum_{i=1}^{N} D_i$, where $D_i = O_i - E_i$, O_i is the indicator that the ith death occurred in a treatment patient, and $E_i = m_{1i}/(m_{0i} + m_{1i})$ is the null expectation of O_i given the respective numbers, m_{0i} and m_{1i}, of control and treatment patients at risk just prior to the ith death. Conditioned on m_{0i} and m_{1i}, O_i has a Bernoulli distribution with parameter E_i. The null conditional mean and variance of D_i are 0 and $V_i = E_i(1 - E_i)$, respectively.

We show in Section 2.9.3 that, unconditionally, the D_i are uncorrelated, mean 0 random variables with variance $E(V_i)$ under the null hypothesis. Thus, conditioned on N, $v_N = \text{var}(S_N) = \sum_{i=1}^{N} \text{var}(D_i) = \sum_{i=1}^{N} E(V_i) = E(\sum_{i=1}^{N} V_i)$. The logrank statistic is given by (2.1), where v_N is replaced by its estimate $\sum_{i=1}^{N} V_i$.

In the setting of survival, we should define the trial fraction in terms of patients with events rather than patients evaluated. Suppose we examine the data after n deaths. If we condition on N and n and define the trial fraction by (2.3), the covariance structure of Brownian motion holds. For now, assume that the joint distribution of $B(t_1), \ldots, B(t_k)$ is approximately multivariate normal. Then Brownian motion is again a good approximation to the process $B(t)$. A practical problem is that at the interim analysis, we would not know v_N even if we knew with certainty the number, N, of patients with an event by the end of the trial. We can, however, approximate v_N as follows. Under the null hypothesis, $E(V_i) = E\{E_i(1 - E_i)\} \approx (1/2)(1 - 1/2) = 1/4$. We find this result quite remarkable—without making any assumption about the form of the survival curve, this simple argument shows that the variance of D_i is approximately $1/4$. It follows that $v_N \approx N/4$. This calculation leads to the familar estimate $t = n/N$. In other words, for the logrank test, the trial fraction is the ratio of the number of patients with an event thus far to the number expected by trial's end.

Example 2.3. Consider a trial comparing mortality of lung cancer patients on a new treatment plus the standard treatment compared to placebo plus the standard treatment. Assume 200 deaths expected over the 2-year trial, and monitoring every 6 months. The total numbers of deaths at the first three looks were 20, 50, and 122, so the estimated trial fractions were $t_1 = 20/200 = 0.10$, $t_2 = 50/200 = 0.25$, and $t_3 = 122/200 = 0.61$. The values of the logrank statistic at these looks were $Z(0.10) = -0.162$, $Z(0.25) = 0.258$, and $Z(0.61) = 1.384$, so the B-values were $(0.10)^{1/2}(-0.162) = -0.051$, $B(0.25) = (0.25)^{1/2}(0.258) = 0.129$, and $B(0.61) = (0.61)^{1/2}(1.384) = 1.081$. Under the null hypothesis, these B-values behave like Brownian motion. Suppose we constructed boundaries c_1, c_2, and c_3 such that

$$\Pr(Z(0.10) \geq c_1 \cup Z(0.25) \geq c_2 \cup Z(0.61) \geq c_3) = 0.01.$$

But imagine that when we reached the end of the trial, we had 190 instead of the expected 200 deaths. Thus, the "right" trial fractions at earlier looks should have been $t_1 = 20/190 = 0.105$, $t_2 = 50/190 = 0.263$, and $t_3 = 122/190 = 0.642$. The actual probability of crossing at least one earlier boundary should have been

$$\Pr(Z(0.105) \geq c_1 \cup Z(0.263) \geq c_2 \cup Z(0.642) \geq c_3). \tag{2.8}$$

Fortunately, this discrepancy does not present a problem because the null joint distribution of $Z(t_1), Z(t_2), Z(t_3)$ is multivariate normal with marginal mean 0 and variance 1, and $\text{cov}\{Z(t_i)/Z(t_j)\} = (t_i/t_j)^{1/2}$. This distribution depends on the trial fractions only through their ratios. The ratio of trial fractions is invariant to how many events we thought there would be at the end; e.g., $(20/200)/(50/200) = (20/190)/(50/190) = 20/50$. Thus, the correct probability of crossing an earlier boundary, (2.8), is also 0.01. We will see this invariance property many more times.

We used some sleight of hand in concluding that $(B(t_1), \ldots, B(t_k))$ is approximately multivariate normal in the survival setting. Because $\sum_{i=1}^{N} D_i$ is a sum of uncorrelated but not independent observations, we can no longer rely on the central limit theorem to conclude that the asymptotic marginal distribution of $\sum_{i=1}^{N} D_i$ is normal. Furthermore, asymptotic marginal normality of $\sum_{i=1}^{N} D_i$ does not necessarily imply asymptotic multivariate normality of $(\sum_{i=1}^{n_1} D_i, \ldots, \sum_{i=1}^{n_k} D_i)$, as it did in the clinical trial scenarios in which the D_is were independent. Things get even more complicated if we account for the fact that in most trials participants are recruited over time (staggered entry) instead of all at once. A more rigorous treatment accounting for these factors requires a stochastic process formulation. Using such a formulation, one can show that the simple result obtained above holds under staggered entry as well. That is, $B(t) = t^{1/2} Z(t)$ behaves asymptotically like Brownian motion, where the trial fraction t is the ratio of the number of patients with an event thus far to the number expected by trial's end, and $Z(t)$ is the logrank statistic at trial fraction t.

2.1.4 Summary of Sums

In the clinical trial scenarios considered thus far, the test statistic was a sum of either independent or uncorrelated observations. In either case, we adopted the following approach to convert the statistic to a B-value:

Approach 1. *We transform a sum of independent or uncorrelated random variables to a B-value $B(t)$ having the same correlation structure as Brownian* *motion by dividing the current sum S_n by the standard deviation of the sum S_N at the end of the trial. The time parameter t of $B(t)$ is the trial fraction $t = \mathrm{var}(S_n)/\mathrm{var}(S_N)$.*

If the random variables are i.i.d., the same force that causes the z-statistic to be asymptotically standard normal—namely the central limit theorem—also causes the asymptotic joint distribution of B-values to be that of Brownian motion. In fact, the result holds even if the random variables are independent but not identically distributed (proof in Section 2.9.2).

Result 2.1 *Let S_N be a sum of independent (not necessarily identically distributed) random variables with mean 0, and let $n_i \to \infty$ and $N \to \infty$ such that $v_{n_i}/v_N \to t_i$, $i = 1, \ldots, k$. Then the joint distribution of the B-values from Approach 1 is asymptotically that of Brownian motion if and only if the marginal distribution of the z-statistic is asymptotically standard normal.*

2.2 An Estimation Perspective

2.2.1 Information

In each scenario above, we were able to write the test statistic in terms of a sum $S_n = \sum_{i=1}^{n} D_i$, but testing whether the treatment effect is 0 is only one facet of inference; we are also interested in estimating the size of the treatment effect. Thus, we must determine the joint distribution of the treatment effect estimator $\hat{\delta}$ across different interim analyses. In the simplest setting, which involves paired data $D_1, \ldots, D_n$, the treatment effect estimator $\hat{\delta}$ is a sample mean $\bar{D}$. The joint distribution of $\hat{\delta}_1, \ldots, \hat{\delta}_k$ with $n_1, \ldots, n_k$ pairs is multivariate normal with marginal mean δ and covariance

$$
\begin{aligned}
\mathrm{cov}(\hat{\delta}_i, \hat{\delta}_j) &= (n_i n_j)^{-1}\mathrm{cov}\left(\sum_{r=1}^{n_i} D_r, \sum_{r=1}^{n_j} D_r\right) \\
&= (n_i n_j)^{-1}\mathrm{cov}\left(\sum_{r=1}^{n_i} D_r, \sum_{r=1}^{n_i} D_r + \sum_{r=n_i+1}^{n_j} D_r\right) \\
&= (n_i n_j)^{-1}\left\{\mathrm{cov}\left(\sum_{r=1}^{n_i} D_r, \sum_{r=1}^{n_i} D_r\right) + \mathrm{cov}\left(\sum_{r=1}^{n_i} D_r, \sum_{r=n_i+1}^{n_j} D_r\right)\right\} \\
&= (n_i n_j)^{-1}\left\{\mathrm{var}\left(\sum_{r=1}^{n_i} D_r\right) + 0\right\} \\
&= (n_i n_j)^{-1} n_i \sigma^2 = \sigma^2/n_j \\
&= \mathrm{var}(\hat{\delta}_j).
\end{aligned}
\tag{2.9}
$$

Equation (2.9) shows the covariance of $\hat{\delta}$ over time when $\hat{\delta}$ is a sample mean; however, when the treatment and control sample sizes differ, the treatment effect estimator $\hat{\delta} = \bar{Y}_T - \bar{X}_T$ is not a sample mean. Can we nonetheless view $\hat{\delta}$ as being *like* a sample mean even when the numbers n_T and n_C of treatment and control observations differ? If so, then a mean of how many observations? Let us assume that $\hat{\delta}$ behaves like a sample mean of, say, I i.i.d. observations with mean δ and variance 1. Then $E(\hat{\delta}) = \delta$ and $\text{var}(\hat{\delta}) = 1/I$. Solving for I yields

$$I = 1/\text{var}(\hat{\delta}). \tag{2.10}$$

Think of $\hat{\delta}$ as a sample mean and I as its sample size, even though I need not be an integer. Note that $\hat{\delta}$ has the same expectation and variance as a sample mean of I i.i.d. observations with mean δ and variance 1. We will show later that $\hat{\delta}$ computed at different interim analyses also has the same covariance as a sample mean computed at those analysis times. I defined by (2.10) is called the *information* contained in $\hat{\delta}$, which can be interpreted as the number of independent observations with expectation δ and variance 1 whose sample mean has the same precision as $\hat{\delta}$.

In the continuous outcome scenario with treatment and control sample sizes n_T and n_C, the information contained in $\hat{\delta} = \bar{Y} - \bar{X}$ is

$$I = \{\sigma^2(1/n_T + 1/n_C)\}^{-1} = n_T n_C / \{(n_T + n_C)\sigma^2\}.$$

I decreases as σ^2 increases, and for a fixed total sample size $n_T + n_C$, I increases as the disparity between n_T and n_C decreases.

Although information is interesting in its own right, we return to our goal of showing that $\hat{\delta}$ behaves like a sample mean of I i.i.d. random variables with mean δ and variance 1. We showed that this holds marginally, but we now show that the covariance over time of $\hat{\delta}$ is also that of a sample mean. The covariance over time for a sample mean was given by (2.9), which in view of (2.10) may be rewritten as

$$\text{cov}(\hat{\delta}_i, \hat{\delta}_j) = 1/I_j. \tag{2.11}$$

That is, the covariance between sample means at two different times is the inverse of the information at the later time.

Returning to the estimator $\hat{\delta} = \bar{Y} - \bar{X}$, let (n_{Ti}, n_{Ci}) and I_i be the (Treatment, Control) sample sizes and information, respectively, at the ith interim analysis. Then for $i \le j$,

$$
\begin{aligned}
\text{cov}(\hat{\delta}_i, \hat{\delta}_j) &= \text{cov}\left\{ \frac{1}{n_{Ti}}\sum_{r=1}^{n_{Ti}} Y_r - \frac{1}{n_{Ci}}\sum_{r=1}^{n_{Ci}} X_r, \frac{1}{n_{Tj}}\sum_{r=1}^{n_{Tj}} Y_r - \frac{1}{n_{Cj}}\sum_{r=1}^{n_{Cj}} X_r \right\} \\
&= \frac{1}{n_{Ti}n_{Tj}}\text{cov}\left\{ \sum_{r=1}^{n_{Ti}} Y_r, \sum_{r=1}^{n_{Tj}} Y_r \right\} - \frac{1}{n_{Ti}n_{Cj}}\text{cov}\left\{ \sum_{r=1}^{n_{Ti}} Y_r, \sum_{r=1}^{n_{Cj}} X_r \right\} \\
&\quad - \frac{1}{n_{Ci}n_{Tj}}\text{cov}\left\{ \sum_{r=1}^{n_{Ci}} X_r, \sum_{r=1}^{n_{Tj}} Y_r \right\} + \frac{1}{n_{Ci}n_{Cj}}\text{cov}\left\{ \sum_{r=1}^{n_{Ci}} X_r, \sum_{r=1}^{n_{Cj}} X_r \right\}
\end{aligned}
$$

$$= \frac{n_{Ti}\sigma^2}{n_{Ti}n_{Tj}} - 0 - 0 + \frac{n_{Ci}\sigma^2}{n_{Ci}n_{Cj}}$$

$$= \sigma^2 \left(\frac{1}{n_{Tj}} + \frac{1}{n_{Cj}} \right)$$

$$= \text{var}(\hat{\delta}_j)$$

$$= 1/I_j. \tag{2.12}$$

Equation (2.12) shows that, just as with a sample mean, the covariance of $\hat{\delta}$ computed at different times is the inverse of the information at the later time.

The same thing happens with binary data (Section 2.1.2), where the information in $\hat{\delta} = \hat{p}_T - \hat{p}_C$ is $\{p_T(1 - p_T)/n_T + p_C(1 - p_C)/n_C\}^{-1} = n_T n_C/\{n_C p_T(1 - p_T) + n_T p_C(1 - p_C)\}$. Again, (2.11) holds.

No estimator was immediately apparent for survival data (Section 2.1.3), but one was actually lurking in the background. For each i, $(O_i - E_i)/V_i$ is an estimate of the log hazard ratio (see the Statistical Appendix of Yusuf et al., 1985 [YPL85] for a heuristic justification of a closely related odds ratio estimate) with estimated variance $1/V_i$. We combine these uncorrelated estimates by weighting inversely proportionally to their variance:

$$\hat{\delta} = \frac{\sum_{r=1}^{n} V_r\{(O_r - E_r)/V_r\}}{\sum_{r=1}^{n} V_r} = S_n/\hat{v}_n,$$

where $S_n = \sum_r (O_r - E_r)$ and $\hat{v}_n = \sum_{r=1}^{n} V_r$ is an estimate of $v_n = \sum_{r=1}^{n} \text{E}(V_r)$. It can be shown that $\hat{v}_n/n$ converges to a constant just as in Sections 2.1.1 and 2.1.2. Thus, we can treat $\hat{v}_n$ as if it were v_n;

$$\text{var}(\hat{\delta}) \approx v_n^{-2}\text{var}(S_n) = v_n^{-2}v_n = 1/v_n,$$

and information is approximately $I = v_n$, estimated by $\hat{v}_n$. Again $\hat{\delta}$ behaves like a mean of I i.i.d. observations with expectation δ and variance 1; $\hat{\delta}$ has mean δ and variance $1/I$. Furthermore, for $I_i = v_{n_i} \leq I_j = v_{n_j}$,

$$\text{cov}(\hat{\delta}_i, \hat{\delta}_j) = \text{cov}\left((1/I_i)\sum_{r=1}^{n_i} D_r, (1/I_j)\sum_{r=1}^{n_j} D_r \right)$$

$$= (I_i I_j)^{-1}\text{cov}\left(\sum_{r=1}^{n_i} D_r, \sum_{r=1}^{n_i} D_r + \sum_{r=n_i+1}^{n_j} D_r \right)$$

$$= (I_i I_j)^{-1}\left\{ \text{var}\left(\sum_{r=1}^{n_i} D_r \right) + \text{cov}\left(\sum_{r=1}^{n_i} D_r, \sum_{r=n_i+1}^{n_j} D_r \right) \right\}$$

$$\approx (I_i I_j)^{-1}\{v_{n_i} + 0\}$$

$$= (I_i I_j)^{-1}I_i$$

$$= 1/I_j. \tag{2.13}$$

Equation (2.13) shows that the covariance of log hazard ratio estimators computed at two different times is the same as for a sample mean, namely the inverse of the information at the later time.

The reason for the $\approx$ in the fourth line of the derivation of (2.13) is that we are no longer assuming the null hypothesis, and the D_r are not uncorrelated under the alternative hypothesis. Still, under a local alternative (loosely speaking, an alternative "near" the null hypothesis—see Section 2.9.4), the D_r are approximately uncorrelated.

2.2.2 Summary of Treatment Effect Estimators

With the t-test, the test of proportions, or the logrank test, the treatment effect estimator computed at k different interim analyses behaves just like cumulative sample means. It is cumbersome and vague to repeat each time we discuss estimation that the treatment effect estimator "behaves like" a sample mean of i.i.d. observations with expectation δ and variance 1. Instead, we follow the approach of Lan and Zucker (1993) [LZ93], spelling out precisely what we mean by "behaves like" a sample mean, and attaching a name to processes with these properties. Let τ be any measure of how far through the trial we are, scaled such that $\tau = 0$ and $\tau = 1$ at the beginning and end of the trial, respectively. For example, τ may be the calendar fraction (e.g., the 6-month point of a 5-year trial corresponds to $\tau = 1/10$). Let the increasing function $I(\tau)$ denote the information at time τ. What we mean when we say that $\hat{\delta}(\tau)$ "behaves like" a sample mean of $I(\tau)$ random variables with expectation δ and variance 1 is that $\hat{\delta}(\tau)$ satisfies—at least asymptotically—the following properties:

- E1: $\hat{\delta}(\tau_1), \ldots, \hat{\delta}(\tau_k)$ have a multivariate normal distribution,
- E2: $\mathrm{E}\{\hat{\delta}(\tau)\} = \delta$, and
- E3: $\mathrm{cov}\{\hat{\delta}(\tau_i), \hat{\delta}(\tau_j)\} = \mathrm{var}\{\hat{\delta}(\tau_j)\} = 1/I(\tau_j)$ for $i \leq j$.

Lan and Zucker called an estimator satisfying E1-E3 an *E-process* (E standing for estimator or estimation) with parameter δ and information function $I(\tau)$. An arguably better term might be *sample mean process* because properties E1-E3 are those of cumulative sample means of $I(\tau_1), \ldots, I(\tau_k)$ observations. We will soon see that many other estimators are also E-processes.

2.3 Connection Between Estimators, Sums, Z-Scores, and Brownian Motion

Because the treatment effect estimator for the comparison of means, proportions, or log hazard ratios behaves like a sample mean of I i.i.d. random variables with expectation δ and variance 1, it stands to reason that $I\hat{\delta}$ should behave like a sum of I i.i.d. observations with expectation δ and variance 1. That is, if $\hat{\delta}(\tau)$ is an E-process, then $S(\tau) = I(\tau)\hat{\delta}(\tau)$ "behaves like" a sum of $I(\tau)$ i.i.d. random variables with expectation δ and variance 1. By "behaves like" a sum of $I(\tau)$ i.i.d. random variables with expectation δ and variance 1, we mean that $S(\tau)$ satisfies—at least asymptotically—

- S1: $S(\tau_1), \ldots, S(\tau_k)$ have a multivariate normal distribution.
- S2: $\mathrm{E}\{S(\tau)\} = I(\tau)\delta$.
- S3: For $\tau_i \le \tau_j$, $\mathrm{cov}\{S(\tau_i), S(\tau_j)\} = \mathrm{var}\{S(\tau_i)\} = I(\tau_i)$.

Lan and Zucker (1993) [LZ93] termed $S(\tau)$ an *S-Process* because it behaves like a sum. The following result formalizes the notion that the estimator $\hat{\delta}(\tau)$ behaves like a sample mean if and only if $I(\tau)\hat{\delta}(\tau)$ behaves like a sum. We omit the straightforward proof.

Result 2.2 *If $\hat{\delta}$ is an unbiased estimator with information $0 < I(\tau) < \infty$ for $\tau > 0$, then $\hat{\delta}$ is an E-process iff $I(\tau)\hat{\delta}$ is an S-process.*

To emphasize that $I\hat{\delta}(\tau)$ behaves like a sum of $I(\tau)$ random variables, we use the more suggestive notation $S_{I(\tau)}$ for $I(\tau)\hat{\delta}(\tau)$. Because $S_{I(\tau)}$ behaves like a sum, we try to use Approach 1 to convert to Brownian motion, where $I(\tau)$ plays the role of the sample size. In Approach 1 we divide the current "sum" $S_{I(\tau)} = I(\tau)\hat{\delta}(\tau)$ by the standard deviation of the "sum" $S_{I(1)}$ at the end of the trial: $\{\mathrm{var}(S_{I(1)})\}^{1/2} = \{I(1)\}^{1/2}$. The trial fraction and B-value are

$$\begin{aligned} t &= \mathrm{var}\{S_{I(\tau)}\}/\mathrm{var}\{S_{I(1)}\} \\ &= I(\tau)/I(1) \end{aligned} \tag{2.14}$$

and

$$B(t) = I(\tau)\hat{\delta}(\tau)/\{I(1)\}^{1/2}. \tag{2.15}$$

We call expression (2.14) the *information fraction* or *information time*. It is a generalization of the trial fraction, which was defined only for actual sums, not S-processes. Henceforth, we dispense with the notion of trial fraction in favor of the more general information fraction.

We next show that $B(t)$ defined by (2.15) has the properties of Brownian motion, except that its mean is not 0 under the alternative hypothesis. To see that $B(t)$ has the covariance structure of Brownian motion, note that for $t_i = I(\tau_i)/I(1) \le t_j = I(\tau_j)/I(1)$,

$$\begin{aligned} \mathrm{cov}\{B(t_i), B(t_j)\} &= \mathrm{cov}[S_{I(\tau_i)}/\{I(1)\}^{1/2}, S_{I(\tau_j)}/\{I(1)\}^{1/2}] \\ &= \{I(1)\}^{-1}\mathrm{cov}(S_{I(\tau_i)}, S_{I(\tau_j)}) \\ &= \{I(1)\}^{-1}I(\tau_i) \\ &= t_i. \end{aligned}$$

The mean of $B(t)$ is different from the mean under the null hypothesis. Under the alternative hypothesis,

$$\begin{aligned} \mathrm{E}\{B(t)\} &= \mathrm{E}[I(\tau)\hat{\delta}(\tau)/\{I(1)\}^{1/2}] \\ &= I(\tau)\delta/\{I(1)\}^{1/2} \\ &= [\{I(1)\}^{1/2}\delta]\{I(\tau)/I(1)\} \\ &= \theta t, \end{aligned}$$

where $\theta = \{I(1)\}^{1/2}\delta$ is the expected value of the z-score $\hat{\delta}(1)/[\mathrm{var}\{\hat{\delta}(1)\}]^{1/2} = \{I(1)\}^{1/2}\hat{\delta}(1)$ at the end of the trial. $B(t)$ is said to be a Brownian motion with *drift* θ. The standard Brownian motion has drift 0.

Instead of beginning with the estimator $\hat{\delta}(\tau)$, transforming to a sum, then transforming to Brownian motion, we could have begun with the z-score $Z(t) = \hat{\delta}(\tau)/[\mathrm{var}\{\hat{\delta}(\tau)\}]^{1/2} = \{I(\tau)\}^{1/2}\hat{\delta}(\tau)$ and multiplied by $t^{1/2} = \{I(\tau)/I(1)\}^{1/2}$ to obtain (2.15). We have essentially proven the following result.

Result 2.3 *(Summary) Let $I(\tau)/I(1)$ be the information fraction. We can convert an E-process, S-process, or Z-process to Brownian motion with drift θ, the expected value of the z-score at the end of the trial, as follows:*

$$\text{E to B}: B(t) = I(\tau)\hat{\delta}(\tau)/\{I(1)\}^{1/2}$$

$$\text{S to B}: B(t) = S(\tau)/\{I(1)\}^{1/2}$$

$$\text{Z to B}: B(t) = t^{1/2}Z(t).$$

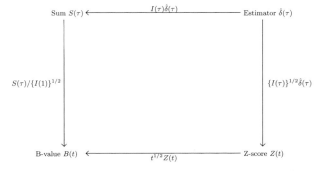

Fig. 2.2. Relationship between S-processes, E-processes, z-scores, and Brownian motion with drift θ, where θ is the expected value of the z-score at the end of the trial, $I(\tau)$ is the information function, and t is the information fraction $I(\tau)/I(1)$.

Figure 2.2 summarizes the relationships between S-processes, E-processes, z-scores, and Brownian motion.

Now that we are not restricting ourselves to the null hypothesis, we see the advantage of using the B-value instead of the z-score to monitor data. Because $\mathrm{E}\{B(t)\} = \theta t$, it follows that $B(t)/t$ estimates the drift parameter, a simple transformation of the treatment effect estimate. Geometrically, $B(t)/t$ is the slope of the line joining the origin to $(t, B(t))$ (Figure 2.3). We can easily see whether the treatment effect estimate increases from one interim look to the next by seeing whether the slope of the line increases. Chapter 3 on conditional power uses the B-value approach extensively.

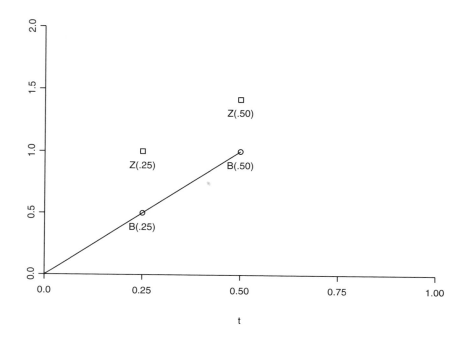

Fig. 2.3. Summarizing data with $B(t)$ instead of $Z(t)$ makes it easy to see whether results are improving over time. The slope of the line segment connecting the origin to $(t, B(t))$ is the drift parameter estimate, which is a simple transformation of the treatment effect estimate; the treatment effect estimate is larger at t_{i+1} than at t_i if and only if the slope of the line connecting the origin to $(t_{i+1}, B(t_{i+1}))$ is larger than the slope of the line connecting the origin to $(t_i, B(t_i))$. For the data shown in this graph, the line segments joining the origin to the circle at $(0.50, B(0.50))$ and the origin to the circle at $(0.25, B(0.25))$ have the same slope, so the treatment effect estimate at $t = 0.50$ is the same as at $t = 0.25$. Deducing this information from the z-scores (squares) is more difficult.

2.4 Maximum Likelihood Estimation

As discussed previously, many clinical trials use a difference in means or proportions to compare treatments; in other trials, the treatment effect is estimated by maximum likelihood in a model that adjusts for covariates. Analysis of covariance and logistic regression are the covariate-adjusted analogs of differences in means or proportions. To deal with these situations, assume that we have independent observations $X_1, \ldots, X_n$ from a distribution with density $f(x, \delta)$. We will show that that the maximum likelihood estimator (MLE)

$\hat{\delta}$ of the treatment effect is asymptotically an E-process, and therefore can be converted to Brownian motion. This allows us to apply the results of Sections 2.1 through 2.3. In fact, as we shall demonstrate below, for the same set of information times, the monitoring boundaries for a trial that uses an MLE as the outcome are the same as the boundaries of the t-test, a test of proportions, or the logrank test.

First we review the arguments leading to asymptotic normality of an MLE at a single time point. Let $L(\delta)$ be the log likelihood function:

$$L(\delta) = \sum_{i=1}^{n}(\partial/\partial\delta)\{\ln f(X_i, \delta)\}.$$

Using a familiar technique, we expand the log likelihood in a Taylor series:

$$\begin{aligned}
0 = L(\hat{\delta}) &\approx L(\delta) + L'(\delta)(\hat{\delta} - \delta) \\
&= L(\delta) + \sum_{i=1}^{n}(\partial^2/\partial\delta^2)\{\ln f(X_i, \delta)\}(\hat{\delta} - \delta),
\end{aligned}$$

and hence

$$\begin{aligned}
\hat{\delta} - \delta &\approx \frac{-L(\delta)}{\sum_{i=1}^{n}(\partial^2/\partial\delta^2)\{\ln f(X_i, \delta)\}} \\
&= \frac{\sum_{i=1}^{n}(\partial/\partial\delta)\{\ln f(X_i, \delta)\}}{\sum_{i=1}^{n}-(\partial^2/\partial\delta^2)\{\ln f(X_i, \delta)\}} \\
&\approx \frac{\sum_{i=1}^{n}(\partial/\partial\delta)\{\ln f(X_i, \delta)\}}{\mathcal{I}_n}.
\end{aligned} \tag{2.16}$$

In the last step, we replaced the denominator by its expectation, $\mathcal{I}_n = -n\mathrm{E}[(\partial^2/\partial\delta^2)\{\ln f(X, \delta)\}]$, the Fisher information contained in $X_1, \ldots, X_n$. Multiplying both sides of (2.16) by $\mathcal{I}_n$ results in

$$\mathcal{I}_n(\hat{\delta} - \delta) = S_n + R_n, \tag{2.17}$$

where $S_n = L(\delta) = \sum_{i=1}^{n}(\partial/\partial\delta)\{\ln f(X_i, \delta)\}$ is a sum of i.i.d. mean 0 random variables and R_n is a remainder term. It is not difficult to show that, under mild conditions, $\mathrm{var}(S_n) = \mathcal{I}_n$. Thus, from (2.17),

$$\begin{aligned}
\frac{\mathcal{I}_n(\hat{\delta} - \delta)}{\mathcal{I}_n^{1/2}} &= \frac{S_n}{\mathcal{I}_n^{1/2}} + \frac{R_n}{\mathcal{I}_n^{1/2}} \\
\mathcal{I}_n^{1/2}(\hat{\delta} - \delta) &= \frac{S_n}{\sqrt{\mathrm{var}(S_n)}} + \mathcal{I}_n^{-1/2}R_n.
\end{aligned} \tag{2.18}$$

The first term on the right side of (2.18) is asymptotically standard normal by the central limit theorem, while the second term tends to 0 in probability under regularity conditions, so $\mathcal{I}_n^{1/2}(\hat{\delta} - \delta)$ is asymptotically standard normal. In other words, $\hat{\delta}$ is asymptotically normal with mean δ and variance $1/\mathcal{I}_n$. Marginally at least, $\hat{\delta}$ and $\mathcal{I}_n\hat{\delta}$ behave like an E-process and S-process, respectively, with mean δ and information $I_n = \mathcal{I}_n$.

Now consider the MLE monitored over time. Equation (2.17) shows that $\mathcal{I}_n(\hat{\delta} - \delta)$ is essentially a sum, and Approach 1 suggests we can convert it to Brownian motion by dividing by the standard deviation of the sum at the end of the trial, $I_N^{1/2} = \{\text{var}(S_N)\}^{1/2}$. Let $\hat{\delta}_i$ denote the MLE at look i, $i = 1, \ldots, k$. By (2.17),

$$\frac{\mathcal{I}_{n_i}(\hat{\delta}_i - \delta)}{I_N^{1/2}} = \frac{S_{n_i}}{\sqrt{\text{var}(S_N)}} + I_N^{-1/2}R_{n_i}. \tag{2.19}$$

Now let $n_i \to \infty$ and $N \to \infty$ such that $n_i/N \to t_i$, $i = 1, \ldots, k$. Each remainder term $I_N^{-1/2}R_{n_i}$ of (2.19) converges to 0 in probability because

$$I_N^{-1/2}R_{n_i} = (I_{n_i}/I_N)^{1/2}I_{n_i}^{-1/2}R_n$$

$$= (n_i/N)^{1/2}I_{n_i}^{-1/2}R_{n_i}$$

$$\to (t_i^{1/2})(0) = 0$$

in probability. Thus, $\mathcal{I}_{n_1}(\hat{\delta}_1 - \delta)/I_N^{1/2}, \ldots, \mathcal{I}_{n_k}(\hat{\delta}_k - \delta)/I_N^{1/2}$ behaves asymptotically like $S_{n_1}/\{\text{var}(S_N)\}^{1/2}, \ldots, S_{n_k}/\{\text{var}(S_N)\}^{1/2}$, which, in turn, behaves asymptotically like standard Brownian motion by Result 2.1 and the central limit theorem. Note that we can rewrite $\mathcal{I}_{n_i}(\hat{\delta}_i - \delta)/I_N^{1/2}$ as $t_i^{1/2}(\hat{\delta}_i - \delta)/\hat{\sigma}_{\hat{\delta}_i}$.

In summary:

Result 2.4 *(Brownian motion for MLEs with i.i.d. data) Let X_j be i.i.d. with density $f(x_j; \delta)$, and let $\hat{\delta}_i$ and $\hat{\sigma}_{\hat{\delta}_i}$ denote the MLE and its estimated standard error, respectively, after n_i patients are evaluated, $i = 1, \ldots, k$. Suppose that $n_i \to \infty$ and $N \to \infty$ such that $n_i/N \to t_i$. Under the same regularity conditions that imply marginal asymptotic normality of the MLE, $t_1^{1/2}(\hat{\delta}_1 - \delta)/\hat{\sigma}_{\hat{\delta}_1}, \ldots, t_k^{1/2}(\hat{\delta}_k - \delta)/\hat{\sigma}_{\hat{\delta}_k}$ have the asymptotic distribution of standard Brownian motion at $t_1, \ldots, t_k$. Equivalently, the B-values $B(t_i) = t_i^{1/2}\hat{\delta}_i/\hat{\sigma}_{\hat{\delta}_i}$ behave approximately like Brownian motion with drift θ, where $\theta = I_N^{1/2}\delta$ is the expected z-score at the end of the trial.*

Essentially the same arguments leading to Result 2.4 can be used even if the underlying observations X_i are independent but not identically distributed because Result 2.1 does not require identical distributions. A result analogous to Result 2.4 holds when the parameter is a vector (Jennison and Turnbull, 1997 [JT97] or Jennison and Turnbull, 2000 [JT00]).

Example 2.4. Consider a trial in which the outcome was the presence of at least one episode of cardiac ischemia on a Holter monitor—a device recording the electrical activity of the heart over a 24-hour period—12 weeks following randomization. Patients were also monitored with the Holter at baseline, and investigators wanted to use logistic regression to adjust the 12-week results for differences in the baseline number of ischemic episodes. The model is

$$\ln\{p/(1-p)\} = \alpha + \beta u + \delta x,$$

where p is the probability of having ischemia at 12 weeks, u is the baseline number of episiodes, and x is the treatment indicator. We parameterize such that positive z-scores indicate that the treatment is beneficial, so we take $x = 1$ to mean the control condition. We are interested in testing whether $\delta = 0$ (no treatment effect). After 200 of the planned 600 patients are evaluated, the estimated information fraction is $t = 200/600 = 1/3$. For simplicity, rather than using two different time scales τ and t for calendar fraction and information fraction, we use only information fraction. Thus, we denote the current treatment effect estimator and its estimated standard error by $\hat{\delta}(1/3)$ and $\hat{\sigma}_{\hat{\delta}(1/3)}$. Suppose that $\hat{\delta}(1/3) = 0.180$ and $\hat{\sigma}_{\hat{\delta}(1/3)} = 0.153$. The z-score and B-value are $Z(1/3) = 0.180/0.153 = 1.176$ and $B(1/3) = (1/3)^{1/2}(1.176) = 0.679$. Because $Z(1/3)$ has a standard normal distribution under the null hypothesis, we can easily determine a critical value c_1 such that $P_0\{|Z(1/3)| \geq c_1)\} = 0.01$, where P_0 denotes a probability computed under the null hypothesis. We find that $c_1 = 2.576$. Suppose that at the end of the trial, the estimated slope and standard error are $\hat{\delta}(1) = 0.120$ and $\hat{\sigma}_{\hat{\delta}(1)} = 0.095$. The approximate joint distribution of the interim and final B-values under true log odds ratio δ is that of $B(1/3)$ and $B(1)$, where $B(t)$ is Brownian motion with drift $\theta = \mathrm{E}\{Z(1)\} = \delta/\sigma_{\hat{\delta}(1)}$. We estimate θ by $\delta/0.095$, where δ is the true log odds ratio.

Having reached the end of the trial, we can obtain a more precise estimate of the information fraction at the first look: $t_1 = \{\mathrm{var}(\hat{\delta}(\frac{1}{3}))\}^{-1}/\{\mathrm{var}(\hat{\delta}(1))\}^{-1} = (0.153)^{-2}/(0.095)^{-2} = 0.386$ rather than $1/3$. Thus, the approximate joint distribution of the interim and final B-values is that of $B(0.386)$ and $B(1)$, where $B(t)$ is Brownian motion with drift θ. As we have seen before, this correcting of information fractions does not cause a problem for previous boundaries because the z-score at previous analyses has the same null distribution whether or not we correct the information times. Thus, the correct null probability of crossing the boundary at the first look, $P_0\{|Z(0.386)| \geq 2.576)\} = 0.01$, is the same as $P_0\{|Z(1/3)| \geq 2.576)\}$. The advantage of using the slightly more accurate estimate $t_1 = 0.386$ lies in computation of the boundary at the next look at the end of the trial. We determine c_2 such that $P_0\{(|Z(0.386)| \geq 2.576) \cup (|Z(1)| \geq c_2)\} = 0.05$. Numerical integration can be used to obtain $c_2 = 2.014$.

Importantly, the boundaries $c_1 = 2.576$ and $c_2 = 2.014$ for the z-scores associated with the MLE are the same as for a t-test, test of proportions, or logrank test at information fractions $t_1 = 0.386$ and $t_2 = 1$.

2.5 Other Settings Leading to E-Processes and Brownian Motion

We have seen that many estimators frequently used in clinical trials are E-processes when monitored over time. Other broad classes of estimators monitored over time are also E-processes, and can therefore be transformed to Brownian motion using Result 2.3. Sometimes it is possible to argue directly that $\hat{\delta}(\tau)$ satisfies E3, as we now show.

2.5.1 Minimum Variance Unbiased Estimators

Consider a minimum variance unbiased estimator $\hat{\delta}$ in a nonmonitoring setting (i.e., $\hat{\delta}$ has the smallest variance among all unbiased estimators of δ). Let $\hat{\delta}(\tau)$ denote the corresponding minimum variance unbiased estimator monitored over time τ, $0 \leq \tau \leq 1$. Jennison and Turnbull (1997) [JT97] gave a simple argument by contradiction that $\hat{\delta}$ must satisfy E3. Note first that condition E3 can be written in the equivalent way

$$
\begin{aligned}
0 &= 1/I(\tau_j) - \text{cov}\{\hat{\delta}(\tau_j), \hat{\delta}(\tau_i)\} \\
&= \text{var}\{\hat{\delta}(\tau_j)\} - \text{cov}\{\hat{\delta}(\tau_j), \hat{\delta}(\tau_i)\} \\
&= \text{cov}\{\hat{\delta}(\tau_j), \hat{\delta}(\tau_j)\} - \text{cov}\{\hat{\delta}(\tau_j), \hat{\delta}(\tau_i)\} \\
&= \text{cov}\{\hat{\delta}(\tau_j), \hat{\delta}(\tau_j) - \hat{\delta}(\tau_i)\}.
\end{aligned}
\tag{2.20}
$$

Thus, E3 is equivalent to

$$
\text{E3}' : \text{cov}\{\hat{\delta}(\tau_j), \hat{\delta}(\tau_j) - \hat{\delta}(\tau_i)\} = 0.
$$

Suppose E3$'$ did not hold for a minimum variance unbiased estimator $\hat{\delta}$ monitored over time. For example, suppose that $\text{cov}\{\hat{\delta}(\tau_j), \hat{\delta}(\tau_j) - \hat{\delta}(\tau_i)\} > 0$. Jennison and Turnbull argued that for small $\epsilon > 0$, the estimator $\tilde{\delta}_\epsilon(\tau_j) = \hat{\delta}(\tau_j) - \epsilon\{\hat{\delta}(\tau_j) - \hat{\delta}(\tau_i)\}$ has smaller variance than $\hat{\delta}(\tau_j)$. To see this, note that $\text{var}\{\tilde{\delta}_\epsilon(\tau_j)\} = \text{var}\{\hat{\delta}(\tau_j)\} + \epsilon^2 \text{var}\{\hat{\delta}(\tau_j) - \hat{\delta}(\tau_i)\} - 2\epsilon\,\text{cov}\{\hat{\delta}(\tau_j), \hat{\delta}(\tau_j) - \hat{\delta}(\tau_i)\}$, so

$$
\begin{aligned}
\lim_{\epsilon \to 0}[\text{var}\{\tilde{\delta}_\epsilon(\tau_j)\} &- \text{var}\{\hat{\delta}(\tau_j)\}]/\epsilon \\
&= \lim_{\epsilon \to 0} \epsilon\,\text{var}\{\hat{\delta}(\tau_j) - \hat{\delta}(\tau_i)\} - 2\lim_{\epsilon \to 0}\text{cov}\{\hat{\delta}(\tau_j), \hat{\delta}(\tau_j) - \hat{\delta}(\tau_i)\} \\
&= 0 - 2\,\text{cov}\{\hat{\delta}(\tau_j), \hat{\delta}(\tau_j) - \hat{\delta}(\tau_i)\} \\
&= -2\,\text{cov}\{\hat{\delta}(\tau_j), \hat{\delta}(\tau_j) - \hat{\delta}(\tau_i)\} \\
&< 0.
\end{aligned}
$$

But this implies that $\text{var}\{\tilde{\delta}_\epsilon(\tau_j)\} < \text{var}\{\hat{\delta}(\tau_j)\}$ for sufficiently small ϵ, which contradicts the fact that $\hat{\delta}(\tau_j)$ is a minimum variance unbiased estimator. Similarly, if we had begun with the assumption that $\text{cov}\{\hat{\delta}(\tau_j), \hat{\delta}(\tau_j) - \hat{\delta}(\tau_i)\} < 0$, we could show that the estimator $\hat{\delta}(\tau_j) + \epsilon\{\hat{\delta}(\tau_j) - \hat{\delta}(\tau_i)\}$ has smaller variance than the minimum variance unbiased estimator $\hat{\delta}(\tau_j)$ for sufficiently small ϵ. This would again be a contradiction. In other words, we can find a contradiction whenever $\text{cov}\{\hat{\delta}(\tau_j), \hat{\delta}(\tau_j) - \hat{\delta}(\tau_i)\} \neq 0$. Thus, property E3′, and therefore E3, must hold.

Implicit in the above argument is the assumption that $\text{cov}\{\hat{\delta}(\tau_i), \hat{\delta}(\tau_j)\}$ does not depend on the parameter δ. If it did, then $\tilde{\delta}_\epsilon(\tau_j)$ would depend on δ. The fact that it has smaller variance than $\hat{\delta}(\tau_j)$ would not cause a contradiction because $\tilde{\delta}_\epsilon(\tau_j)$ would not be a bona-fide estimator. The arguments above prove the following result.

Result 2.5 *Let $\hat{\delta}$ be a minimum variance unbiased estimator of δ in a non-monitoring setting, and let $\hat{\delta}(\tau)$ denote $\hat{\delta}$ monitored at time τ, $0 \leq \tau \leq 1$. If $\text{cov}\{\hat{\delta}(\tau_i), \hat{\delta}(\tau_j)\}$ does not depend on δ for any $\tau_i < \tau_j$, then $\hat{\delta}(\tau)$ satisfies E3.*

While Result 2.5 does not establish condition E1 (multivariate normality) for a minimum variance unbiased estimator $\hat{\delta}(\tau)$ over time, it does show that $\hat{\delta}(\tau)$ must have the same mean and covariance structure of an E-process. Thus, if we can establish through other arguments that $\hat{\delta}(\tau)$ has an approximate multivariate normal distribution, we can convert to Brownian motion as we did for other estimators.

2.5.2 Complete Sufficient Statistics

This subsection concerns complete sufficient statistics, so we we briefly review the concepts of sufficiency and completeness. If a vector $(X_1, \ldots, X_n)$ of observations has distribution function $F(x_1, \ldots, x_n; \delta)$ depending on a parameter δ, a statistic $S(X_1, \ldots, X_n)$ (which could be a vector) is called *sufficient* if the conditional distribution of the data $X_1, \ldots, X_n$ given $S = s$ does not depend on δ. We could generate data $X_1, \ldots, X_n$ from $F(x_1, \ldots, x_n; \delta)$ by first generating a value of S from its distribution—which depends on δ—and then generating $(X_1, \ldots, X_n)$ from its conditional distribution given $S = s$. The latter generation is a random draw of n numbers from a distribution that has nothing to do with δ. In that sense, once we condition on the value of the sufficient statistic S, no further information about δ can be gleaned from the data.

A statistic S is called *complete* if the condition $\text{E}\{f(S)\} = 0$ for all δ implies that $f(S) = 0$ with probability 1 for all δ. Completeness is typically used to show that there is at most one unbiased function of S, for if both $g_1(S)$ and $g_2(S)$ were unbiased for δ, then $\text{E}\{g_2(S) - g_1(S)\} = 0$, which would mean that $g_2(S) - g_1(S) = 0$; i.e., $g_2(S) = g_1(S)$ with probability 1 for all δ.

We now consider condition E3 of an E-process and relate it to a complete sufficient statistic. By (2.20), we can consider the equivalent condition E3′. Note that condition E3′ would be satisfied if $\hat{\delta}(\tau_j)$ and $\hat{\delta}(\tau_j) - \hat{\delta}(\tau_i)$ were independent. Moreover, under E1, E3′ is equivalent to $\hat{\delta}(\tau_j)$ being independent of $\hat{\delta}(\tau_j) - \hat{\delta}(\tau_i)$. Independence of $\hat{\delta}(\tau_j)$ and $\hat{\delta}(\tau_j) - \hat{\delta}(\tau_i)$ is in some sense natural. Think of the comparison of means: $\hat{\delta}(\tau_j)$ is complete and sufficient for δ, whereas $\hat{\delta}(\tau_j) - \hat{\delta}(\tau_i)$ is *ancillary*, meaning that its distribution does not depend on δ. In a sense, $\hat{\delta}_j$ and $\hat{\delta}_j - \hat{\delta}_i$ contain all of the information and none of the information, respectively, about δ. Not surprisingly, $\hat{\delta}(\tau_j)$ is independent of $\hat{\delta}(\tau_j) - \hat{\delta}(\tau_i)$. In fact, this is a special case of a beautiful theorem due to Basu (1955) [B55]. Basu's theorem states that if $\hat{\delta}$ is sufficient and complete and A is ancillary, then $\hat{\delta}$ and A are independent (see Section 2.9.5 for proof). Thus, condition E3 will hold for any complete sufficient statistic such that $\hat{\delta}(\tau_j) - \hat{\delta}(\tau_i)$ is ancillary.

Result 2.6 *Let $\hat{\delta}$ be a complete sufficient statistic in a nonmonitoring setting, and let $\hat{\delta}(\tau)$ denote $\hat{\delta}$ monitored over time, $0 \le \tau \le 1$. If $\hat{\delta}(\tau_j) - \hat{\delta}(\tau_i)$ is ancillary for every $\tau_i \le \tau_j$, then*

1. *E3 holds.*
2. *E1 holds iff $\hat{\delta}$ is marginally normal.*
3. *E1 holds asymptotically iff $\hat{\delta}$ is asymptotically marginally normal.*

2.6 The Normal Linear and Mixed Models

2.6.1 The Linear Model

Some clinical trials analyze results using a normal linear model. For example, in the nonmonitoring setting, the analysis of covariance model that adjusts the end of study blood pressure Y for baseline blood pressure x may be written as

$$
\underline{Y} = \begin{pmatrix} 1 & 0 & x_1 \\ \vdots & \vdots & \vdots \\ 1 & 0 & x_n \\ 1 & 1 & x_{n+1} \\ \vdots & \vdots & \vdots \\ 1 & 1 & x_{2n} \end{pmatrix} \begin{pmatrix} \alpha_C \\ \delta \\ \lambda \end{pmatrix} + \underline{\epsilon},
$$

where α_C is the intercept in the control arm, $\delta = \alpha_T - \alpha_C$ is the difference between treatment and control intercepts (i.e., δ is the treatment effect), and λ is the slope—assumed the same in the treatment and control arms—of the relationship between baseline and end of study blood pressure. ($Y_1, \ldots, Y_n$ and $Y_{n+1}, \ldots, Y_{2n}$ are end-of-study blood pressures for control and treatment patients, respectively.) More generally, the normal linear model may be written as $\underline{Y} = X\beta + \underline{\epsilon}$, where X is a design matrix of dimension $n \times p$, β is a p-dimensional parameter vector, and $\underline{\epsilon}$ is an n-dimensional vector of i.i.d. $N(0, \sigma^2)$ errors.

Now consider monitoring. At the first interim analysis with n_1 observations per arm, the dimension of $\underline{Y}$ and the number of rows of the design matrix is

$2n_1$. At future interim analyses, $\underline{Y}$ will be appended by additional observations and the design matrix will be appended by additional rows; each new patient contributes a new Y and a new row to the design matrix.

We now argue that the treatment effect estimator is an E-process. To see this, assume for the moment that σ^2 is known. The least squares estimators at different interim analyses are linear combinations of the Ys, and therefore have a multivariate normal distribution. Furthermore, in a nonmonitoring setting, the least squares estimator $\hat{\beta}$ is complete and sufficient (Arnold, 1981 [A81] contains a similar result when σ^2 is unknown). Moreover, if $\hat{\underline{\beta}}(\tau_i)$ and $\hat{\underline{\beta}}(\tau_j)$ denote the least squares estimators at interim analyses at times τ_i and τ_j, then $\hat{\underline{\beta}}(\tau_j) - \hat{\underline{\beta}}(\tau_i)$ is ancillary because it has a multivariate normal distribution with zero mean vector (because both estimators are unbiased) and covariance matrix not depending on $\underline{\beta}$. It follows from Basu's theorem that $\hat{\underline{\beta}}(\tau_j)$ and $\hat{\underline{\beta}}(\tau_j) - \hat{\underline{\beta}}(\tau_i)$ are independent.

Now consider the case when σ^2 is unknown. The least squares estimator $\hat{\underline{\beta}}$ is exactly the same as in the case of known σ^2. It follows that $\hat{\underline{\beta}}(\tau_j)$ and $\hat{\underline{\beta}}(\tau_j) - \hat{\underline{\beta}}(\tau_i)$ are independent in the case of unknown σ^2 as well. In summary:

Result 2.7 *In the normal linear model, $\hat{\underline{\beta}}(\tau_1), \ldots, \hat{\underline{\beta}}(\tau_k)$ are multivariate normal and $\hat{\underline{\beta}}(\tau_j)$ is independent of $\hat{\underline{\beta}}(\tau_j) - \hat{\underline{\beta}}(\tau_i)$, $i = 2, \ldots, k$. Consequently, the treatment effect estimator, its associated z-score, and its associated B-value behave like E-, Z-, and B-processes, respectively.*

A consequence of Result 2.7 is that we may use the same boundaries for the z-scores (treatment effect estimators divided by their standard errors) from a linear model that we used for the t-test.

2.6.2 The Mixed Model

Thus far we have dealt with either independent or uncorrelated observations Y, but sometimes data from clinical trials are correlated. Common examples are trials with continuous, longitudinal data reflecting each patient's progression of disease over time. For example, the model for an observation Y_{ij} at time x_j for patient i might be

$$Y_{ij} = \alpha_C + \beta_C x_j + (\gamma + \delta x_j)u_i + a_i + b_i x_j + \epsilon_{ij}, \qquad (2.21)$$

where α_C and β_C are the mean intercept and slope in the control arm, $u_i = 0, 1$ is the treatment indicator, $\gamma = \alpha_T - \alpha_C$ and $\delta = \beta_T - \beta_C$ are differences between treatment and control mean intercepts and slopes, respectively, and a_i and b_i are random, patient-specific intercepts and slopes. The patient-specific intercepts reflect the fact that patients have different baseline values, whereas the patient-specific slopes measure the patients' improvement or deterioration over time. The quantity $\gamma = \alpha_T - \alpha_C$ reflects the between-arm difference in baseline values. The parameter on which we gauge the success of the treatment is the between-arm difference in slopes, $\delta = \beta_T - \beta_C$.

More generally, for an arbitrary mixed model, the observation vector $\underline{Y}$ is normally distributed with mean vector $X\underline{\beta}$, where $\underline{\beta} = (\beta_1, \ldots, \beta_p)^T$ is the vector of fixed effects and X its design matrix. The design matrix is similar to that of the linear model of the preceding subsection except that each patient contributes multiple rows. Each additional time point for a patient contributes a new row to the design matrix.

Now consider monitoring. Both the number of patients and the number of time points per patient may differ from one interim analysis to the next. The effect of incorporating data between successive analyses is to append observations to the $\underline{Y}$ vector and rows to the design matrix. Observations from one patient to the next are independent, but observations on the same patient over time are correlated. Nonetheless, we shall see that the Brownian motion paradigm still holds if the covariance matrix of $\underline{Y}$ is known.

In the known Σ case, we can transform to the model of the preceding subsection:

$$\Sigma^{-1/2}\underline{Y} = \Sigma^{-1/2}\underline{\beta} + \Sigma^{-1/2}\underline{\epsilon}$$
$$\underline{Y}' = X'\underline{\beta} + \underline{\epsilon}',$$

where $\underline{\epsilon}' = \Sigma^{-1/2}\underline{\epsilon}$ has covariance matrix $\Sigma^{-1/2}\Sigma\Sigma^{-1/2} = I$ (Arnold, 1981 [A81]). As noted earlier, the least squares estimator in this transformed model is complete and sufficient. The arguments of the preceding subsection imply that $\underline{\hat{\beta}}(\tau_j)$ and $\underline{\hat{\beta}}(\tau_j) - \underline{\hat{\beta}}(\tau_i)$ are independent.

Result 2.8 *Result 2.7 holds for the mixed model if the covariance between every pair of Y observations is known.*

A similar result holds in the unknown covariance case provided that the number of distinct covariances to be estimated is small compared to the number of participants.

Result 2.8 means that the null joint distribution of z-statistics (treatment effect estimates divided by their estimated standard errors) at different information fractions $t_i = [\text{var}\{\hat{\delta}(\tau_i)\}]^{-1}/[\text{var}\{\hat{\delta}(1)\}]^{-1}$ in a trial analyzed with a mixed model is the same as for a simple t-test. Therefore, any z-score boundaries developed for continuous outcome trials can be applied to trials employing a mixed model. We have not yet addressed how to estimate $\text{var}\{\hat{\delta}(1)\}$, but as we saw for other clinical trial scenarios, accurate estimation of $\text{var}\{\hat{\delta}(1)\}$ is not important for calculating probabilities under the null hypothesis. Accurate estimation of $\text{var}\{\hat{\delta}(1)\}$ does become important for probability calculations assuming the alternative hypothesis.

Because tests of treatment effects from mixed models are more complicated than t-tests and tests of proportions, we give a more detailed explanation of probability calculations assuming the alternative hypothesis is true. To use Brownian motion we must know the drift parameter $\theta = \text{E}\{Z(1)\}$, which means we must have a representation for the z-statistic at the end of the trial, $Z(1)$. Suppose participant i has observations at M_i time points $x_{i1}, \ldots, x_{iM_i}$ by the time the trial ends, and let $\bar{x}_i(1) = (1/M_i)\sum_{j=1}^{M_i} x_{ij}$. Assuming the M_i are similar across participants (which they typically are in trials that use longitudinal models), the z-statistic using the mixed model is approximately the same as the z-statistic for a test of means applied to participants' end of study least squares slope estimates $b_i(1)$,

$$\hat{b}_i(1) = SSXY_i(1)/SSX_i(1),$$

where $SSXY_i(1) = \sum_{j=1}^{M_i}(x_{ij} - \bar{x}_i(1))(Y_{ij} - \bar{Y}_i(1))$ and $SSX_i(1) = \sum(x_{ij} - \bar{x}_i(1))^2$. The expected z-score at the end of the trial is roughly $\mathrm{E}\{Z(1)\} = \delta/[2\mathrm{var}\{\hat{b}_i(1)\}/N]^{1/2}$, where δ is the difference between treatment and control population mean slopes. We can determine the variance of $\hat{b}_i(1)$ by first conditioning on the patient's true intercept and slope, a_i and b_i, and then using the formula $\mathrm{var}(U \mid \underline{V}) = \mathrm{E}\{\mathrm{var}(U \mid \underline{V})\} + \mathrm{var}\{\mathrm{E}(U \mid \underline{V})\}$, valid for any random variable U (with finite variance) and random vector $\underline{V}$. The conditional variance of $\hat{b}_i(1)$ given the patient-specific intercept and slope is $\sigma_e^2/SSX_i(1)$. The unconditional variance of $\hat{b}_i(1)$ is $\mathrm{E}\{\mathrm{var}(\hat{b}_i(1) \mid a_i, b_i)\} + \mathrm{var}\{\mathrm{E}(\hat{b}_i(1) \mid a_i, b_i)\} = \sigma_e^2/SSX_i + \sigma_b^2$, where σ_e^2 is the within-patient residual variability about his/her regression line and σ_b^2 is the variability of the patient-specific true slopes b_i. We can estimate σ_e^2 and σ_b^2 from the data at an interim analysis. For example, suppose at an interim analysis at information fraction t (we will show how to estimate the information fraction shortly) there are n patients, patient i having measurements at times $x_{i1}, \ldots, x_{im}$, and let $\bar{x}_i(t) = (1/m_i)\sum_{j=1}^{m_i} x_{ij}$. Then $\mathrm{var}\{\hat{b}_i(t)\} = \sigma_e^2/SSX_i(t) + \sigma_b^2$. Averaging over the number of patients gives us an estimate of $\mathrm{var}\{\hat{b}(t)\}$ for a randomly selected patient:

$$\mathrm{var}\{\hat{b}(t)\} = \sigma_e^2(1/n)\sum_{i=1}^{n} 1/SSX_i(t) + \sigma_b^2. \qquad (2.22)$$

We can estimate σ_e^2 as follows. For patient i, we perform least squares regression and compute the residual sum of squares $RSS_i(t) = \sum_{j=1}^{m_i}\{Y_{ij} - (\hat{a}_i + \hat{b}_i x_{ij})\}^2$. We estimate σ_e^2 by pooling over patients:

$$\hat{\sigma}_e^2 = \frac{\sum_{i=1}^{n} RSS_i(t)}{\sum_{i=1}^{n}(m_i - 2)}. \qquad (2.23)$$

We can substitute this $\hat{\sigma}_e^2$ into the right side of (2.22) and the sample variance of the $\hat{b}_i$ pooled across arms into the left side. We estimate σ_b^2 by subtraction: pooled $\mathrm{var}(\hat{b}_i) - \hat{\sigma}_e^2(1/n)\sum_{i=1}^{n} 1/SSX_i$. Because this estimate can be negative, we take the maximum of this estimate and 0:

$$\hat{\sigma}_b^2 = \max\left(0, \text{pooled var}(\hat{b}_i) - \hat{\sigma}_e^2(1/n)\sum_{i=1}^{n} 1/SSX_i(t)\right), \qquad (2.24)$$

where $\hat{\sigma}_e^2$ is given by (2.23). We use $\hat{\sigma}_e^2$ and $\hat{\sigma}_b^2$ to estimate $\mathrm{var}\{\hat{b}(1)\}$. Once we have $\mathrm{var}\{\hat{b}(1)\}$, we estimate $\mathrm{var}\{\hat{\delta}(1)\}$ and $I(1)$ by

$$\hat{\mathrm{var}}\{\hat{\delta}(1)\} = 2\mathrm{var}\{\hat{b}(1)\}/N, \quad I(1) = 1/\hat{\mathrm{var}}\{\hat{\delta}(1)\}$$

The current information is much easier. It is simply the inverse of the variance of the treatment effect estimator at the interim analysis, which we can compute from the standard output of a mixed model program. Specific details of these calculations are given in the following example:

Example 2.5. Consider a trial randomizing overweight patients to an advice-only control arm versus a treatment arm with advice plus an exercise program. Each patient is followed for 7 weeks. Weights are recorded at baseline and weekly thereafter (eight weights total). Data are analyzed according to the mixed model (2.21), where Y_{ij} is the weight of participant i at week x_{ij} (week 0 denotes the baseline period). The planned sample size is 80 patients, 40 in each treatment group.

The interim analysis is to include data from the first 4 weeks of follow-up for the first 20 patients randomized. Table 2.1 shows the data for this cohort. The weights $\underline{y}_i$ for participant i are regressed on the participant's times $\underline{x}_i$, and a least squares line is fit. The table shows, for each participant's data $\underline{x}_i$, $\underline{y}_i$, the slope estimate $\hat{b}_i$, the residual sum of squares RSS_i, $1/SSX_i = [\sum_j \{x_{ij} - (1/m_i)\sum_{r=1}^{m_i} x_{ir}\}^2]^{-1}$, and the degrees of freedom $m_i - 2$. We estimate σ_e^2 by $\sum_{i=1}^{20} RSS_i / \sum_{i=1}^{20}(m_i - 2)$. From Table 2.1, $\sum_{i=1}^{20} RSS_i = 45.6373$ and $\sum_{i=1}^{20}(m_i - 2) = 42$, so

$$\hat{\sigma}_e^2 = 45.6373/42 = 1.0866.$$

The sample variances of the slopes in column 5 for control and treatment patients are 1.1628 and 1.4957, for a pooled variance of $\{9(1.1628) + 9(1.4957)\}/18 = 1.3293$. From (2.24), we estimate σ_b^2 by

$$\hat{\sigma}_b^2 = 1.3293 - 1.0866(1/20)(2.2666) = 1.2062.$$

At the end of the trial, participants will have data for a maximum of 8 weeks, though some data may be missing. At the interim analysis, everyone had a baseline value, but 18 of the 80 possible follow-up weights for the 20 participants were missing (22.5 percent). If we assume the same percentage missing for the seven follow-up weights by the end of the trial as for the follow-up weights thus far, participants will have an average of $0.225(7) = 1.575$ missing observations among the 7 follow-up weeks. Thus, the average participant will have one baseline measurement and $7 - 1.575 = 5.425$ follow-up measurements, for a total of 6.425 measurements. The variance of x values (using M instead of $M - 1$ in the denominator) for a participant with no missing data will be $(1/8)\sum_{j=0}^{7}\{j - (0 + 1 + \ldots + 7)/8\}^2 = 5.25$. We expect

Table 2.1. Interim data from a trial using a mixed model. Twenty patients have been randomized, and up to five measurements (the baseline and first four follow-up measurements) are available. For participant i, vector $\underline{x}_i$ is the number of weeks since randomization and $\underline{y}_i$ contains the weights at weeks $\underline{x}_i$. Ordinary least squares regression is used for each participant's data, and the intercept $\hat{a}_i$ and slope $\hat{b}_i$ are computed. Shown are the slope estimate $\hat{b}_i$, $RSS_i = \sum_j (y_{ij} - a_i - b_i x_{ij})^2$, and $SSX_i = \sum_j (x_{ij} - (1/m_i) \sum_{j=1}^{m_i} x_i)^2$, where m_i is the number of observations per participant. Also shown are the degrees of freedom for each participant, namely $df_i = m_i - 2$.

Patient	Arm	$\underline{x}_i$	$\underline{y}_i$	$\hat{b}_i$	RSS_i	$1/SSX_i$	$m_i - 2$
1	C	$(0, 2, 3, 4)$	$(248, 250, 251, 251)$	0.8000	0.4000	0.1143	2
2	C	$(0, 1, 2, 3, 4)$	$(216, 214, 215, 214, 213)$	−0.6000	1.6000	0.1000	3
3	C	$(0, 1, 2, 3, 4)$	$(217, 218, 220, 217, 216)$	−0.3000	8.3000	0.1000	3
4	C	$(0, 1, 4)$	$(195, 195, 191)$	−1.0769	0.6154	0.1154	1
5	C	$(0, 2, 3, 4)$	$(197, 200, 200, 199)$	0.5714	3.1429	0.1143	2
6	C	$(0, 1, 2, 3, 4)$	$(251, 250, 252, 253, 254)$	0.9000	1.9000	0.1000	3
7	C	$(0, 1, 2, 3, 4)$	$(187, 187, 187, 188, 186)$	−0.1000	1.9000	0.1000	3
8	C	$(0, 1, 2, 4)$	$(208, 208, 207, 206)$	−0.5429	0.1714	0.1143	2
9	C	$(0, 1, 3)$	$(231, 234, 239)$	2.6429	0.0714	0.2143	1
10	C	$(0, 1, 3, 4)$	$(188, 190, 191, 192)$	0.9000	0.6500	0.1000	2
11	T	$(0, 1, 3, 4)$	$(231, 228, 224, 222)$	−2.2000	0.3500	0.1000	2
12	T	$(0, 1, 2, 4)$	$(200, 200, 202, 203)$	0.8286	0.7429	0.1143	2
13	T	$(0, 1, 2, 3, 4)$	$(271, 269, 267, 262, 261)$	−2.7000	3.1000	0.1000	3
14	T	$(0, 1, 2, 3, 4)$	$(226, 227, 225, 222, 226)$	−0.5000	12.3000	0.1000	3
15	T	$(0, 1, 2, 3, 4)$	$(182, 178, 176, 175, 170)$	−2.7000	3.9000	0.1000	3
16	T	$(0, 2, 4)$	$(212, 213, 213)$	0.2500	0.1667	0.1250	1
17	T	$(0, 1, 2, 4)$	$(208, 203, 201, 198)$	−2.3429	4.9714	0.1143	2
18	T	$(0, 3, 4)$	$(178, 174, 173)$	−1.2692	0.0385	0.1154	1
19	T	$(0, 2, 4)$	$(257, 255, 252)$	−1.2500	0.1667	0.1250	1
20	T	$(0, 1, 3, 4)$	$(203, 200, 198, 196)$	−1.6000	1.1500	0.1000	2
					45.6373	2.2666	42

the variance for a patient with missing data to be similar. Thus, a typical participant's SSX at the end of the trial will be

$$SSX(1) = 6.425(5.25) = 33.7313.$$

Thus, we estimate the variance of $\hat{b}(1)$ for a typical participant to be

$$\text{var}\{\hat{b}(1)\} = \hat{\sigma}_e^2/33.7313 + \hat{\sigma}_b^2 = 1.0866/33.7313 + 1.2062 = 1.2384.$$

We estimate the variance of the treatment effect estimate at the end of the trial with 40 participants per arm by

$$\text{var}\{\hat{\delta}(1)\} = 2(1.2384)/40 = 0.0619.$$

From this we calculate the information at the end of the trial to be

$$I(1) = 1/0.0619 = 16.1551.$$

The fitted linear model using SAS's Proc Mixed is $y = 214.0587+2.5513u+(0.3008 - 1.6544u)x$, where u is 1 for a treatment patient and 0 for a control patient. Thus, the control slope minus the treatment slope is estimated to be $\hat{\delta} = 1.6544$, with an estimated standard error of 0.5078. We estimate the current information and information fraction to be

$$I(t) = 1/(0.5078)^2 = 3.8781, \quad t = 3.8781/16.1551 = 0.24.$$

The current z-score and B-value are $Z(0.24) = 1.6544/0.5078 = 3.258$ and $B(0.24) = (0.24)^{1/2}(3.258) = 1.596$.

Calculations like these are useful for computing the conditional probability that the final z-score will be at least 1.96. This probability, called *conditional power*, is very useful for deciding whether there is any hope of seeing a significant treatment benefit by trial's end (see Chapter 3).

This example was instructive because although the interim analysis occurred with data from only one quarter of the patients, each with only between three and five of the eight observations expected by trial's end, the estimated information fraction was 0.24. In other words, the information fraction was almost the same as the fraction of participants evaluated, even though participants had data for only about half the total number of weeks. This occurred because the variance of $\hat{\delta}(t)$ depends on, in addition to the sample size, 1) the number of observations per participant (reflected through SSX_i) and 2) the random effects variance of the true slopes of different participants. If the random effects variance is large enough, it will dominate, and we will not appreciably decrease the variance of $\hat{\delta}(t)$ regardless of the number of weeks of data. That is what occurred in this example. If the random effects variance had been very small, then the number of weeks of data would have contributed mightily to the amount of information.

2.7 When Is Brownian Motion Not Appropriate?

Sometimes observations in clinical trials are not i.i.d. For example, early in a trial clinicians or laboratories may not completely understand the protocol. Early patients may differ from later patients because once certain patient sources (e.g., a catheterization laboratory) are exhausted, other sources for patients must be used. These changes could make the drift nonlinear in t. Nonlinear drift also occurs with survival analysis when the proportional hazards model does not hold. Nonetheless, these things have little to no effect on the null distribution of the test statistic over time. Clinical trialists are most concerned about threats to type 1 error rate, so they do not worry much about the effect of drift.

In almost all realistic settings, we must estimate standard errors from the data. When the sample size is large, we can treat estimated standard errors as though they were constants (see Section 2.9.1). We cannot do this with a small sample size even in a nonmonitoring setting. For example, we know that the t-distribution differs substantially from the standard normal distribution if the number of degrees of freedom is small. Generally speaking, we need large sample sizes to use Brownian motion, although Chapter 8 shows that applying boundaries to p-values instead of z-scores works well unless the sample size is extremely small.

It is not immediately clear what a large sample size means in a complicated mixed model. Consider Example 2.5. Does the number of patients or the number of observations per patient need to be large? Suppose we had only two observations per patient, one at baseline and one at the end. Then each patient's slope would essentially reduce to a change in score from baseline to end of study. With enough patients, the Brownian motion paradigm would still apply. On the other hand, suppose the trial included only two patients per arm, each with a huge number of observations. We would be very confident about slopes of the four individuals in the study, but not at all about the mean slopes in the entire populations. Because we aim to make inferences about all patients in the population, we need a large number of patients, not a large number of observations per patient.

Another way to determine what must be large in Example 2.5 is to examine the expression for the variance of the treatment effect estimate. The variance contains parameters such as σ_e^2 and σ_b^2 that must be estimated from the data. The weakest link is the random effect variance σ_b^2. Consider a best case scenario with an infinite number of observations per participant, so we could estimate each participant's slope perfectly. In that case the best estimate of σ_b^2 would be the sample variance of those n patient-specific slopes. If n were small, that sample variance would be a very poor estimate of σ_b^2, and so the Brownian motion approximation would also be poor.

Example 2.6. The Rapid Early Action for Coronary Treatment (REACT) [LRO00] was a trial that randomized communities instead of individual patients. The intervention consisted of a media campaign intended to reduce the delay time between the onset of symptoms of a heart attack and the patient's arrival at the hospital emergency room. Control communities received no intervention. The data within each community consisted of delay times as a function of calendar time, and the slope of the relationship between calendar time and the logarithm of delay time time summarized the trend in a given community.

This example is similar to Example 2.5 in certain respects. Both involved multiple correlated observations on the same randomized unit. The difference is that the number of randomized units is necessarily small in a community randomized trial. The primary analysis in REACT was a paired t-test with only 9 degrees of freedom. Brownian motion provides a very poor approximation to the joint distribution of this paired t-statistic over time. Indeed, the Brownian motion approximation would treat the B-value $B(1)$ at the end of the trial as a standard normal deviate instead of a t-deviate with only 9 degrees of freedom.

2.8 Summary

This chapter showed that commonly used test statistics of the form $\hat{\delta}/\{\text{var}(\hat{\delta})\}^{\frac{1}{2}}$ behave like standardized sums of independent random variables with mean δ and variance 1. In these settings we measure the proportion of the trial completed in terms of information rather than chronological time. Information, the inverse of the variance of the treatment effect estimator $\hat{\delta}$, can be interpreted as the number of i.i.d. observations with expectation δ and variance 1 whose average has the same variance as $\hat{\delta}$. The information fraction t, the ratio of the current information to that at the end of the trial, is used to define the B-value $B(t) = t^{1/2}Z(t)$. The B-value is used to monitor the trial. Tables 2.2 and 2.3 summarize the B-value approach to monitoring.

Table 2.2. Brownian motion framework for four testing scenarios. For survival, n and N are the numbers of patients with an event at calendar fraction τ and the end of the trial ($\tau = 1$), respectively. For the other three scenarios, they are the numbers of patients evaluated at those times. The expressions given for information and information fraction assume equal per-arm sample sizes for means, proportions, and survival.

	Means	Proportions	Survival	MLE
Parameter δ	$\mu_T - \mu_C$	$p_T - p_C$	$\ln(\lambda_T/\lambda_C)$	arbitrary
Estimator $\hat{\delta}(\tau)$	$\bar{Y}_T - \bar{Y}_C$	$\hat{p}_T - \hat{p}_C$	$\dfrac{\sum_{i=1}^{n}(O_i - E_i)}{\sum_{i=1}^{n} V_i}$	MLE
$I(\tau) = [\text{var}\{\hat{\delta}(\tau)\}]^{-1}$	$\dfrac{n}{2\sigma^2}$	$\dfrac{n}{2p(1-p)}$	$\sum_{i=1}^{n} V_i$	Fisher info.
Info. fraction t	n/N	n/N	$\approx n/N$	$\approx n/N$
$Z(t)$	$\{I(\tau)\}^{1/2}\hat{\delta}(\tau)$	$\{I(\tau)\}^{1/2}\hat{\delta}(\tau)$	$\{I(\tau)\}^{1/2}\hat{\delta}(\tau)$	$\{I(\tau)\}^{1/2}\hat{\delta}(\tau)$
Drift $\theta = \text{E}\{Z(1)\}$	$\{I(1)\}^{1/2}\delta$	$\{I(1)\}^{1/2}\delta$	$\{I(1)\}^{1/2}\delta$	$\{I(1)\}^{1/2}\delta$

The advantage of monitoring the trial using the B-value instead of the more commonly used z-score is that its mean is a linear function of t. In fact, $\text{E}\{B(t)\} = \theta t$, where $\theta = \text{E}\{Z(1)\}$ is the expected z-score at the end of the

Table 2.3. Distribution and relationship between $B(t)$ and $Z(t)$.

B-value		Relationship	Z-score	
$E\{B(t)\}$	$\mathrm{cov}\{B(s), B(t)\}$ $s \leq t$	between $B(t)$ and $Z(t)$	$E\{Z(t)\}$	$\mathrm{cov}\{Z(s), Z(t)\}$ $s \leq t$
θt	s	$B(t) = t^{1/2} Z(t)$	$\theta t^{1/2}$	$(s/t)^{1/2}$

trial. Plotting the B-value against θt makes it very easy to see whether, and to what degree, the current trend in the data is better or worse than expected.

2.9 Appendix

2.9.1 Asymptotic Validity of Using Estimated Standard Errors

In Section 2.1.1, the variance of $\hat{\delta}$ depended on σ^2, which we treated as known. In practice we estimate σ^2 by the sample variance s^2. We know that in a nonmonitoring setting, we can substitute s^2 for σ^2 and treat it as fixed if the sample size is large because $\hat{\delta}/(2s^2/N)^{1/2} = Z_N + R_N$, where $Z_N = \hat{\delta}/(2\sigma^2/N)^{1/2}$ converges in distribution to a standard normal deviate Z and $R_N = \{\hat{\delta}/(2\sigma^2/N)^{1/2}\}(\sigma/s - 1)$ converges in probability to 0. Similarly, in a nonmonitoring situation we treat the standard error of the MLE as if it were a fixed constant instead of being estimated from the data because $\hat{\delta}/\hat{\sigma}_{\hat{\delta}} = Z_N + R_N$, where $Z_N = \hat{\delta}/\sigma_{\hat{\delta}}$ converges in distribution to a standard normal deviate and $R_N = (\hat{\delta}/\sigma_{\hat{\delta}})(\sigma_{\hat{\delta}}/\hat{\sigma}_{\hat{\delta}} - 1)$ converges in probability to 0. Both these cases relied on Slutsky's theorem (Cramér, 1946 [C46]), which says that if Z_N converges in distribution to Z and R_N converges in probability to 0, then $Z_N + R_N$ converges in distribution to Z.

With monitoring, we know that $(\hat{\delta}_1/\sigma_{\hat{\delta}_1}, \ldots, \hat{\delta}_k/\sigma_{\hat{\delta}_k})$ converges in distribution, and we want to show that $(\hat{\delta}_1/\hat{\sigma}_{\hat{\delta}_1}, \ldots, \hat{\delta}_k/\hat{\sigma}_{\hat{\delta}_k})$ converges in distribution to the same thing. We need the following generalization of Slutsky's theorem.

Result 2.9 *Suppose that $\underline{X}_n = (X_{n1}, \ldots, X_{np})$ converges in distribution to $\underline{X} = (X_1, \ldots X_p)$.*

1. *If $\underline{Y}_n = (Y_{n1}, \ldots, Y_{np})$ converges to $\underline{0}$ in probability, then $\underline{X}_n + \underline{Y}_n$ converges in distribution to $\underline{X}$.*
2. *If A_n is an $m \times p$ dimensional matrix of random variables, each converging in probability to the corresponding element of the constant matrix A, then $A_n \underline{X}_n$ converges in distribution to $A\underline{X}$.*

Proof of 1: By the Cramer-Wold device (see, for example, page 18 of Serfling, 1980 [S80]), it suffices to prove that $\underline{a} \cdot (\underline{X}_n + \underline{Y}_n)$ converges in distribution to $\underline{a} \cdot \underline{X}$ for every p-dimensional nonrandom vector $\underline{a}$. But $\underline{a} \cdot \underline{X}_n$ converges in distribution to $\underline{a} \cdot \underline{X}$, and $\underline{a} \cdot \underline{Y}_n$ converges to 0 in probability. By Slutsky's theorem for one-dimensional random variables, $\underline{a} \cdot (\underline{X}_n + \underline{Y}_n)$ converges in distribution to $\underline{a} \cdot \underline{X}$, completing the proof of 1. $||$

Proof of 2: $A_n \underline{X}_n = A\underline{X}_n + (A_n - A)\underline{X}_n$. It is clear that $A\underline{X}_n$ converges in distribution to $A\underline{X}$ because $f(\underline{x}) = A\underline{x}$ is a continuous function of $\underline{x}$. Furthermore, because each element of the matrix $A_n - A$ converges in probability to 0 and X_n converges in distribution, $(A_n - A)\underline{X}_n$ converges in probability to the m-dimensional zero vector. It follows from part 1 that $A_n \underline{X}_n$ converges in distribution to $A\underline{X}$. $||$

Result 2.9 shows that when the sample sizes are large, we can treat the estimated standard errors of $\hat{\delta}_1, \ldots, \hat{\delta}_k$ as if they were exact because

$$\left(\frac{\hat{\delta}_1}{\hat{\sigma}_{\hat{\delta}_1}}, \ldots, \frac{\hat{\delta}_k}{\hat{\sigma}_{\hat{\delta}_k}} \right) = \left(\frac{\hat{\delta}_1}{\sigma_{\hat{\delta}_1}}, \ldots, \frac{\hat{\delta}_k}{\sigma_{\hat{\delta}_k}} \right) \left(\frac{\sigma_{\hat{\delta}_1}}{\hat{\sigma}_{\hat{\delta}_1}} - 1, \ldots, \frac{\sigma_{\hat{\delta}_k}}{\hat{\sigma}_{\hat{\delta}_k}} - 1 \right) + \left(\frac{\hat{\delta}_1}{\sigma_{\hat{\delta}_1}}, \ldots, \frac{\hat{\delta}_k}{\sigma_{\hat{\delta}_k}} \right)$$

$$(2.25)$$

and each $\sigma_{\hat{\delta}_i}/\hat{\sigma}_{\hat{\delta}_i} - 1$ converges to 0 in probability.

2.9.2 Proof of Result 2.1

One direction is obvious, so we prove that if $S_N/v_N^{1/2}$ is asymptotically standard normal, then the asymptotic distribution of $(S_{n_1}/v_N^{1/2}, \ldots, S_{n_k}/v_N^{1/2})$ is that of $B(t_1), \ldots, B(t_k)$.

We first prove that the asymptotic distribution of $(S_M - S_m)/(v_M - v_m)^{1/2}$ is standard normal for $m < M$, $m \to \infty$, $M \to \infty$ such that $v_m/v_M \to t$. Write

$$(S_M/v_M^{1/2}) \left(\frac{v_M}{v_M - v_m} \right)^{1/2} = \frac{S_M - S_m}{(v_M - v_m)^{1/2}} + (S_m/v_m^{1/2}) \left(\frac{v_m}{v_M - v_m} \right)^{1/2}$$

$$W_{m,M} = U_{m,M} + V_{m,M},$$

where $U_{m,M}$ and $V_{m,M}$ are independent, $W_{m,M}$ converges in distribution to $N(0, (1-t)^{-1})$ and $V_{m,M}$ converges in distribution to $N(0, t/(1-t))$. Because $U_{m,M}$ is independent of $V_{m,M}$,

$$E(e^{isW_{m,M}}) = E(e^{isU_{m,M}})E(e^{isV_{m,M}}). \qquad (2.26)$$

The left side of (2.26) converges to $\exp[-s^2/\{2(1-t)\}]$, while $E(e^{isV_{m,M}})$ converges to $\exp[-s^2 t/\{2(1-t)\}]$. It follows that $E(e^{isU_{m,M}})$ converges to $\exp[(-s^2/2)\{1/(1-t)-t/(1-t)\}] = \exp(-s^2/2)$, the characteristic function of a standard normal deviate. Hence, $(S_M - S_m)/(v_M - v_m)^{1/2}$ is asymptotically standard normal as $m \to \infty$, $M \to \infty$, $v_m/v_M \to t$.

Let $n = 10^{n_1} + \ldots + 10^{n_k}$, so that each $(n_1, \ldots, n_k)$ corresponds to a unique integer n. Let $\underline{Z}_n^T = (S_{n_1}/v_{n_1}, (S_{n_2} - S_{n_1})/(v_{n_2} - v_{n_1})^{1/2}, \ldots, (S_{n_k} - S_{n_{k-1}})/(v_{n_k} - v_{n_{k-1}})^{1/2})$. The Z_{ni} are independent, and we have shown that each converges in distribution to a standard normal, so the asymptotic distribution of $\underline{Z}_n$ is that of i.i.d. standard normals $\underline{Z} = (Z_1, \ldots, Z_k)^T$. Moreover, $(S_{n_1}/v_N^{1/2}, \ldots S_{n_k}/v_N^{1/2})^T = A_n \underline{Z}_n$, where the (i,j)th element of the $k \times k$ matrix A_n is $\{(v_{n_j} - v_{n_{j-1}})/v_N\}^{1/2}$ if $j \leq i$ and 0 if $j > i$, where $v_{n_0} = 0$. The (i,j)th element of A_n converges to $A_{ij} = (t_j - t_{j-1})^{1/2}$ for $j \leq i$ and 0 for $j > i$, where $t_0 = 0$, so by Result 2.9, $(S_{n_1}/v_N^{1/2}, \ldots S_{n_k}/v_N^{1/2})^T$ converges in distribution to $A\underline{Z}$. The joint distribution of $A\underline{Z}$ is multivariate normal with zero means and covariance matrix AA^T. Direct calculation shows that (i,j)th component of AA^T is t_j for $j \leq i$ and t_i for $j > i$. Thus, $(S_{n_1}/v_N^{1/2}, \ldots S_{n_k}/v_N^{1/2})$ converges in distribution to $(B(t_1), \ldots, B(t_k))$. ||

2.9.3 Proof that for the Logrank Test, $D_i = O_i - E_i$ Are Uncorrelated Under H_0

To show that the D_i are uncorrelated, mean 0 random variables, we use the identity $\mathrm{var}(Y) = \mathrm{E}\{\mathrm{var}(Y \mid \underline{X})\} + \mathrm{var}\{\mathrm{E}(Y \mid \underline{X})\}$ for a random variable Y with finite variance and a random vector $\underline{X}$. The unconditional mean and variance of D_i are $\mathrm{E}(D_i) = \mathrm{E}\{\mathrm{E}(D_i \mid m_{0i}, m_{1i})\} = \mathrm{E}(0) = 0$ and $\mathrm{var}(D_i) = \mathrm{E}\{\mathrm{var}(D_i \mid m_{0i}, m_{1i})\} + \mathrm{var}\{\mathrm{E}(D_i \mid m_{0i}, m_{1i})\} = \mathrm{E}(V_i) + \mathrm{var}(0) = \mathrm{E}(V_i)$. The D_i are uncorrelated because $\mathrm{cov}(D_i, D_j) = \mathrm{E}(D_i D_j) = \mathrm{E}\{\mathrm{E}(D_i D_j \mid D_i, m_{0j}, m_{1j})\} = \mathrm{E}\{D_i \mathrm{E}(D_j \mid D_i, m_{0j}, m_{1j})\}$.

Now consider $\mathrm{E}\{D_i \mathrm{E}(D_j \mid D_i, m_{0j}, m_{1j})\}$. Just prior to the jth death, D_i is relevant only in that it provides information about the numbers m_{0j} and m_{1j} of patients at risk at that time. Therefore, once we condition on m_{0j} and m_{1j}, the additional variable D_i becomes irrelevant so $\mathrm{E}(D_j \mid D_i, m_{0j}, m_{1j}) = \mathrm{E}(D_j \mid m_{0j}, m_{1j}) = 0$.

2.9.4 A Rigorous Justification of Brownian Motion with Drift: Local Alternatives

Up to now we have not been completely rigorous in our use of Brownian motion with drift. Consider the t-test for a continuous outcome trial. Ordinarily, we think of the treatment effect δ as a fixed constant (e.g., a 3 mm Hg blood pressure difference between the treatment and control arms). But then the expected final z-score,

$$\theta = \frac{\delta}{\sqrt{2\sigma^2/N}},$$

would tend to ∞ as $N \to \infty$, reflecting the obvious fact that power tends to 1 as the sample size tends to ∞. To avoid having the power tend to 1, we must consider local alternatives (i.e., treatment effects δ_N that approach 0 as $N \to \infty$). The situation is analogous to the Poisson approximation to the binomial (n, p) distribution; for fixed p, the number of successes tends to ∞ as $n \to \infty$, but if $p = p_n$ tends to 0 such that $np_n \to \lambda$, the number of successes has an approximate Poisson distribution with mean λ.

Returning to the t-test, consider the location shift setting in which the $2N$ observations at the end of the trial in the control and treatment arms are i.i.d. $F(x)$ and i.i.d. $F(x - \delta_N)$, respectively, for some distribution function $F(x)$ and location parameter δ_N. We can imagine generating such data by generating $2N$ i.i.d. observations $Y_1, \ldots, Y_{2N}$ from F and adding δ_N to the first N. The interim z-statistic after n observations/arm is

$$Z_n = \frac{\sum_{i=1}^n (Y_i + \delta_N) - \sum_{i=1}^n Y_{N+i}}{\sqrt{2n\sigma^2}}$$

$$= \frac{\sum_{i=1}^n Y_i - \sum_{i=1}^n Y_{N+i}}{\sqrt{2n\sigma^2}} + \sqrt{\frac{n}{2\sigma^2}} \delta_N.$$

Converting to B-values gives

$$B_n = \frac{\sum_{i=1}^n Y_i - \sum_{i=1}^n Y_{N+i}}{\sqrt{2N\sigma^2}} + \sqrt{\frac{N}{2\sigma^2}} \delta_N (n/N) \qquad (2.27)$$

The first term of (2.27) is the B-value under the null hypothesis, whose joint distribution over information time is asymptotically standard Brownian motion. Let $\theta_N = \{N/(2\sigma^2)\}^{1/2} \delta_N$ and suppose that as $N \to \infty$, $n/N \to t$ and $\delta_N \to 0$ such that $\theta_N \to \theta$ for some constant θ. The rightmost term of the right side of (2.27) converges in probability to θt, so the multivariate version of Slutsky's theorem implies that the joint distribution of $B_{n_1}, \ldots, B_{n_k}$ is that of a Brownian motion with drift θ.

A similar technique can be used with dichotomous outcome trials. A rigorous justification of local alternatives in survival analysis is beyond the scope of this book. An excellent reference for the required martingale approach is Helland (1982) [H82].

2.9.5 Basu's Theorem

Result 2.10 *Basu (1955) [B55]. If $\hat{\underline{\delta}} = (\hat{\delta}_1, \ldots, \hat{\delta}_p)$ is a complete sufficient statistic for $(\delta_1, \ldots, \delta_p)$ and $\underline{A} = (A_1, \ldots, A_m)$ is ancillary, then $\hat{\underline{\delta}}$ and $\underline{A}$ are independent.*

Proof: Let $f(\underline{A})$ be any function with finite expectation, and let $\psi(\hat{\underline{\delta}}) = \mathrm{E}\{f(\underline{A}) \,|\, \hat{\underline{\delta}}\}$. Then $\mathrm{E}\{\psi(\hat{\underline{\delta}})\} = \mathrm{E}\{f(\underline{A})\}$, so $\mathrm{E}[\psi(\hat{\underline{\delta}}) - \mathrm{E}\{f(\underline{A})\}] = 0$. Because $\underline{A}$ is ancillary, $\mathrm{E}\{f(\underline{A})\}$ does not depend on δ, so $\psi(\hat{\underline{\delta}}) - \mathrm{E}\{f(\underline{A})\}$ is a statistic and a function of $\hat{\underline{\delta}}$. Completeness of $\hat{\underline{\delta}}$ implies that $\psi(\hat{\underline{\delta}}) = \mathrm{E}\{f(\underline{A})\}$. Thus, $\mathrm{E}\{f(\underline{A}) \,|\, \hat{\underline{\delta}}\} = \mathrm{E}\{f(\underline{A})\}$ for any function f with finite expectation. Taking $f(\underline{A}) = I(A_1 \leq a_1, \ldots, A_m \leq a_m)$ shows that $\underline{A}$ and $\hat{\underline{\delta}}$ are independent. ||

3

Power: Conditional, Unconditional, and Predictive

Having developed a unified statistical framework for the monitoring of trials involving different kinds of endpoints, we apply it to the calculation of different types of power. We focus primarily on trials not designed to allow early stopping for benefit. For example, in a short-term feeding trial in people with mild hypertension, we do not feel ethically compelled to stop early for benefit even if the intervention is superior to the control. On the other hand, if it becomes clear that the new diet is not worthwhile, we may not want to continue the expensive feeding. Thus, stopping for futility may still be important.

3.1 Unconditional Power

Adequate sample size and power are essential for a well-designed clinical trial. The necessary calculations are easy for any of the z-statistics discussed in the previous chapter, for all are asymptotically normal with mean θ and variance 1 (Figure 3.1).

We equate θ, the expected z-score of Table 2.2, to $z_{\alpha/2} + z_\beta$ and solve for either the sample size or power. For example, power is obtained as follows:

$$\theta = z_{\alpha/2} + z_\beta \qquad (3.1)$$
$$\Rightarrow \Phi(\theta - z_{\alpha/2}) = 1 - \beta = \text{power} \qquad (3.2)$$

Hence, for a two-sided level .05 test with 80 percent power, the expected z-score is $1.96 + 0.84 = 2.80$; its associated two-sided p-value is $2\{1 - \Phi(2.80)\} = .005$. With 90 percent power, the expected z-score and associated two-sided p-value are $1.96 + 1.28 = 3.24$ and $2\{1 - \Phi(3.24)\} = .001$, respectively. The p-value corresponding to the expected z-score for a study with 50 percent power ($z_\beta = 0$) is .05. Often when we statisticians present the results of a sample size calculation, the clinicians with whom we work protest that they have been able to find statistical significance with much smaller sample sizes. Although they do not conceptualize their argument in terms of power, we believe their

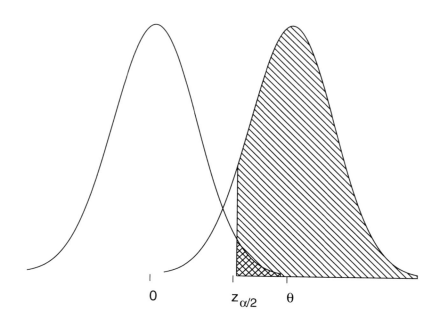

Fig. 3.1. The null (left curve) and alternative (right curve) distributions of the z-statistic are normal with variance 1 and respective means 0 and θ. The areas of the crosshatched regions correspond to type 1 error rate and power. Power $1 - \beta$ is achieved when $z_{\alpha/2}$ is the βth percentile of the distribution on the right. Because the distribution on the right is a shift (by θ units) of the standard normal density on the left, its βth percentile is a shift (by θ units) of $-z_\beta$, the βth percentile of the standard normal density. In summary, $z_{\alpha/2} = \theta - z_\beta$. That is, $\theta = z_{\alpha/2} + z_\beta$.

experience comes from an intuitive feel for 50 percent power. We have found that showing them Equation (3.1) and explaining its consequences in terms of sample size and power helps them understand the risk of small sample sizes and the fact that a large sample size buys them the ability to declare a small observed treatment effect statistically significant. In some cases a treatment may be onerous enough that only if it had a relatively large effect would it be considered viable. Ninety percent power to detect a very large effect might equate to roughly 50 percent power for a more traditional effect size.

Example 3.1. Consider a trial with a short-term dichotomous outcome such as 28-day mortality analyzed using a test of proportions. The proportion of deaths in the control arm is expected to be 0.60, and we wish to have 85 percent power to detect a 25 percent reduction (from 0.60 to 0.45) in the treatment arm.

The expected z-score with N per arm is $\theta = \delta/\{2p(1-p)/N\}^{1/2}$, where $\delta = 0.60 - 0.45 = 0.15$ and $p = (0.60 + 0.45)/2 = 0.525$. A sample size of $N = 150$ per arm yields $\theta = 2.60$ and power $\Phi(2.60 - 1.96) = \Phi(0.64) = 0.74$. To achieve 85 percent power, we set $\theta = 1.96 + 1.04 = 3$ and solve for N, which yields $N = 2p(1-p)(1.96 + 1.04)^2/\delta^2 \approx 200$ per treatment arm.

3.2 Conditional Power for Futility

Power tells whether a clinical trial is likely to yield useful, interpretable data given the available sample size. Very low power means the trial is futile, that is, unlikely to reach statistical significance even if the alternative hypothesis is true. One should not begin a trial believed to be futile. But sometimes futility becomes apparent only after a trial is well under way.

Suppose the interim data in example 3.1 with 191 and 193 patients evaluated in the control and treatment arms were as given in Table 3.1.

Table 3.1. Interim data for Example 3.1.

	Event		
	Yes	No	
Control	75	116	191
Treatment	75	118	193
	150	234	384

Even if all nine remaining control patients had events and all 7 remaining treatment patients were event-free, the final results would not show a statistically significant benefit: $\hat{p}_C = 84/200$, $\hat{p}_T = 75/200$, $Z = 0.92$. If our aim for that trial were simply to declare, or not declare, statistical significance, we could choose to stop now. Stopping a trial because the final result is completely determined at an interim analysis is called *curtailment*. As in this example, curtailment can only happen near the end of the trial.

Though the result was completely determined only very close to the end of the trial, it must have been "almost" determined earlier. For example, suppose that after 180 patients per arm, the results had been as shown in Table 3.2. A statistically significant benefit at the end is possible only if all 20 remaining control patients have events and all 20 remaining treatment patients are event-free. This is extremely unlikely given that about 39 percent of all patients have had events thus far. In fact, we can quantify how unlikely a statistically significant final result is by computing *conditional power*, the

Table 3.2. Data for Example 3.1 at an earlier time.

	Event Yes	Event No	
Control	71	109	180
Treatment	71	109	180
	142	218	360

conditional probability of a statistically significant benefit at the end given the current data. In this example, because the only way to get a statistically significant benefit is for all 20 remaining control patients to have an event and all 20 remaining treatment patients not to have one, conditional power is $p_C^{20}(1 - p_T)^{20} \approx 0$ to several decimal places under any reasonable assumption about the event probabilities p_C and p_T for future patients in the control and treatment arms. Thus, we might stop the trial because the final result is known with high probability. This stochastic version of curtailment is called *stochastic curtailment*.

We are able to compute exact conditional power in this example because only one outcome leads to a statistically significant final result. Usually, however, many possible outcomes lead to a significant result, and we approximate conditional power using the B-value formulation of the previous chapter. Conditional power is the conditional probability that $B(1) > z_{\alpha/2}$ given that $B(t) = b$. Write $B(1)$ as $B(t) + B(1) - B(t)$. The increment $B(1) - B(t)$ is independent of $B(t)$ and has mean and variance

$$E\{B(1) - B(t)\} = \theta \cdot 1 - \theta \cdot t = \theta(1 - t)$$

$$\begin{aligned} \text{var}\{B(1) - B(t)\} &= \text{var}\{B(1)\} + \text{var}\{B(t)\} - 2\text{cov}\{B(1), B(t)\} \\ &= 1 + t - 2t = 1 - t. \end{aligned}$$

Thus, given $B(t) = b$, the quantity $B(1) = b + B(1) - B(t)$ is normally distributed with variance $1 - t$ and mean:

$$E_\theta\{B(1) \mid B(t) = b\} = b + \theta(1 - t), \tag{3.3}$$

where the drift parameter θ is the expected z-score at the end of the trial. It follows that conditional power for a two-tailed test at level α (or one-tailed test at level $\alpha/2$) is

$$CP_\theta(t) = 1 - \Phi\left(\frac{z_{\alpha/2} - E_\theta\{B(1) \mid B(t) = b)\}}{\sqrt{1 - t}}\right), \tag{3.4}$$

where $E_\theta\{B(1) \mid B(t) = b\}$ is given by (3.3).

The conditional mean of $B(1)$ given $B(t) = b$ may be viewed geometrically as the endpoint of a line segment beginning at (t, b) with slope θ. If we superimpose a $N(b + \theta(1 - t), 1 - t)$ distribution "on its side," conditional power is the area above the point $(1, z_{\alpha/2})$ (Figure 3.2).

Under the null hypothesis $\theta = 0$, Equation (3.3) simplifies to

$$E_0\{B(1) \mid B(t) = b\} = b. \tag{3.5}$$

The empirical estimate for θ is $\hat{\theta} = B(t)/t = b/t$. Under this "current trend" hypothesis, Equation (3.3) becomes

$$E_{\hat{\theta}}\{B(1) \mid B(t) = b\} = b/t = \hat{\theta}. \tag{3.6}$$

Formula (3.4) applies to any of the testing situations we considered in Chapter 2, and it shows that conditional power increases as the drift parameter increases. We illustrate the use of formula (3.4) with several examples.

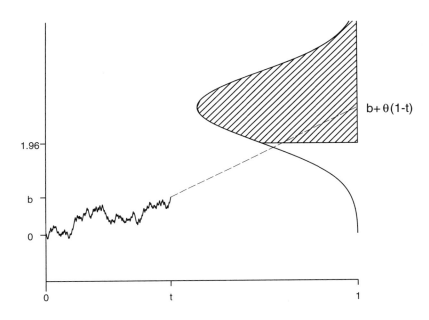

Fig. 3.2. Given $B(t) = b$, $B(1)$ is normal with mean $b + \theta(1 - t)$ and variance $1 - t$. Conditional power is the crosshatched area above 1.96 for a two-tailed test at level .05.

Example 3.2. We initiate a feeding trial to compare the effects of two diets on diastolic blood pressure change from baseline to 8 weeks. We anticipate the standard deviation of change scores to be approximately 5 mm Hg, and we want 90 percent power to detect an effect of 2 mm Hg. Equating the expected z-score, $\theta = \delta/(2\sigma^2/N)^{1/2}$, to $z_{\alpha/2} + z_\beta = 1.96 + 1.28 = 3.24$ and solving for N yields a per-arm sample size of $N = 2(25)(3.24)^2/2^2 \approx 132$ (rounding up to be conservative).

Suppose after 98 and 102 participants are evaluated in the control and treatment diets, the treatment effect and pooled standard deviation are $\hat{\delta} = 0.683$ and $\hat{\sigma} = 7.750$. The current information and information expected by trial's end are $\{\sigma^2(1/98 + 1/102)\}^{-1} = (98)(102)/(200\sigma^2)$ and $(2\sigma^2/132)^{-1} = 66/\sigma^2$, respectively. The information fraction is $(98)(102)/\{(200)(66)\} = 0.757$, virtually the same as if we had used the average sample size $(98 + 102)/2 = 100$ and approximated the information fraction by $100/132$. The z-score and B-value are

$$Z(0.757) = 0.683/\{(7.750)^2(1/98 + 1/102)\}^{1/2} = 0.623,$$

$$B(0.757) = (0.757)^{1/2}Z(0.757) = 0.542.$$

The expected B-value under the originally assumed treatment effect and standard deviation is $E\{B(t)\} = 3.24t$, so the current results are poorer than expected (Figure 3.3). Is there so little benefit of treatment thus far that we should stop the trial?

We first compute conditional power under the originally hypothesized treatment effect of $\delta = 2$ mm Hg and standard deviation of $\sigma = 5$ mm Hg. Because our sample size $N = 132$ was based on 90 percent power, the expected z-score at the end of the trial under the original assumptions is $\theta = 1.96 + 1.28 = 3.24$. That is, if our hypothesized effect size is true, we would expect the two-sided p-value to be .001. Graphically, we form a line segment at $(t, B(t)) = (0.757, 0.542)$ with slope 3.24 (Figure 3.3). The conditional mean of $B(1)$ given $B(0.757) = 0.542$ is the value of the line segment at $t = 1$, namely $0.542 + 3.24(1 - 0.757) = 1.329$. The variance of $B(1)$ given $B(0.757) = 0.542$ is $1 - 0.757 = 0.243$. Conditional power is

$$\mathrm{CP}_{3.24}(0.757) = 1 - \Phi\left\{(1.96 - 1.329)/(0.243)^{1/2}\right\}$$
$$= 1 - \Phi(1.28) = 0.10.$$

That is, conditional power is only 10 percent under the original assumptions about the treatment effect and standard deviation.

The original assumptions appear very optimistic because the observed standard deviation is larger than expected (7.750 instead of 5) and the observed treatment effect is smaller than expected (0.683 instead of 2). We could incorporate these estimates by computing conditional power under the empirical (i.e., observed) drift parameter $\hat{\theta} = B(t)/t = 0.542/0.757 = 0.716$. We form a line segment beginning at $(0.757, 0.542)$ with slope 0.716. This amounts to extending the line segment joining $(0,0)$ and $(t, B(t))$ to $(1, 0.716)$ (Figure

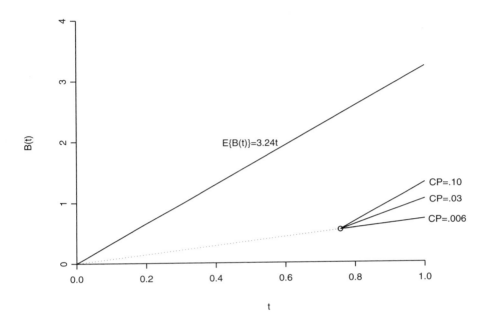

Fig. 3.3. Conditional power (CP) in Example 3.2. The solid line joining the origin to $(1, 3.24)$ shows the expected value of $B(t)$ under the original assumptions. The current B-value (circle) lies below that line, indicating poorer than expected results. Conditional power is computed under 1) the original assumptions (CP = 0.10), 2) the original treatment effect but the empirical standard deviation (CP=0.03), and 3) the empirical treatment effect and standard deviation (CP=0.006).

3.3). Conditional power under the empirical treatment effect and standard deviation is

$$CP_{0.716}(0.757) = 1 - \Phi\{(1.96 - 0.716)/(0.243)^{1/2}\}$$
$$= 1 - \Phi(2.52) = 0.006.$$

Thus, if the empirical trend is true, then we have less than a 1 percent chance of a statistically significant benefit at the end of the trial.

Another reasonable choice for the drift parameter is to use the empirical standard deviation estimate 7.750, but maintain the original treatment effect, $\delta = 2$. After all, the study was powered to detect a treatment effect of 2. The drift parameter is $\theta = 2/\{2(7.75)^2/132\}^{1/2} = 2.097$. The conditional mean of $B(1)$ is $0.542 + 2.097(1 - 0.757) = 1.052$. Conditional power is

$$CP_{2.097}(0.757) = 1 - \Phi\{(1.96 - 1.052)/(0.243)^{1/2}\}$$
$$= 1 - \Phi(1.84) = 0.03$$

(Figure 3.3). Conditional power is less than 5 percent under this realistic standard deviation estimate and the original treatment effect.

In this example, any reasonable assumption yields very low conditional power. Whether we should stop a trial that has low conditional power depends on whether the precision at the end would be sufficient to exclude the originally hypothesized treatment effect. We determine that by computing the *un*conditional power to detect the originally hypothesized treatment effect $\delta = 2$ using the revised standard deviation estimate $\sigma = 7.75$. The expected z-score is 2.097 instead of 3.24. Plugging $\theta = 2.097$ into the unconditional power formula (3.2) yields $\Phi(2.097 - 1.96) = 0.55$. This low unconditional power lends more support for abandoning the trial for futility. Not only is there a high probability of reaching a nonsignificant result at the end, but a nonsignificant result will not rule out the originally hypothesized treatment effect because unconditional power is so low.

Suppose instead the interim results had been $\hat{\delta} = 0.441, \hat{\sigma} = 5.000$. The current z-statistic would still have been $Z(0.757) = 0.623$, so conditional power under $\delta = 2$ and $\sigma = 5$ would be 0.10 as above, but unconditional power would now be $UP = \Phi\left(\frac{2}{\sqrt{2(5)^2/132}} - 1.96\right) = 0.90$. In this case a null result would be meaningful because it would exclude a treatment benefit of 2. Depending on the context of the trial, one might want to continue the trial to demonstrate that treatment is ineffective. For example, in a National Institutes of Health (NIH)-sponsored trial comparing diets designed to lower cholesterol, it might be important to demonstrate that a popular diet does not work.

Example 3.3. Returning to Example 3.1, suppose that at the first interim analysis, 22 of 44 control patients and 24 of 48 treatment patients have events, as shown in Table 3.3. The information fraction is $t = \{p(1-p)(1/44 + 1/48)\}^{-1}/\{p(1-p)(2/200)\}^{-1} = 0.230$.

Table 3.3. Interim data for Example 3.1.

	Event Yes	No	
Control	22	22	44
Treatment	24	24	48
	46	46	92

Because $\hat{p}_T = \hat{p}_C = 0.5$, it follows that $Z(0.230) = B(0.230) = 0$. Under the original event probability assumptions in the two arms, the drift parameter is

$\theta = 1.96 + 1.04 = 3$, so the conditional mean of $B(1)$ given $B(0.230) = 0$ is $0 + 3(1 - 0.230) = 2.310$.

Conditional power under the original assumptions is

$$CP_3(0.230) = 1 - \Phi\left\{(1.96 - 2.310)/(1 - .230)^{1/2}\right\}$$
$$= 1 - \Phi(-0.40) = 0.66.$$

Conditional power is not dismally low even though the observed treatment effect is zero because we are still relatively early in the trial ($t = 0.230$).

Using the empirical estimates of event probabilities in the two arms corresponds to using the empirical drift parameter estimate $B(t)/t = 0$. The conditional mean of $B(1)$ given $B(0.230) = 0$ is $0 + 0(1 - 0.230) = 0$, so conditional power is

$$CP_0(0.230) = 1 - \Phi\{(1.96 - 0)/(1 - 0.230)^{1/2}\}$$
$$= 1 - \Phi(2.23) = 0.01.$$

There is a huge discrepancy between this conditional power value and the one computed under the original assumptions. The empirical estimates of event probabilities and the drift parameter are poor at this early stage, so we should not give too much weight to conditional power under those estimates. Conditional power under empirical estimates becomes more important later in a trial.

For the continuous outcome case in Example 3.2, one of our conditional power calculations assumed the original treatment effect but used the empirical standard deviation estimate. The standard deviation is a nuisance parameter statistically independent of the sample treatment difference. In the dichotomous outcome case, the empirical combined event proportion $\hat{p} = (n_T\hat{p}_T + n_C\hat{p}_C)/(n_T + n_C)$ is a nuisance parameter uncorrelated with, and asymptotically independent of, the sample treatment difference $\hat{p}_C - \hat{p}_T$. The analogous conditional power calculation assumes the original treatment reduction (25 percent) but uses the empirical combined event probability $\hat{p} = (22 + 24)/(44 + 48) = 0.50$ to estimate $(p_C + p_T)/2$. Solving the two equations

$$(p_C + p_T)/2 = 0.50$$
$$p_T/p_C = 0.75$$

yields $p_C = 0.571$, $p_T = 0.429$. The drift parameter and conditional mean of $B(1)$ given $B(0.230) = 0$ are $\theta = (0.571 - 0.429)/\{2(0.5)(1 - 0.5)/200\}^{1/2} = 2.840$ and $E\{B(1) \mid B(0.230) = 0\} = 0 + 2.840(1 - 0.230) = 2.187$. Conditional power is

$$CP_{2.840}(0.230) = 1 - \Phi\{(1.96 - 2.187)/(1 - 0.230)^{1/2}\}$$
$$= 1 - \Phi(-0.26) = 0.60.$$

If conditional power had been very low, say under 20 percent, then it would have made sense to compute unconditional power under the empirical estimate of the combined event probability and the original 25 percent treatment reduction. As in the continuous outcome case, low conditional power but high unconditional power might justify continuing a trial, if ethically feasible, to demonstrate that the treatment does not work.

Example 3.4. Suppose we compare survival for bypass surgery (treatment) versus medicine (control) for patients with coronary artery disease. We expect the control hazard rate to be 0.05/year over an average follow-up of 5 years, and we want 80 percent power to detect a 30 percent lower hazard in the treatment arm. Recall from Chapter 2 that the logrank statistic is

$$
Z = \frac{\sum_{i=1}^{N}(O_i - E_i)}{\sqrt{\sum_{i=1}^{N} V_i}}
$$

$$
= \left\{ \sum_{i=1}^{N} V_i \right\}^{1/2} \left\{ \frac{\sum_{i=1}^{N}(O_i - E_i)}{\sum_{i=1}^{N} V_i} \right\}
$$

$$
\approx (N/4)^{1/2}\hat{\delta},
$$

where N is the total number of deaths and $\hat{\delta} = \sum(O_i - E_i)/\sum V_i$ estimates δ, the log hazard ratio. The expected z-score is

$$
\theta = (N/4)^{1/2}\delta.
$$

Note that in this parameterization of the logrank statistic, negative values for δ and Z indicate that treatment is beneficial. We prefer to make positive values correspond to treatment benefit, so we reverse the treatment labels. The hazard ratio we want to detect then becomes $1/0.7$ instead of 0.7. We obtain the sample size for 80 percent power by first determining the required number of deaths. Equating the expected z-score to $1.96 + 0.84$ and solving for N gives $N = 4(1.96 + 0.84)^2/\{\ln(1/0.7)\}^2 = 247$ deaths.

The next step is to estimate the number of patients needed to produce 247 deaths. For purposes of sample size calculation only, we assume exponential survival, so the 5-year mortality in control and treatment arms is expected to be $1 - \exp\{-5(0.05)\} = 0.221$ and $1 - \exp\{-5(0.7)(0.05)\} = 0.161$. The combined 5-year mortality is $(0.221 + 0.161)/2 = 0.191$. To have 247 events, we need $247/0.191 \approx 1300$ people.

Suppose that at an interim analysis after an average follow-up of 2.6 years, everyone is randomized and we find that 35 of 654 control patients and 25 of 646 treatment patients have died.

We originally expected 247 deaths by the end of the study, but now such a high mortality rate seems unrealistic. We therefore compute conditional power assuming a more realistic figure of, say, 120 deaths by the end of the trial. The current information fraction is $t = (35 + 25)/120 = 0.50$. Suppose the log hazard ratio estimate and logrank statistic are $\hat{\delta} = \ln(1.20) = 0.182$ and $Z(0.50) = 0.706$. The B-value is $B(0.50) = (0.50)^{1/2}(0.706) = 0.499$.

The empirical estimate of the drift parameter is $B(0.50)/0.50 = 0.998$. The expected value of $B(1)$ given $B(0.50) = 0.499$ is also 0.998, so conditional power is

$$CP_{0.998}(0.50) = 1 - \Phi\{(1.96 - 0.998)/(1 - 0.50)^{1/2}\}$$
$$= 1 - \Phi(1.36) = 0.09.$$

Conditional power computed under the empirical drift parameter is quite low.

Under the originally assumed log hazard ratio, the drift parameter is $\theta = (N/4)^{1/2}\delta = (120/4)^{1/2}\ln(1/0.7) = 1.954$, and the expected B-value at the end of the trial is $0.499 + 1.954(1 - 0.50) = 1.476$. Conditional power is

$$CP_{1.954}(0.50) = 1 - \Phi\{(1.96 - 1.476)/(1 - 0.50)^{1/2}\}$$
$$= 1 - \Phi(0.68) = 0.25,$$

higher than CP under the empirical drift, but still fairly low.

Conditional power is low in this example because the total number of deaths is markedly lower than expected. Unless the mortality rate increases dramatically, there is a fairly high probability of failing to reach a statistically significant result at the end of the trial. An aggravating factor is the low unconditional power $\Phi(1.954 - 1.96) = 0.50$. This means that a nonsignificant final result will not rule out the originally hypothesized 30 percent benefit. The decision whether to stop will likely incorporate conditional and unconditional power, as well as the mitigating factor that all patients have already been randomized and received treatment, so only follow-up remains.

3.3 Varied Uses of Conditional Power

Conditional power has been used to justify stopping several trials. For example, the decision to stop the Cardiac Arrhythmia Suppression Trial (CAST) II because of excess mortality in the two-week drug-titration phase compared to placebo titration was bolstered by conditional power calculations showing little chance (conditional power< 0.08) of establishing longer term benefit.

The estrogen and progesterone trial (PERT) of the Women's Health Initiative stopped early because the treated arm showed an excess of invasive breast cancer and an overall unfavorable balance of risk to benefit. In terms of inference regarding the effect of estrogen/progesterone on the heart, conditional power calculations under a wide variety of scenarios showed a very small chance of ever demonstrating benefit.

Conditional power is also a convenient tool for evaluating the impact of missing or unadjudicated observations.

Example 3.5. The Asymptomatic Cardiac Ischemia Pilot (ACIP) [KBP94] study evaluated three treatment strategies for patients with cardiac ischemia:

1) an angina-guided arm in which patients received medication when they experienced angina, 2) an ischemia-guided arm in which patients received medicine when they experienced angina or when 24-hour ambulatory electrocardiograms (AECGs) administered 4 and 8 weeks after randomization detected silent ischemia, and 3) a revascularization arm in which patients received either angioplasty or bypass surgery, at the discretion of the treating physician. The primary outcome measure was absence of ischemia on an AECG administered 12 weeks after randomization. A Bonferroni adjustment was made to account for the three paired comparisons. Because ACIP was a pilot study, the overall type 1 error rate was set at .10, meaning that each pairwise comparison required $p < .033$, $(|Z| > 2.13)$.

Table 3.4. ACIP data.

	Ischemia-free?		
	Yes	No	
Angina-guided	75	118	193+11 missing=204
Ischemia-guided	78	111	189+13 missing=202
Revascularization	105	87	192+20 missing=212
	258	316	574+44 missing=618

Table 3.4 shows that ACIP had 11 and 20 missing observations in the angina-guided and revascularization arms, respectively. The comparison of nonmissing data in these arms is statistically significant ($Z = 3.112, p = .002$). Might the results be biased? There are, after all, more missing data in the revascularization arm.

One way to assess the impact of missing data is to try to predict what the results would have been had all data been observed. We could treat the numbers of ischemia-free patients among missing data in the angina-guided and revascularization arms as binomials with respective parameters $(11, p_0)$ and $(20, p_1)$. We make conservative assumptions about p_0 and p_1 and calculate the conditional probability of a statistically significant result if all the data were observed. For example, Proschan et al. (2001) [PMS01] showed that under the quite pessimistic case that p_0 and p_1 equaled the observed proportions ischemia-free in the opposite arms, the conditional probability of a significant result would be about 0.99.

Though their calculations were based on binomial $(11, p_0)$ and binomial $(20, p_1)$ distributions, the B-value approximation gives nearly the same answer. The information fraction and B-value are

$$t = (1/193 + 1/192)^{-1}/(1/204 + 1/212)^{-1} = 0.926$$

and

$$B(0.926) = (0.926)^{1/2}(3.112) = 2.995.$$

The opposite arm imputation scheme assumes $p_0 = 105/192 = 0.547$ and $p_1 = 75/193 = 0.389$, so $p = (p_0 + p_1)/2 = 0.468$ and the drift parameter is

$$\theta = (0.389 - 0.547)/\{(0.468)(1 - 0.468)(1/204 + 1/212)\}^{1/2} = -3.229.$$

The conditional mean of $B(1)$ given $B(0.926) = 2.995$ is $2.995 - 3.229(1 - 0.926) = 2.756$. Conditional power is approximately

$$
\begin{aligned}
\mathrm{CP}_{-3.229}(0.926) &= 1 - \Phi\{(2.13 - 2.756)/(1 - 0.926)^{1/2}\} \\
&= 1 - \Phi(-2.30) \approx 0.99.
\end{aligned}
$$

This analysis reinforces the conclusion that revascularization is superior to angina-guided therapy.

A similar idea can be applied at an interim analysis when some potential events have not yet been officially classified. A data monitoring committee faced with such uncertainty is usually concerned that it might recommend stopping a trial because the z-score for the adjudicated data crosses a pre-specified stopping boundary, only to find that the z-score drops under the boundary once all the data have been adjudicated.

The Multicenter Study of Hydroxyurea in Sickle Cell Anemia (MSH) trial [CTM95] compared the rates of painful crises during 2 years of follow-up in 299 patients assigned randomly to hydroxyurea or placebo. A participant's crisis rate was defined as the number of painful crises divided by the participant's follow-up time. Because of the expected skewed distribution of rates of crises (some people experience very many crises, while others experience none), the primary analysis used a rank test, the van der Waerden normal scores test. The combined (treatment and control) crisis rates were ranked, the actual data were replaced by the corresponding expected order statistics from a standard normal distribution, and a t-test was performed on these "normal scores." Another advantage of the normal scores test is that deaths were used in the analysis by assigning them the worst ranks, with earlier deaths given a worse rank than later deaths.

Because the trial used a rank test whose joint distribution over time was not known, a simple method known as the Haybittle-Peto procedure (see Chapter 4) was used to monitor over four interim looks and one final look. Statistically significant benefit could be declared if the p-value at any of the first four looks were .001 or less, while the p-value at the last look would have to be $.05 - 4(.001) = .046$ or less to be declared significant.

Ascertaining whether a patient actually had a painful crisis required time-consuming adjudication by the Crisis Review Committee. Though the boundary for efficacy was crossed at the third interim analysis, approximately 22 percent of episodes had not yet been classified. The Data and Safety Monitoring Board (DSMB) wanted to know whether results would change once these episodes were classified, and whether results at the planned end of the trial with all current and future episodes classified would change. Therefore, the board asked for conditional power calculations at the fourth interim analysis.

Conditional power was complicated by the nonstandard rank test, so simulation was used. The study was divided by calendar time into three periods: Period I, at which time documentation and classification of medical contacts was complete; Period II, the time between the end of Period I and the last interim analysis (approximately 7 months); and Period III, the time between the last interim analysis and the planned end of the trial (approximately 7 months). Pooled data from Period I were used to estimate the probability that an episode would be classified as a crisis, as well as the future number of crises. Using pooled data to estimate these parameters assumes the null hypothesis for the remaining data. To account for patient differences in event rates, contact and crisis rates in Period I were stratified by the number of crises reported in the year prior to study entry. Thus, for a given patient, a number of crises was assigned as follows. Any past crises that had been classified were counted. For the n episodes not yet classified, the number that would ultimately be declared crises was simulated from a binomial distribution. The number of future episodes was simulated using a Poisson distribution. Thus, if the remaining follow-up time for a given patient were t, the number of future episodes was simulated from a Poisson distribution with mean λt (with the binomial again being used to simulate the number of those episodes that would be declared crises). Once each patient's data was simulated, the normal scores statistic and its p-value were computed. This process of simulating the rest of the trial was repeated 2,000 times, and the proportion of trials reaching a p-value of .046 or less was computed. Approximately 99.9 percent of simulated trials produced $p < .046$. The mean p-value was .007, leading the DSMB to feel comfortable about recommending stopping the trial at the fourth interim analaysis. See [MWG97] for further details of the conditional power calculations used.

The applications of conditional power in ACIP and MSH differed markedly from previous applications in that conditional power was very high even under pessimistic assumptions. Just as low conditional power under optimistic assumptions might justify stopping a trial for futility, high conditional power under pessimistic assumptions might justify stopping for benefit. For example, we could compute conditional power under the null hypothesis. If conditional power computed under the null hypothesis is sufficiently high, one can be confident that the current statistically significant benefit will be sustained at the end of the trial. Stochastic curtailment for benefit means stopping the trial when conditional power computed under the null hypothesis exceeds a prespecified threshold.

Example 3.6. A trial comparing two treatments for opiate addiction administers a drug test 60 days postrandomization. Participants who fail to take the test are counted as positive (i.e., on drugs). The outcome is binary, but investigators want to use logistic regression to adjust for baseline covariates such as number of years of drug use. The sample size is set at 70 per arm. At an interim analysis after 55 arm A participants and 57 arm B participants are eveluted, the treatment effect estimate and estimated standard error are $\hat{\delta} = 0.693$ (arm A to arm B odds ratio of $\exp(0.693) = 2.0$) and $\hat{\sigma}_{\hat{\delta}} = 0.212$, respectively.

The information fraction, z-score, and B-value are $t = (\frac{1}{55}+\frac{1}{57})^{-1}/(\frac{2}{70})^{-1} = 0.800$, $Z(t) = 0.693/0.212 = 3.269$, and $B(t) = (0.800)^{1/2}(3.269) = 2.924$. If we very conservatively assume the null hypothesis, then $E\{B(1)\,|\,B(0.800) = 2.924\} = 2.924$ and conditional power is

$$CP_0(0.800) = 1 - \Phi\{(1.96 - 2.924)/(1 - 0.800)^{1/2}\}$$
$$= 1 - \Phi(-2.16) \approx 0.98.$$

Conditional power is overwhelming even under a very pessimistic assumption (the null hypothesis) that is completely unsupported by the data. We can stop the study and declare with confidence the superiority of arm B.

3.4 Properties of Conditional Power

It is instructive to rewrite the conditional power formula (3.4) as

$$CP_\theta(t) = \Phi\left(\frac{E_\theta\{Z(1)\,|\,B(t) = b\} - z_{\alpha/2}}{\sqrt{1-t}}\right) \tag{3.7}$$

because it facilitates comparison of conditional power and unconditional power. Conditional power formula (3.7) is just like unconditional power formula (3.2) except that 1) the unconditional mean of $Z(1)$ is replaced by its conditional mean given $B(t) = b$ and 2) there is a $(1 - t)^{1/2}$ term in the denominator. At the start of a trial, $t = 0$ and the conditional and unconditional means of $Z(1)$ are the same. Thus, conditional power at the beginning of the trial equals its unconditional power. If results proceed as expected (i.e., the empirical drift parameter estimate equals the prior hypothesized value $\theta = z_{\alpha/2} + z_\beta$), the conditional mean of $Z(1)$ will equal its unconditional mean, so the only difference between conditional and unconditional power will be the term $(1 - t)^{1/2}$ in the denominator of conditional power. The result is that conditional power will increase over time if the originally hypothesized treatment effect is observed.

Because conditional and unconditional power are equal at $t = 0$, conditional power under the originally hypothesized treatment effect will be high near the beginning of the trial even if early results are negative. This makes it nearly impossible to use conditional power to stop for futility very early in a trial. In fact, one can sometimes stop for harm without demonstrating futility. An example of this apparent paradox comes from CAST. Recall that the early results of CAST showed three of 576 placebo patients and 19 of 571 treated patients with events. Because 425 events were expected by trial's end, the information fraction was $22/425 = 0.052$. The logrank statistic and B-value were approximately $Z(0.052) = -3.47$ and

$B(0.052) = (0.052)^{1/2}Z(0.052) = -0.79$, respectively. Suppose we assume, contrary to the observed data, that treatment reduces the hazard by 30 percent relative to placebo. The drift parameter assuming 425 events by the end of the trial is approximately $\ln(1/0.70)(425/4)^{1/2} = 3.68$. The conditional mean of $B(1)$ given $B(0.052) = -0.79$ is $-0.79 + 3.68(1 - 0.052) = 2.70$. Conditional power is therefore

$$CP_{3.68}(0.052) = 1 - \Phi\{(1.96 - 2.70)/(1 - 0.052)^{1/2}\}$$
$$= 1 - \Phi(-0.76) = 0.78.$$

Thus, even in the face of strong evidence of harm, conditional power assuming a 30 percent benefit is almost 80 percent because it is so early in the trial.

Table 3.5. Conditional power boundaries for $Z(t)$ for five equally spaced looks. The interim z-score must exceed the tabled value to stop early for benefit using stochastic curtailment.

Info. Time	$CP_0 = 0.50$	$CP_0 = 0.80$
0.20	4.38	6.06
0.40	3.10	4.13
0.60	2.53	3.22
0.80	2.19	2.61
1.00	1.96	1.96
	$\alpha = 0.031$	$\alpha = 0.026$

Table 3.5 quantifies the difficulty of stopping early using stochastic curtailment for benefit. It shows the interim z-score necessary for conditional power to drop under a 50 percent or 80 percent threshold at each of five equally spaced looks. Note that even the 50 percent boundaries are quite high early in the trial.

As always, there is no such thing as a free lunch. We must pay for stochastic curtailment through the increased probability of a type 1 error if used for benefit, or increased probability of a type 2 error if used for futility. Surprisingly, the effects on the type 1 and 2 error rates are not very large. We prove the following result due to Lan, Simon, and Halperin (1982) [LSH82] in Section 3.7.1.

Result 3.1 *(Lan, Simon, and Halperin, 1982 [LSH82]).*

1. *If a trial with no monitoring has type 1 error rate α, and stochastic curtailment is used to stop for benefit if conditional power under the null hypothesis exceeds $1 - \epsilon$, the type 1 error rate is at most $\alpha/(1 - \epsilon)$ irrespective of the number of interim analyses. It is exactly $\alpha/(1 - \epsilon)$ under continuous monitoring.*

2. *If a trial with no monitoring has type 2 error rate β, and stochastic cur-*
tailment is used to stop for futility if conditional power under the origi-
nally hypothesized treatment effect falls below ϵ, the type 2 error rate is at
most $\beta/(1-\epsilon)$ irrespective of the number of interim analyses. It is exactly
$\beta/(1-\epsilon)$ under continuous monitoring.

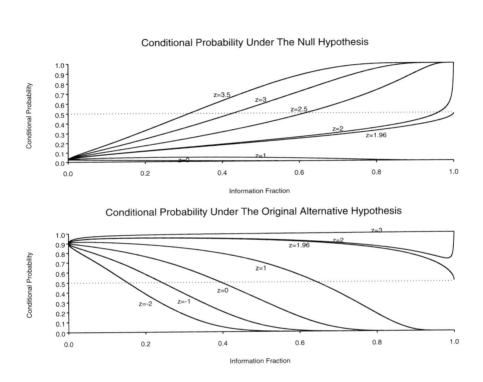

Fig. 3.4. Conditional power as a function of information fraction and observed z-score under the null (top panel) and alternative (bottom panel) hypotheses. Note that conditional power under a given hypothesis need not be a monotone function of the information fraction t. Furthemore, for z-scores close to $z_{\alpha/2}$, conditional power near $t = 1$ is highly sensitive to small changes in the z-score.

Conditional power sometimes has unusual properties. Figure 3.4 shows conditional power as a function of the information fraction for different z-scores. We see that for some z-scores, conditional power is not a monotone function of information fraction. Furthermore, if the current z-score is close to $z_{\alpha/2}$, conditional power for t close to 1 is very sensitive to small changes in the z-score. This makes sense; for fixed $z > z_{\alpha/2}$, conditional power approaches 1 as $t \to 1$, whereas it approaches 0 as $t \to 1$ for fixed $z < z_{\alpha/2}$. One role of a statistician on a DSMB using conditional power is to explain this nonmonotonicity to other members of the board; otherwise, the results at successive meetings can be confusing to the nonstatistician members.

3.5 A Bayesian Alternative: Predictive Power

We have seen that conditional power is quite sensitive to the drift parameter, which is not well estimated at interim analyses. This has prompted some to suggest a Bayesian alternative (Spiegelhalter, Freedman, and Blackburn, 1986 [SFB86]) to conditional power. Before the trial begins one specifies a prior distribution for the treatment effect, or equivalently, a prior distribution for the drift parameter, θ. At an interim analysis, conditional power $CP_\theta(t)$ is averaged over the posterior distribution $\pi(\theta \mid B(t))$ of θ given the B-value. This average conditional power is called *predictive power* $PP(t)$,

$$
\begin{aligned}
PP(t) &= \int CP_\theta(t)\pi\{\theta \mid B(t) = b\}d\theta \\
&= \int_{-\infty}^{\infty} \Phi\left(\frac{b + \theta(1-t) - z_{\alpha/2}}{\sqrt{1-t}}\right) \pi\{\theta \mid B(t) = b\}d\theta. \quad (3.8)
\end{aligned}
$$

Predictive power accounts for the current data $B(t)$ through both $CP(t)$ and $\pi(\theta \mid B(t) = b)$. The difference between $PP(t)$ and $PP(0)$ is used to decide whether to recommend stopping a trial.

We illustrate predictive power when the prior distribution $\pi(\theta)$ is normal with mean θ_0 and variance σ_0^2. The posterior distribution of θ given $B(t) = b$ is normal with mean a weighted combination of the prior mean θ_0 and the data estimate $B(t)/t$:

$$
\begin{aligned}
E(\theta \mid B(t) = b) &= \frac{(1/\sigma_0^2)\theta_0 + t(b/t)}{1/\sigma_0^2 + t} \\
&= \frac{\theta_0 + b\sigma_0^2}{1 + t\sigma_0^2}. \quad (3.9)
\end{aligned}
$$

The variance of the posterior distribution is $\sigma_0^2(1 - \rho^2)$, where ρ is the correlation between $B(t)$ and θ. As seen in Section 3.7.2, $\rho = t^{1/2}\sigma_0/(1 + t\sigma_0^2)^{1/2}$, $\text{var}(\theta \mid B(t) = b) = \sigma_0^2/(1 + t\sigma_0^2)$, and predictive power is

$$
PP(t) = \Phi\left[\frac{(b - z_{\alpha/2})(1 + t\sigma_0^2) + (1-t)(\theta_0 + b\sigma_0^2)}{\sqrt{(1-t)(1 + \sigma_0^2)(1 + t\sigma_0^2)}}\right]. \quad (3.10)
$$

Note that for $\sigma_0^2 = 0$, predictive power reduces to conditional power under the originally hypothesized treatment effect (3.4). At the beginning of the trial, $b = 0$ and $t = 0$, so predictive power reduces to

$$PP(0) = \Phi\left(\frac{\theta_0 - z_{\alpha/2}}{\sqrt{1 + \sigma_0^2}}\right). \tag{3.11}$$

Here is an appealing way to choose the mean and variance of the normal prior distribution. Take prior mean θ_0 to be the treatment effect upon which the sample size calculation was based. Determination of the prior variance is based on how much weight we choose to give the prior treatment estimate relative to the estimate from the trial. Recall that the posterior mean of θ at the end of the trial is a weighted combination $\{(1/\sigma_0^2)\theta_0 + B(1)\}/\{1/\sigma_0^2 + 1\}$ of the two drift parameter estimates θ_0 and $B(1)$. If we feel that our prior opinion should carry about 20 percent weight, we choose σ_0^2 such that $(1/\sigma_0^2)/(1/\sigma_0^2 + 1) = 0.20$. In other words, $\sigma_0^2 = 4$.

We return to Example 3.2, a feeding trial in which we expected the blood pressure difference between arms to be 2 mm Hg. We compute predictive power assuming a normal prior distribution for δ with mean 2. This translates to a prior distribution for θ that has mean 3.24. Suppose we want the prior information to carry about 10 percent weight compared to the data at the end of the current trial. Then we set $(1/\sigma_0^2)/(1/\sigma_0^2 + 1) = 0.10$ and solve for σ_0^2, yielding $\sigma_0^2 = 9$.

Before the trial begins, predictive power is, from (3.11):

$$PP(0) = \Phi\left(\frac{3.24 - 1.96}{\sqrt{1 + 9}}\right) = \Phi(0.405) = 0.66. \tag{3.12}$$

Recall that the unconditional power when $\delta = 2$ was 0.90; however, here the predictive power at the beginning of the trial is only 0.66. Predictive power is the average conditional power over the posterior distribution of θ given the data; at the beginning of the trial, we have no data, so the posterior distribution of θ is the prior distribution of θ, and conditional power is the same as unconditional power. Thus, at the beginning of the trial, predictive power is unconditional power averaged over the prior distribution for θ. Because our prior information was worth so little (recall that we selected the prior variance to give our prior information about 10 percent weight relative to the data at the end of the trial), the prior distribution was quite diffuse. The more diffuse the prior, the more predictive power reflects averaging over a uniform distribution on the entire line (see Figure 3.5). As $\sigma_0 \to \infty$, predictive power tends to 0.50.

Suppose the results at the interim analysis after evaluating 52 and 50 patients in the treatment and control arms were $\hat{\delta} = 1$ and $\hat{\sigma} = 6.1$. The information fraction, z-score, and B-value are $t = (1/52 + 1/50)^{-1}/(2/132)^{-1} = 0.386$ $Z(t) = 1/\{6.1^2(1/50 + 1/52)\}^{1/2} = 0.828$, $B(t) = (0.386)^{1/2}(0.828) = 0.514$. From (3.10), predictive power is

$$PP(0.386) = \Phi\left[\frac{(0.514 - 1.96)(1 + 0.386(9)) + (1 - 0.386)(3.24 + 0.514(9))}{\sqrt{(1 - 0.386)(1 + 9)(1 + 0.386(9))}}\right].$$

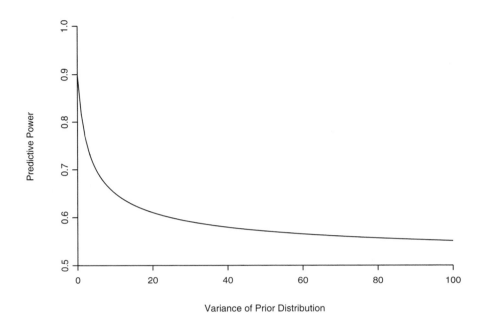

Fig. 3.5. Predictive power at the beginning of the trial as a function of the variance σ_0^2 of the normal prior distribution. The prior mean θ_0 is such that power under θ_0 is 0.90. When $\sigma_0^2 = 0$, the prior distribution is a point mass at θ_0, and predictive power is 0.90. When σ_0^2 is very large, predictive power has an asymptote at 0.50.

$$= \Phi(-0.313) = 0.38.$$

Thus, predictive power has dropped from 66 percent at the beginning of the trial to 38 percent now. The drop is a result of two factors: 1) the current B-value is lower than expected, so we need a steeper trajectory from now to the end to reach statistical significance; and 2) the poorer than expected results have caused us to revise our opinion about the likely value of the drift parameter. The first factor would apply to both conditional and predictive power, but the second factor is unique to predictive power. Proponents of predictive power base the decision of whether to stop a trial on the change in predictive power from the beginning of the trial to the interim analysis.

3.6 Summary

Conditional power, the conditional probability of a significant result at the end of the trial given the data observed thus far, is a useful tool when considering whether to stop a trial for futility. Low conditional power means that a null result is likely. Whether that null result is meaningful depends on unconditional power revised to incorporate the current estimate of the overall probability of event or the variance for a continuous outcome trial. If both conditional and revised unconditional power are low, the trial is doomed because a null result is both likely and uninformative. On the other hand, if conditional power is low but revised unconditional power high, continuing the trial might provide an estimate of effect precise enough to rule out the originally hypothesized value.

Conditional power has other uses, including assessing the likely impact of missing or unadjudicated data on results.

Conditional power is usually computed under different hypotheses that translate into different values of the drift parameter θ (see Table 3.6). Geometrically, having observed B-value $B(t)$ at current information time t, we draw a line segment with slope θ beginning at $(t, B(t))$; its ordinate at information time 1 is the conditional mean of the z-score at the end of the trial given the current data (Figure 3.6). The best estimate of θ from the data itself is $\hat{\theta} = B(t)/t$, which is the slope of the line connecting the origin to $(t, B(t))$.

Table 3.6. Some hypotheses under which to compute conditional power. "Original" denotes the original assumptions for both the treatment effect and nuisance parameters such as the variance or overall treatment effect, whereas "Original trt" denotes the original assumption for the treatment effect but the empirical estimate of nuisance parameters. For a survival outcome, "HR" stands for hazard ratio and N is the total number of patients with events.

Assumptions	Continuous Outcome	Dichotomous Outcome	Survival Outcome
Original	$\theta = z_{\alpha/2} + z_\beta$	$\theta = z_{\alpha/2} + z_\beta$	$\theta = z_{\alpha/2} + z_\beta$
Original trt.	$\delta = \delta_0,\ \sigma = s$	RR= RR_0, $p = \hat{p}$	HR $= HR_0$, $N = \hat{N}$
Empirical	$\theta = B(t)/t$	$\theta = B(t)/t$	$\theta = B(t)/t$
Null	$\theta = 0$	$\theta = 0$	$\theta = 0$

Stopping a trial when conditional power under the originally assumed treatment effect falls below a fixed threshold (typically $0.10 - 0.15$), or when conditional power under the null hypothesis exceeds a fixed threshold (typically at least 0.80), is called stochastic curtailment for futility or benefit, respectively. Though stochastic curtailment increases error rates, the magnitude of increase is relatively small even if we monitor the data continuously.

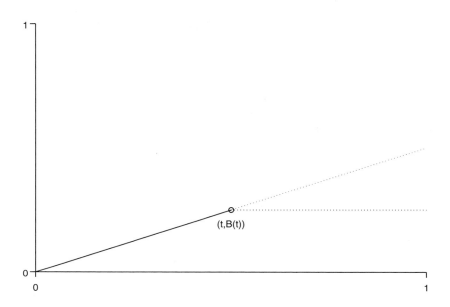

Fig. 3.6. The geometry of conditional power. The best estimate of the treatment effect at information time t is $B(t)/t$, the slope of the line segment joining the origin to $(t, B(t))$. To compute conditional power under drift θ, append a line segment with slope θ to $(t, B(t))$; its ordinate at information time 1 is $E\{Z(1) \mid B(t)\}$, which determines conditional power. To calculate conditional power under the null hypothesis, use a flat line from now until the end of the trial. To calculate conditional power under the current trend, extend, to the end of the trial, the segment joining the origin to $(t, B(t))$.

Predictive power, a Bayesian alternative to conditional power, averages conditional power over the posterior distribution of the drift parameter given the data.

3.7 Appendix

3.7.1 Proof of Result 3.1

We prove part 2 because stochastic curtailment is used most often for futility. The proof of part 1 is very similar. Consider a worst case scenario—continuous monitoring. Let $A = \{Z(1) < z_{\alpha/2}\}$ be the event that a type 2 error is made at the end of the trial. If A occurs, there must be some t for which $CP(t) < \epsilon$ because $CP(t)$ is continuous, $CP(0) = 1 - \beta$, and $CP(1) = 0$ if A occurs. Let τ be the first time conditional power drops below ϵ; $\tau = \inf\{t \leq 1 : CP(t) < \epsilon\}$, and set $\tau = 2$ if $CP(t) \geq \epsilon$ for all $t \leq 1$. Let $F(t)$ be the distribution function for τ. Then

$$
\begin{aligned}
\beta &= \Pr\{B(1) < z_{\alpha/2}\} \\
&= \int_{(0,1]} \Pr\{B(1) < z_{\alpha/2} | \tau = t\} dF(t) \\
&= \int_{(0,1]} (1 - \epsilon) \, dF(t) \\
&= (1 - \epsilon) \Pr(\tau \leq 1) \\
&= (1 - \epsilon) \Pr(\text{type 2 error}),
\end{aligned}
$$

from which $\Pr(\text{type 2 error}) = \beta/(1 - \epsilon)$.

The heuristic reasoning behind the third step is as follows. The event $\tau = t$ depends only on $B(s)$, $s \leq t$, and it implies $B(t) = b_\epsilon(t)$, where $b_\epsilon(t)$ is the value such that $CP(t) = \epsilon$. Once we know $B(t) = b_\epsilon(t)$, the implication of $\tau = t$ on $B(s)$ for $s < t$ becomes irrelevant. Thus $\Pr(B(1) < z_{\alpha/2} | \tau = t) = 1 - CP(t) = 1 - \epsilon$. A more careful treatment partitions the interval $(0, 1]$ into $I_m = ((m-1)/M, m/M]$, $m = 1, \ldots, M$ and replaces $\int_{(0,1]}$ by $\sum_{m=1}^{M}$, and the event $\{\tau = t\}$ by $\tau \in I_m$. We can then take the limit as $M \to \infty$ and use the uniform continuity of $CP(t)$ on $[0, 1]$.

3.7.2 Formula for $\text{corr}\{B(t), \theta\}$ and $\text{var}\{\theta \,|\, B(t) = b\}$

Note that

$$
\begin{aligned}
E\{B(t)\theta\} &= E[E\{B(t)\theta \,|\, \theta\}] = E[\theta E\{B(t) \,|\, \theta\}] \\
&= E\{\theta(\theta t)\} = t E(\theta^2) \\
&= t[\text{var}(\theta) + \{E(\theta)\}^2] \\
&= t(\sigma_0^2 + \theta_0^2),
\end{aligned}
$$

$$
E\{B(t)\} = E[E\{B(t) \,|\, \theta\}] = t E(\theta) = t\theta_0,
$$

and $E(\theta) = \theta_0$, so

$$
\begin{aligned}
\text{cov}\{B(t), \theta\} &= E\{B(t)\theta\} - E\{B(t)\}E(\theta) \\
&= t(\sigma_0^2 + \theta_0^2) - t\theta_0^2 = t\sigma_0^2.
\end{aligned}
$$

Also,

$$
\begin{aligned}
\text{var}\{B(t)\} &= E[\text{var}\{B(t) \,|\, \theta\}] + \text{var}[E\{B(t) \,|\, \theta\}] \\
&= E(t) + \text{var}(\theta t) = t + t^2 \sigma_0^2 \\
&= t(1 + t\sigma_0^2)
\end{aligned}
$$

and $\text{var}(\theta) = \sigma_0^2$, so

$$\rho = \frac{\text{cov}\{B(t), \theta\}}{\sqrt{\text{var}\{B(t)\}\text{var}(\theta)}} = \frac{t\sigma_0^2}{\sqrt{t(1 + t\sigma_0^2)\sigma_0^2}}$$

$$= \frac{t^{1/2}\sigma_0}{\sqrt{1 + t\sigma_0^2}}.$$

Finally, because $B(t)$ and θ have a bivariate normal distribution,

$$\text{var}(\theta \mid B(t) = b) = \text{var}(\theta)(1 - \rho^2) = \sigma_0^2 \left(1 - \frac{t\sigma_0^2}{1 + t\sigma_0^2}\right)$$

$$= \frac{\sigma_0^2}{1 + t\sigma_0^2}.$$

3.7.3 Simplification of Formula (3.8)

To simplify (3.8), let Z be a standard normal deviate independent of $(B(t), \theta)$. Note that $\Pr[Z \leq \{B(t) + \theta(1 - t) - z_{\alpha/2}\}/(1 - t)^{1/2} \mid B(t) = b]$ is given by (3.8). In other words, (3.8) is equivalent to $\Pr\{(1 - t)^{1/2}Z - \theta(1 - t) \leq B(t) - z_{\alpha/2} \mid B(t) = b\}$. Conditioned on $B(t) = b$, $(1 - t)^{1/2}Z - \theta(1 - t)$ is normally distributed with mean

$$\text{E}\{(1 - t)^{1/2}Z - \theta(1 - t) \mid B(t) = b\} = -(1 - t)\text{E}\{\theta \mid B(t) = b\}$$

$$= -(1 - t)\left(\frac{\theta_0 + b\sigma_0^2}{1 + t\sigma_0^2}\right)$$

(the last step used Equation (3.9)) and variance

$$\text{var}\{(1 - t)^{1/2}Z - \theta(1 - t) \mid B(t) = b\} = 1 - t + (1 - t)^2\text{var}\{\theta \mid B(t) = b\}$$

$$= 1 - t + \frac{(1 - t)^2\sigma_0^2}{1 + t\sigma_0^2}$$

$$= (1 - t)\left\{1 + \frac{(1 - t)\sigma_0^2}{1 + t\sigma_0^2}\right\}.$$

Thus

$$PP(t) = \Phi\left[\frac{b - z_{\alpha/2} + \frac{(1-t)(\theta_0 + b\sigma_0^2)}{(1 + t\sigma_0^2)}}{\sqrt{(1 - t)\left\{1 + \frac{(1-t)\sigma_0^2}{(1 + t\sigma_0^2)}\right\}}}\right]$$

$$= \Phi\left[\frac{(b - z_{\alpha/2})(1 + t\sigma_0^2) + (1 - t)(\theta_0 + b\sigma_0^2)}{\sqrt{(1 - t)(1 + \sigma_0^2)(1 + t\sigma_0^2)}}\right].$$

4

Historical Monitoring Boundaries

The last chapter focused primarily on stopping a trial for futility, but in many trials we have an ethical obligation to stop if evidence for benefit of treatment becomes unequivocal. A statistical naif might compute the z-score at each interim analysis and declare benefit if it ever exceeds 1.96. But just as our confidence in a dart thrower's ability is eroded if he takes 10 throws to hit the target, so too is our confidence when one of many z-scores reaches the targeted 1.96. The probability of eventually hitting the target is high even for an unskilled dart thrower. So too is the probability of eventually reaching a z-score of 1.96 even if the treatment has no real effect.

4.1 How Bad Can the Naive Approach Be?

First consider interim analyses with equally spaced information. The probability that the absolute value of at least one z-score exceeds 1.96 can be estimated either through simulation or by numerical integration. Section 4.7 gives the numerical integration approach of Armitage, McPherson, and Rowe (1969) [AMR69]. The second and fourth columns of Table 4.1 show the type 1 error rate rejecting the null hypothesis when $|Z(i/k)| > z_\alpha$ for some $i = 1, \ldots, k$ and $\alpha = .01$ and $.05$. With only five equally spaced looks, the type 1 error rate has already reached .142 instead of .05. As the number of looks approaches ∞, the type 1 error rate very slowly approaches 1.

The situation can worsen with unequally spaced interim analyses. To bound the worst case type 1 error rate we note that for $t_1 < \ldots < t_k$, the z-scores $Z(t_1), \ldots, Z(t_k)$ are multivariate normal with $\mathrm{corr}\{Z(t_i), Z(t_j)\} = (t_i/t_j)^{1/2} > 0$. Intuitively, these z-statistics are more likely all to be large or all small than if they were independent. The same is true if we replace $Z(t_i)$ by $|Z(t_i)|$. In fact, Hochberg and Tamhane (1987) [HT87] show that $\Pr(\cap_i Z_{t_i} \leq c_i) \geq \prod_i \Pr\{Z(t_i) \leq c_i\}$ and $\Pr(\cap_i |Z_{t_i}| \leq c_i) \geq \prod_i \Pr\{|Z(t_i)| \leq c_i\}$. It follows that

$$\Pr(\cup_{i=1}^{k} Z(t_i) > z_\alpha) \leq 1 - (1 - \alpha)^k \text{ and}$$

$$\Pr(\cup_{i=1}^{k} |Z(t_i)| > z_{\alpha_2}) \leq 1 - (1 - \alpha)^k. \tag{4.1}$$

The worst case sequence of information times $t_1, \ldots, t_k$ is as follows. Let ϵ be a small positive number and suppose that $t_1 = \epsilon^{k-1}, t_2 = \epsilon^{k-2}, \ldots, t_k = \epsilon^0 = 1$. Then $\text{corr}\{Z(t_i), Z(t_j)\} = (t_i/t_j)^{1/2} \leq \epsilon^{1/2}$ for each i, j. In other words, $Z(t_1), \ldots, Z(t_k)$ are arbitrarily close to being independent, so the bound (4.1) is approached as $\epsilon \to 0$ (Proschan, Follmann, and Waclawiw, 1992 [PFW92]).

The third and fifth columns of Table 4.1 give the worst case type 1 error rate for two-tailed tests at $\alpha = 0.01$ and $\alpha = 0.05$. With only five looks the type 1 error rate can be nearly 0.226 instead of 0.05. Note how much more quickly the type 1 error rate approaches 1 under the worst case timing of looks than under equal spacing.

Table 4.1. Type 1 error rate by the number and timing of looks for a two-tailed test at $\alpha = 0.01$ and $\alpha = 0.05$ obtained by numerical integration for $k \leq 20$ and simulation of a million trials for $k > 20$.

# Looks (k)	$\alpha = 0.01$		$\alpha = 0.05$	
	Equally Spaced	Worst Case	Equally Spaced	Worst Case
2	.018	.020	.083	.098
3	.024	.030	.107	.143
4	.029	.039	.126	.185
5	.033	.049	.142	.226
6	.036	.059	.155	.265
7	.040	.068	.166	.302
8	.042	.077	.176	.337
9	.045	.086	.185	.370
10	.047	.096	.193	.401
11	.050	.105	.201	.431
12	.052	.114	.207	.460
13	.053	.122	.214	.487
14	.055	.131	.220	.512
15	.057	.140	.225	.537
16	.058	.149	.230	.560
17	.060	.157	.235	.582
18	.061	.165	.239	.603
19	.063	.174	.244	.623
20	.064	.182	.248	.642
50	.088	.395	.319	.923
100	.107	.634	.373	.994
1000	.172	1	.531	1
∞	1	1	1	1

What causes most of the trouble is very early monitoring. In fact, because the joint distribution of the z-statistics depends only on ratios of information fractions, the type 1 error rate for k equally spaced looks on the unit interval is exactly the same as for k equally spaced looks on $[0, \epsilon]$ for arbitrarily small ϵ. Thus, for example, the type 1 error rate used during the first half of an eight-look trial is the same as over the entire duration of a four-look trial. This is another way of seeing that the type 1 error rate for continuous monitoring using a constant z-score boundary is 1; it is clear that $\Pr(Z(t) > c$ for some $t \leq 1)$ must be strictly greater than $\Pr(Z(t) > c$ for some $t \leq \epsilon)$ unless $\Pr(Z(t) > c$ for some $t \leq \epsilon) = 1$. Thus, continuous monitoring for any length of time beginning at time 0 produces a type 1 error rate of 1 if we use a constant z-score boundary. If we agree to refrain from monitoring before, say, information fraction 0.20, the type 1 error rate is not nearly so inflated. Delong (1981) [D81] developed formulas and presented a table for $\Pr(Z(t) > c$ for some $t \geq \gamma)$ for different values of γ.

4.2 The Pocock Procedure

A natural solution to the problem of inflation of the type 1 error rate is to monitor at equally spaced information times and "raise the bar" for the z-statistics. For a two-tailed test, the Pocock procedure (Pocock, 1977 [P77]) rejects at the ith of k interim looks if $|Z(i/k)| > c_P(k)$, where $c_P(k)$ is such that $\Pr(\cup_{i=1}^{k} |Z(i/k)| > c_P(k)) = \alpha$.

Table 4.2 gives the constants $c_P(k)$ for a two-tailed test at level 0.01, 0.05, and 0.10. For example, with $\alpha = 0.05$ and five analyses, the absolute value of the z-score at a given analysis would have to exceed 2.413 to be declared significant. That includes the final analysis, and therein lies the practical problem. The use of 2.413 instead of 1.96 at the end of the trial is a high price to pay for monitoring. A z-score of 2.413 translates to a two-tailed "nominal p-value" of $2\{1 - \Phi(2.413)\} = 0.016$. That is, we require the nominal p-value at the end of the trial to be 0.016 or less to reject the null hypothesis. As $k \to \infty$, $c_P(k) \to \infty$, albeit slowly. The problem arises from the fact that the Pocock procedure requires the same level of evidence for early and late looks at the data. Clinical trialists prefer to require a greater level of evidence early in a trial. A less serious drawback to Pocock's procedure is that it requires equally spaced looks. Pocock himself now cautions against using his procedure, though some people use the method for monitoring safety (see Chapter 9).

4.3 The Haybittle Procedure and Variants

An even earlier approach than Pocock's was less well known to statisticians because it first appeared in a radiology journal rather than a statistics journal.

Table 4.2. Two-tailed boundaries for the Pocock procedure

# Looks (k)	$\alpha = 0.01$	$\alpha = 0.05$	$\alpha = 0.10$
1	2.576	1.960	1.645
2	2.772	2.178	1.875
3	2.873	2.289	1.992
4	2.939	2.361	2.067
5	2.986	2.413	2.122
6	3.023	2.453	2.164
7	3.053	2.485	2.197
8	3.078	2.512	2.225
9	3.099	2.535	2.249
10	3.117	2.555	2.270
11	3.133	2.572	2.288
12	3.147	2.588	2.304
13	3.160	2.602	2.319
14	3.172	2.614	2.332
15	3.182	2.626	2.344
16	3.192	2.637	2.355
17	3.201	2.646	2.365
18	3.210	2.656	2.375
19	3.217	2.664	2.384
20	3.225	2.672	2.392
∞	∞	∞	∞

Haybittle (1971) [H71] suggested using a z-score boundary of 3 at interim analyses and retaining 1.96 at the final analysis. Because the boundary at interim analyses is so high, the degree of inflation of the type 1 error rate is small unless the number of analyses is large.

The Haybittle procedure is simple to implement. The test it uses at the end of the trial is identical to the one that would have been used without monitoring. These two advantages make the procedure attractive; however, the second advantage is not quite fair to claim because the procedure in fact does inflate the type 1 error rate slightly. We could eliminate the inflation through a Bonferroni adjustment. In this modified Haybittle procedure, we would require $p < .001$ to declare significance at all but the final analysis, but at the final analysis we would require $p < .05 - .001(k - 1)$. Here p is the "nominal p-value" computed the usual way without taking monitoring into consideration. For example, with 5 looks we require $p < .001$ at any of the first 4 looks, and $p < .05 - 4(.001) = .046$ at the final look. The Bonferroni fix, like Pocock's procedure, requires prespecification of the number of analyses. Unlike Pocock's procedure, the Bonferroni fix does not require them to be equally spaced in terms of information. It also is valid regardless of the joint distribution of $Z(t_1), \ldots, Z(t_k)$. Thus, we can use the Bonferroni-adjusted Haybittle method for any test statistic, not just for those that can be transformed to Brownian motion.

Some users of Haybittle-type procedures informally deal with inflation of type 1 error rate by modifying the boundary in other ways. They may demand a z-score of 4 for the first half of the study and 3 thereafter or they may require crossing the boundary at two successive looks.

One problem with the Haybittle procedure and its various fixes is the precipitous drop in the boundary at the end of the study, or, for those modifications that change the boundary from 4 to 3, at the halfway point. This can lead to a logical inconsistency. For example, suppose in a study with five equally spaced looks, the z-score at the fourth look is 2.8. Suppose the trend is completely reversed between the fourth and fifth analyses so that the z-score for the incremental data is $(1/5)^{1/2}\{B(5/5) - B(4/5)\} = -1$. Then the cumulative z-score at the final analysis, $(4/5)^{1/2}(2.8) + (1/5)^{1/2}(-1) = 2.06$, is now significant. In other words, the evidence was not deemed sufficient at the fourth analysis with a z-score of 2.8, but the observed subsequent negative trend convinces us that the effect is real. That does not make sense.

4.4 The O'Brien-Fleming Procedure

That the Haybittle boundary is high very early and close to 1.96 at the end is an asset. We want to resist stopping early when there is large variability, both statistical and nonstatistical (e.g., it may take clinicians some time to learn the protocol). We also do not want to pay as high a price at the end as the Pocock procedure does. Thus, we would like to retain these two properties while avoiding the logical inconsistency encountered at the end of the last section.

Assume our looks are equally spaced with respect to information, and let $a_1, \ldots, a_k$ denote the boundary for the B-value process. We wish to avoid the possibility that $B(i/k) < a_i$, $B((i+1)/k) - B(i/k) < 0$, and $B((i+1)/k) > a_{i+1}$. This clearly requires $a_1 \geq a_2 \geq \ldots \geq a_k$. Among all such boundaries that avoid the logical inconsistency, the one that makes it the most difficult to stop early is $a_{i+1} = a_i$, $i = 1, \ldots, k-1$. O'Brien and Fleming (1979) [OF79] proposed this constant boundary for the B-value process.

Table 4.3 gives the O'Brien-Fleming boundary $a(k)$ for the B-value for a two-tailed test at $\alpha = .01, .05$, and .10 and different numbers of looks. The O'Brien-Fleming z-value boundary $c_{O-F}(i/k)$ at the ith analysis is $a(k)/(i/k)^{1/2}$. For example, the tabled value for five looks and $\alpha = .05$ is $a(5) = 2.040$. Accordingly, the boundaries for $Z(1/k), \ldots, Z(5/5)$ are $2.040/(1/5)^{1/2} = 4.562$, $2.040/(2/5)^{1/2} = 3.226, \ldots, 2.040/(5/5)^{1/2} = 2.040$.

We can look at the O'Brien-Fleming boundary in a different way. Think of a one-tailed test. We saw at the end of the last chapter that conditional power for benefit also makes it very difficult to stop early. In fact, the boundary

Table 4.3. Two-tailed B-value boundaries $a(k)$ for the O'Brien-Fleming procedure. Boundaries for the z-score $Z(i/k)$ are $a(k)/(i/k)^{1/2}$.

# Looks (k)	$\alpha = .01$	$\alpha = .05$	$\alpha = .10$
1	2.576	1.960	1.645
2	2.580	1.977	1.678
3	2.595	2.004	1.710
4	2.609	2.024	1.733
5	2.621	2.040	1.751
6	2.631	2.053	1.765
7	2.640	2.063	1.776
8	2.648	2.072	1.786
9	2.654	2.080	1.794
10	2.660	2.087	1.801
11	2.665	2.092	1.807
12	2.670	2.098	1.813
13	2.674	2.103	1.818
14	2.677	2.106	1.822
15	2.681	2.110	1.826
16	2.684	2.114	1.830
17	2.687	2.117	1.834
18	2.690	2.120	1.837
19	2.693	2.123	1.840
20	2.695	2.126	1.842
∞	2.807	2.241	1.960

based on 50 percent conditional power under the null hypothesis is very close to the O'Brien-Fleming boundary except that its type 1 error rate exceeds 0.05. We can correct the 50 percent conditional power boundary by using a slightly larger boundary for the final z-score instead of 1.96. Thus, we reject at the end if $B(1) > a$, and we reject earlier if conditional power under the null hypothesis is at least 0.50. But that means we reject at the ith analysis if $B(i/k) > a$. In other words, this corrected conditional power boundary is a constant boundary for the B-value process; in fact, it is identical to the O'Brien-Fleming boundary.

4.5 A Comparison of the Pocock and O'Brien-Fleming Boundaries

Both Pocock and O'Brien-Fleming proposed constant boundaries, Pocock for the z-process and O'Brien-Fleming for the B-process. The two boundaries are, in a sense, the two practical extremes in terms of steepness of z-score boundaries. On the one hand, we want the z-score boundaries to decrease with

t; a z-score of 3 at the end of the trial should be more compelling than a z-score of 3 at the midway point, for example. Thus, Pocock's flat z-score boundary is the smallest descent we would like in a boundary. On the other hand, a B-value boundary that decreases with t might have the logical inconsistency pointed out with the Haybittle procedure. That is, we could see a B-value below the boundary at t_1, observe a negative trend from t_1 to t_2, and have $B(t_2)$ above its boundary (Figure 4.1). Thus, O'Brien-Fleming's flat B-value boundary is the steepest descent we would like in a boundary.

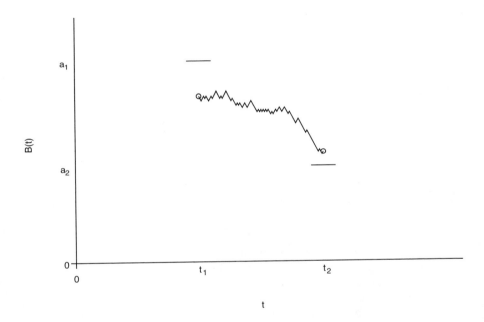

Fig. 4.1. If the B-value boundary decreases from $t = t_1$ to $t = t_2$, we could encounter a logical inconsistency whereby $B(t_1)$ is below its boundary, a negative trend is observed between t_1 and t_2, yet $B(t_2)$ is above its boundary.

The Pocock and O'Brien-Fleming z-value boundaries c_P and c_{O-F} are contrasted in Figure 4.2 for a trial with four equally spaced looks. The O'Brien-Fleming boundary makes it much more difficult to stop early than the Pocock boundary. Accordingly, the O'Brien-Fleming boundary extracts a much smaller price at the end.

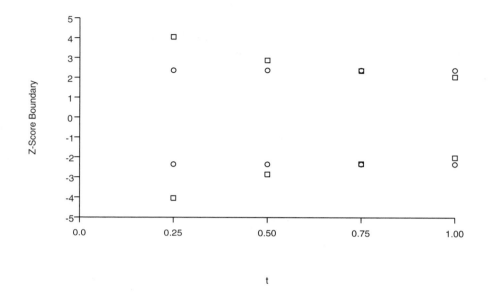

Fig. 4.2. Pocock (circles) and O'Brien-Fleming (squares) z-score boundaries for four looks.

Another way to compare the Pocock and O'Brien-Fleming boundaries is to contrast the cumulative type 1 error rate used up at the different looks. For both boundaries, interim analyses occur at equally spaced information fractions $0/k = 0, 1/k, \ldots, k/k = 1$. The cumulative type 1 error rate used by information fraction j/k is the probability of rejection at or before j/k, $\Pr(\cup_{i=1}^{j}|Z(t_i)| > c_i)$. For both boundaries, the amount of type 1 error rate used by information fractions 0 and 1 is 0 and α, respectively. The cumulative type 1 error rate functions for the Pocock and O'Brien-Fleming boundaries with four looks are shown in Figure 4.3. The Pocock cumulative type 1 error rate increases sharply at first, but much less so toward the end. The O'Brien-Fleming cumulative type 1 error rate function behaves in just the opposite way; it increases very slowly early on, and jumps precipitously at the end.

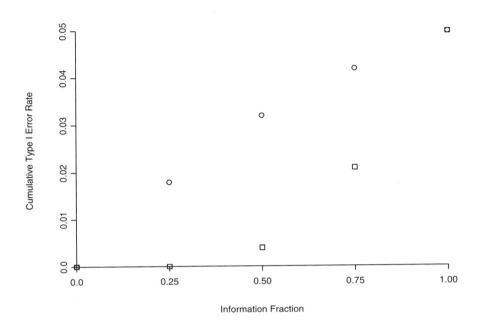

Fig. 4.3. Cumulative type 1 error rate used by the Pocock (circles) and O'Brien-Fleming (squares) procedures with four looks.

4.6 Effect of Monitoring on Power

It is clear that monitoring must decrease power compared to conducting a single test at the end of the trial. After all, the sufficient statistic in a trial without monitoring is the final z-score; conditioned on it, the interim z-scores are ancillary. The flexibility gained by allowing early stopping must therefore cost power, but how much?

We can calculate bounds on power as follows. For a one-tailed test,

$$P_\theta(Z(1) \geq c_k) \leq \text{Power} = P_\theta(\cup_{i=1}^{k} Z(t_i) \geq c_i) \leq P_\theta(Z(1) \geq z_\alpha).$$

That is,

$$1 - \Phi(c_k - \theta) \leq \text{Power} \leq 1 - \Phi(z_\alpha - \theta).$$

Equivalently,

$$\Phi(\theta - c_k) \leq \text{Power} \leq \Phi(\theta - z_\alpha). \tag{4.2}$$

For boundaries such as those of O'Brien-Fleming, the final critical value c_k is very close to z_α, so the left and right sides of (4.2) are almost equal.

For other boundaries, the left and right sides of (4.2) may not be close. For example, even for two looks, the Pocock boundary at the end of the trial is $c_2 = 2.18$, which differs substantially from 1.96. Fortunately, it is easy to calculate power even using a program that computes boundary crossing probabilities only under the null hypothesis. We can generate a Brownian motion with drift θ by $B(t)+\theta t$, where $B(t)$ is a standard (zero-drift) Brownian motion. Thus, power is

$$\Pr(\cup_{i=1}^{k} B(t_i) + \theta t_i \geq a_i) = \Pr(\cup_{i=1}^{k} B(t_i) > a_i - \theta t_i). \qquad (4.3)$$

We can use a computer program that computes boundary crossing probabilities for standard Brownian motion, and supply the boundary $a_i - \theta t_i$.

We can also use free software at www.medsch.wisc.edu/landemets/ to compute the effect of monitoring on power. A complete demonstration of the features of version 2.1 of the program is presented in Chapter 14. For now we show how to compute the power we lose by monitoring a trial. In a clinical trial with no monitoring, to achieve power $1 - \beta$ in a one-tailed test at level $\alpha/2$ or a two-tailed test at level α, we equate the expected z-score to $z_{\alpha/2} + z_{\beta}$ (see Chapter 3). For example, for 85 percent power and a two-tailed test at level 0.05, the expected z-score must be $1.96 + 1.04 = 3$. Suppose we monitor using the Pocock boundary with two looks.

We begin by opening the program winld.exe and clicking on the title page, making it disappear. We then go to the "Compute" menu and select "Probability." From the "**Analysis Parameters**" area we go to "Interim Analyses," type 2, and hit enter. (With this program, one must hit enter after making a choice, otherwise the choice will not register.) The program then shows 0.50 and 1.00 in the "Time" column of the data table at the upper right of the screen. We want to enter our own boundaries, so we go to "**Probability Parameters**," "Determine Bounds," and select "User Input" followed by enter. We then go to the "Upper" column of the data table at the upper right of the screen, and we type the two-look Pocock bounds 2.178 and 2.178. The program automatically supplies symmetrical lower bounds. If we wanted to use a one-tailed test instead, we would have gone to "**Analysis Parameters**," "Test Boundaries," and selected "One-Sided." We then enter 3 under "**Probability Parameters**," "Drift." When we click "Calculate," we see the cumulative exit probabilities 0.47741 and 0.81296 in the last column of the data table at the upper right of the screen. This means that the probability of exceeding the boundary at the first look is 0.47741, while the probability of exceeding the boundary at either the first or second look is 0.81296. In other words, the power drops from about 85 percent in a trial with no monitoring to about 81 percent using the Pocock boundary with only two looks. The loss in power is fairly dramatic considering we took only one interim look and a final look.

Another way of assessing the loss in power using the Pocock boundary is to see how much the drift parameter must be increased to maintain 85 percent power. This time we choose "Drift" from the "Compute" menu. Again we select 2 from the "**Analysis Parameters**," "Interim Analyses," and "User Input" from the "Determine Bounds" box of "**Probability Parameters**." We again enter 2.178, 2.178 under the "Upper" column of the data table at the upper right of the screen. We then go to "Power" from "**Power and Bounds Parameters**" and type 0.85 followed by enter. When we click on "Calculate," we see 3.1503 under **Drift**. In other words, the drift parameter required to maintain 85 percent power increases from 3 with no monitoring to 3.1503 using the Pocock boundary with only two looks. Putting it another way, the relative sample sizes for a two-look trial monitoring using the Pocock boundary and a trial with no monitoring is $(3.1503/3)^2 = 1.10$. We must increase the sample size by 10 percent to maintain 85 percent power, even though we are taking only one interim and one final look.

We can repeat this exercise using the O'Brien-Fleming boundary. We find that a much smaller increase in sample size is required to maintain the same power with the O'Brien-Fleming boundary. Tables 4.4 and 4.5 show the percentage increase for a trial monitoring using the Pocock and O'Brien-Fleming boundaries compared to a trial with no monitoring

Table 4.4. Drift parameter to achieve 80, 85, and 90 percent power using the Pocock boundary for a two-tailed test at $\alpha = 0.05$. The percentage increase in sample size compared to a trial with no monitoring is shown in parentheses.

# Looks (k)	Power= 0.80	Power= 0.85	Power= 0.90
2	2.952 (11)	3.150 (11)	3.399 (10)
3	3.025 (17)	3.225 (16)	3.477 (15)
4	3.072 (20)	3.273 (19)	3.526 (18)
5	3.105 (23)	3.307 (22)	3.561 (21)
6	3.131 (25)	3.334 (24)	3.588 (22)
7	3.151 (26)	3.354 (25)	3.609 (24)
8	3.168 (28)	3.372 (27)	3.627 (25)
9	3.183 (29)	3.387 (28)	3.642 (26)
10	3.196 (30)	3.400 (29)	3.656 (27)
∞	∞	∞	∞

4.7 Appendix: Computation of Boundaries Using Numerical Integration

Armitage, McPherson, and Rowe (1969) [AMR69] showed how to integrate numerically to compute probabilities like $\Pr(Z(t_1) \leq c_1, \ldots, Z(t_k) \leq c_k)$. The $k = 1$ case is simple; $\Pr(Z(t_1) \leq c_1) = \Phi(c_1)$. Now consider $k = 2$. Note that

Table 4.5. Drift parameter to achieve 80, 85, and 90 percent power using the O'Brien-Fleming boundary for a two-tailed test at $\alpha = 0.05$. The percentage increase in sample size compared to a trial with no monitoring is shown in parentheses.

# Looks (k)	Power= 0.80	Power= 0.85	Power= 0.90
2	2.812 (1)	3.007 (1)	3.253 (1)
3	2.826 (2)	3.022 (2)	3.268 (2)
4	2.835 (2)	3.031 (2)	3.277 (2)
5	2.841 (3)	3.037 (3)	3.284 (3)
6	2.846 (3)	3.043 (3)	3.290 (3)
7	2.849 (3)	3.046 (3)	3.293 (3)
8	2.852 (4)	3.049 (4)	3.297 (3)
9	2.855 (4)	3.052 (4)	3.300 (4)
10	2.858 (4)	3.055 (4)	3.302 (4)
∞	∞	∞	∞

$$\Pr(Z(t_1) \leq c_1, Z(t_2) \leq c_2)$$

$$= \int_{-\infty}^{c_1} \Pr\{Z(t_2) \leq c_2 \mid Z(t_1) \in (x, x + dx)\} \Pr\{Z(t_1) \in (x, x + dx)\}$$

$$= \int_{-\infty}^{c_1} \Pr\{B(t_2) \leq c_2 t_2^{1/2} \mid Z(t_1) \in (x, x + dx)\} \Pr\{Z(t_1) \in (x, x + dx)\}$$
$$\times \Pr\{Z(t_1) \in (x, x + dx)\}$$

$$= \int_{-\infty}^{c_1} \Pr\{B(t_2) - B(t_1) \leq c_2 t_2^{1/2} - x t_1^{1/2} \mid Z(t_1) \in (x, x + dx)\}$$
$$\times \Pr\{Z(t_1) \in (x, x + dx)\}$$

$$= \int_{-\infty}^{c_1} \Phi\left(\frac{c_2 t_2^{1/2} - x t_1^{1/2}}{\sqrt{t_2 - t_1}}\right) \phi(x)dx, \tag{4.4}$$

Now think of c_1 as fixed and consider (4.4) as a function $F_{c_1}(c_2)$. Note that $F_{c_1}(c_2)$ is like a distribution function except that $F_{c_1}(\infty) = \Pr(Z(t_1) \leq c_1) < 1$. The derivative

$$\frac{dF_{c_1}(c_2)}{dc_2} = f_{c_1}(c_2) = \int_{-\infty}^{c_1} \sqrt{\frac{t_2}{t_2 - t_1}} \, \phi\left(\frac{c_2 t_2^{1/2} - x t_1^{1/2}}{\sqrt{t_2 - t_1}}\right) \phi(x)dx \tag{4.5}$$

behaves like a density in that $F_{c_1}(c_2) = \int_{-\infty}^{c_2} f_{c_1}(x)dx$. Loosely speaking, $f_{c_1}(x)$ is $\Pr\{Z(t_1) \leq c_1, Z(t_2) = x\}$, meaning that $f_{c_1}(x)dx$ is $\Pr\{Z(t_1) \leq c_1, Z(t_2) \in (x, x + dx)\}$.

For $k = 3$,

$$F_{c_1,c_2}(c_3) = \Pr(Z(t_1) \leq c_1, Z(t_2) \leq c_2, Z(t_3) \leq c_3)$$

$$= \int_{-\infty}^{c_2} \Pr\{Z(t_3) \le c_3 \mid Z(t_1) \le c_1, Z(t_2) \in (x, x + dx)\}$$
$$\times \Pr\{Z(t_1) \le c_1, Z(t_2) \in (x, x + dx)\}$$

$$= \int_{-\infty}^{c_2} \Phi\left(\frac{c_3 t_3^{1/2} - x t_2^{1/2}}{\sqrt{t_3 - t_2}}\right) f_{c_1}(x)dx, \text{ and} \tag{4.6}$$

$$\frac{dF_{c_1,c_2}(c_3)}{dc_3} = f_{c_1,c_2}(c_3) = \int_{-\infty}^{c_2} \sqrt{\frac{t_3}{t_3 - t_2}} \, \phi\left(\frac{c_3 t_3^{1/2} - x t_2^{1/2}}{\sqrt{t_3 - t_2}}\right) f_{c_1}(x)dx \tag{4.7}$$

Continuing in this fashion, we obtain the iterative relationship

$$f_{c_1,\dots,c_{k-1}}(c_k) = \int_{-\infty}^{c_{k-1}} \sqrt{\frac{t_k}{t_k - t_{k-1}}} \, \phi\left(\frac{c_k t_k^{1/2} - x t_{k-1}^{1/2}}{\sqrt{t_k - t_{k-1}}}\right) f_{c_1,\dots,c_{k-2}}(x)dx$$
$$\tag{4.8}$$

for $k \ge 2$, where $f_{c_1,\dots,c_{k-2}}(x)$ is defined to be $\phi(x)$ when $k = 2$.

One simple iterative procedure for computing $\Pr(Z(t_1) \le c_1, \dots, Z(t_k) \le c_k)$ is as follows. Create a grid of say 100 equally spaced points between -7 and 7 and use Simpson's rule to evaluate $f_{c_1}(x)$ of (4.5) for each grid point x, where we replace $-\infty$ by -7. Then use Simpson's rule again to compute $f_{c_1,c_2}(x)$ of (4.7) for each grid point x, where again we replace $-\infty$ by 7. We continue this process and obtain $f_{c_1,\dots,c_{k-1}}(c_k)$ at each grid point x. One final application of Simpson's rule approximates

$$\Pr(Z(t_1) \le c_1, \dots, Z(t_k) \le c_k) = \int_{-\infty}^{c_k} f_{c_1,\dots,c_{k-1}}(x)dx.$$

5

Spending Functions

5.1 Upper Boundaries

The classical Pocock and O'Brien-Fleming boundaries introduced in Chapter 4 require a prespecified number of equally spaced looks, but Data and Safety Monitoring Boards typically want more flexibility. A DSMB may have to postpone a meeting for logistical reasons, or members may want to look at the data more frequently in response to concerns they have. Lan and DeMets (1983) [LD83] showed how to construct boundaries that do not require prespecification of the number or timing of looks. For simplicity, we first consider upper boundaries, deferring discussion of upper and lower boundaries to Section 5.2.

Table 5.1. Cumulative type 1 error rate used by the O'Brien-Fleming procedure with four and eight looks and one-tailed $\alpha = .025$.

	.125	.25	.375	.5	.625	.75	.875	1
4 Looks		.0000		.0021		.0105		.0250
8 Looks	.0000	.0000	.0004	.0018	.0050	.0101	.0168	.0250

The idea introduced in Section 4.5 of considering the cumulative type 1 error rate used by different information times is the key to making boundaries more flexible. Rows 1 and 2 of Table 5.1 show the cumulative type 1 error rate for one-tailed O'Brien-Fleming boundaries with $\alpha = .025$ and four and eight looks, respectively. Notice that the type 1 error rate used by the information fractions common to four and eight looks, namely $t = 0, 1/4, 2/4, 3/4, 1$, are almost the same for row 1 and row 2. Thus, doubling the number of looks doubles the number of points at which the cumulative type 1 error rate function is defined but does not appreciably change its value at previously existing support points. Imagine doubling the number of looks ad infinitum.

The O'Brien-Fleming B-value boundary a_k approaches a as $k \to \infty$, where a is such that $\Pr(B(s) > a$ for some $s \leq 1) = \alpha$. The probability of crossing the boundary by time t is

$$\alpha_1^*(t) = \Pr(B(s) > a \text{ for some } s \leq t). \tag{5.1}$$

Later we will derive a formula for the cumulative crossing probability $\alpha_1^*(t)$

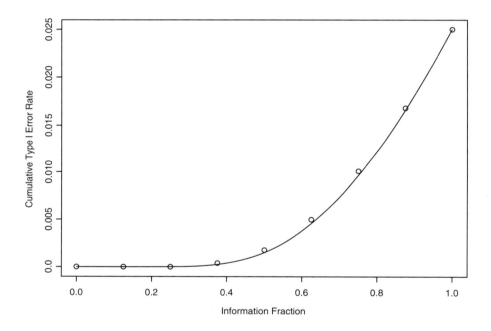

Fig. 5.1. Cumulative type 1 error rate used by the one-tailed O'Brien-Fleming boundary with $\alpha = 0.025$ for eight (circles) versus infinitely many (curve) equally spaced looks. The curve with infinitely many looks is the O'Brien-Fleming-like spending function.

of (5.1); for now note that $\alpha_1^*(t)$ is an increasing function defined on all of $[0, 1]$ with $\alpha_1^*(0) = 0$ and $\alpha_*(1) = \alpha$ (Figure 5.1). A function satisfying these conditions is called a *spending function*. Instead of specifying the number and timing of looks, we can specify a spending function telling how much alpha to use by information time t.

We illustrate the spending function approach using the linear spending function

$$\alpha_2^*(t) = \alpha t$$

with $\alpha = 0.025$ and one-tailed testing. Suppose the first look occurs at information fraction $t = 0.20$. We spend $\alpha_2^*(0.20) = 0.025(0.20) = 0.005$ at the first interim analysis and therefore determine a critical value c_1 such that $\Pr(Z(t_1) > c_1) = 0.005$. The corresponding boundary is $c_1 = \Phi^{-1}(0.995) = 2.576$. We reject the null hypothesis at the first analysis if $Z(0.20) > 2.576$. Suppose this does not happen, and the next interim analysis occurs at information fraction $t = 0.5$. The cumulative type 1 error rate by $t = 0.50$ is $\alpha_2^*(0.5) = 0.025(0.5) = 0.0125$. We determine the boundary c_2 such that $\Pr(Z(0.20) > 2.576 \cup Z(0.5) > c_2) = 0.0125$. This requires numerical integration described in the appendix of Chapter 4. Fortunately, free software for computing boundaries can be downloaded from www.medsch.wisc.edu/landemets/. Chapter 14 contains complete details of how to use version 2.1 of the menu-driven program. Briefly, we specify that we want 1) to compute bounds, 2) two interim analyses, 3) a one-tailed test at $\alpha = 0.025$, 4) to supply information times as user input, and 5) the linear spending function, which the program denotes as a power function with Phi=1. We enter the information times 0.20 and 0.50 at the upper right and find that $c_2 = 2.377$. Thus, we reject the null hypothesis at the second analysis if $Z(0.50) > 2.377$. Suppose this does not happen either and the next analysis occurs at the end of the trial, $t = 1$. The cumulative type 1 error rate at $t = 1$ is $0.025(1) = 0.025$. We determine the value c_3 such that $\Pr(Z(0.20) > 2.576 \cup Z(0.5) > 2.377 \cup Z(1) > c_3) = 0.025$. Another application of the program, this time with three interim analyses at user-specified information times 0.20, 0.50, and 1, yields $c_3 = 2.141$. Thus, we reject the null hypothesis at the end of the trial if $Z(1) > 2.141$.

In this example we found c_i iteratively such that

$$\Pr(\cup_{i=1}^j Z(t_i) > c_i) = \alpha^*(t_j), \quad j = 1, \ldots, k. \tag{5.2}$$

Most computer programs, including the one that can be downloaded from www.medsch.wisc.edu/landemets/, compute boundaries using the slightly easier, but equivalent, first exit formulation rather than the cumulative type 1 error rate formulation. The event $\cup_{i=1}^j Z(t_i) > c_i$ is equivalent to $\{i_f < j\} \cup \{i_f = j\}$, where i_f denotes the first index i such that $Z(t_i) > c_i$; $\{i_f < j\} = \cup_{i=1}^{j-1} Z(t_i) > c_i$ and $\{i_f = j\} = \{(\cap_{i=1}^{j-1} Z(t_i) \le c_i) \cap Z(t_j) > c_j\}$. Thus,

$$\alpha^*(t_j) = \Pr(\cup_{i=1}^j Z(t_i) > c_i)$$

$$= \alpha^*(t_{j-1}) + \Pr\{(\cap_{i=1}^{j-1} Z(t_i) \le c_i) \cap Z(t_j) > c_j\}.$$

It follows that 5.2 is equivalent to 5.3 below.

$$\Pr\{(\cap_{i=1}^{j-1} Z(t_i) \le c_i) \cap Z(t_j) > c_j\} = \alpha^*(t_j) - \alpha^*(t_{j-1}), \quad j = 1, \ldots, k. \tag{5.3}$$

Note that in the above example neither the number nor the timing of the looks needed to be specified in advance. This added flexibility is the advantage of the spending function approach. The example used a linear spending function, but we could have used any other spending function.

We now return to the spending function (5.1) motivated by endlessly doubling the number of looks for the O'Brien-Fleming procedure. The following result is proven in the appendix using Result 3.1 of Chapter 3.

Result 5.1 *The probability that standard Brownian motion crosses the horizontal boundary a* **by** *time t is twice the probability that it crosses* **at** *time t; i.e., $\Pr\{B(s) > a \text{ for some } s \leq t\} = 2\Pr\{B(t) > a\} = 2\{1 - \Phi(a/t^{1/2})\}$.*

If we select a such that $\Pr(B(s) > a \text{ for some } s \leq 1) = \alpha$, Result 5.1 applied to $t = 1$ implies that $a = z_{\alpha/2}$. Thus,

$$\alpha_1^*(t) = \Pr(B(s) > z_{\alpha/2} \text{ for some } s \leq t).$$

Another application of Result 5.1 shows that

$$\alpha_1^*(t) = 2\{1 - \Phi(z_{\alpha/2}/t^{1/2})\} \tag{5.4}$$

(see Figure 5.1). Spending function $\alpha_1^*(t)$ of (5.4) mimics the O'Brien-Fleming boundary when the looks are equally spaced, but we can use it even when looks are not equally spaced.

Next we try to find a spending function that mimics the Pocock boundary for equally spaced looks. We begin as before, looking at the boundaries for the Pocock procedure with a fixed number of looks, k, and letting k become large. But there is a problem; the z-score boundary c_k for the Pocock procedure tends to ∞ as $k \to \infty$. Consequently, the cumulative α spent by information fraction t converges to α as $k \to \infty$ for each $t > 0$. To see this, let A_k (resp. B_k) denote the event that $Z(i/k) > c_k$ for some i such that $i/k \leq t$ (resp., for some i such that $i/k > t$). Note that

$$P(B_k) \leq \Pr(\sup_{0 \leq s \leq 1} B(s)/t^{1/2} > c_k)$$
$$= \Pr(\sup_{0 \leq s \leq 1} B(s) > c_k t^{1/2}).$$

Because $\sup_{0 \leq s \leq 1} B(s)$ converges in distribution and $c_k \to \infty$, $\Pr(B_k) \to 0$ as $k \to \infty$. Thus,

$$\alpha = \Pr(A_k \cup B_k) \leq \Pr(A_k) + \Pr(B_k)$$
$$\Pr(A_k) \geq \alpha - \Pr(B_k) \to \alpha - 0 = \alpha \text{ as } k \to \infty.$$

In other words, the cumulative type 1 error function resulting from this limiting process spends all of the α by information time t for *any* $t > 0$. The trial is over at the first look regardless of when the look occurs. This is not a reasonable spending function. We cannot hope to mimic Pocock boundaries

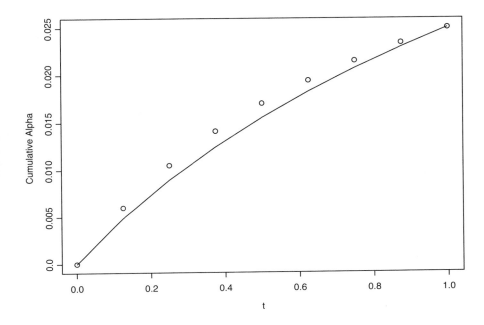

Fig. 5.2. Cumulative type 1 error rate used by the Pocock procedure with a one-tailed test at $\alpha = 0.025$ and eight looks (circles), together with the Pocock-like spending function $0.025 \ln\{1 + (e - 1)t\}$ (curve).

for large k. The best we can hope for is a spending function that mimics the Pocock boundaries for a reasonable number of looks (Table 5.2).

Figure 5.2 shows the cumulative type 1 error rate used by information fraction t for the Pocock procedure at one-tailed $\alpha = .025$ and eight looks. Lan and DeMets (1983) [LD83] noted that its shape is similar to a logarithmic curve, except that it must lie between 0 and α for $0 \leq t \leq 1$. Their approach was first to change the location and scale to force the log function to lie between 0 and 1 for $0 \leq t \leq 1$: $\ln\{1 + (e - 1)t\}$, and then multiply by α to obtain a spending function yielding boundaries similar to Pocock's:

$$\alpha_3^*(t) = \alpha \ln\{1 + (e - 1)t\}.$$

The three spending functions discussed so far are plotted in Figure 5.3. The O'Brien-Fleming-like spending function is convex, spending very little of the α early, but rising steeply at the end. As a result, the critical value at the end

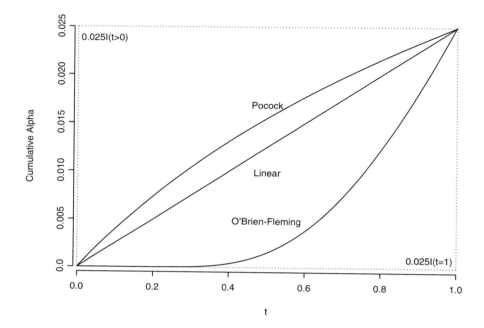

Fig. 5.3. Cumulative type 1 error rate used by the O'Brien-Fleming-like, linear, and Pocock-like spending functions at one-tailed $\alpha = 0.025$, as well as the two extreme spending functions $0.025I(t > 0)$ and $0.025I(t = 1)$.

Table 5.2. Three spending functions.

O'Brien-Fleming-like	Linear	Pocock-like
$\alpha_1^*(t) = 2\{1 - \Phi(z_{\alpha/2}/t^{1/2})\}$	$\alpha_2^*(t) = \alpha t$	$\alpha_3^*(t) = \alpha \ln\{1 + (e - 1)t\}$

of the study is close to what it would have been with no monitoring. Table 5.3 shows that the final critical value is 1.969, only a slight increase from the 1.96 figure with no monitoring. The concave Pocock-like spending function spends a considerable amount of α early. Consequently, using it incurs a much larger penalty at the end of the trial. Table 5.3 shows that the final critical value is 2.225. The linear spending function (which is both concave and convex) lies between the O'Brien-Fleming-like and Pocock-like spending functions. Hence, its final critical value of 2.141 (see Table 5.3) lies between that of the O'Brien-Fleming-like and Pocock-like spending functions. Also shown in Figure 5.3 is the spending function $\alpha^*(t) = \alpha I(t > 0)$ derived as the limiting cumulative type 1 error rate of the Pocock procedure as the number of looks tends to ∞. It can be viewed as a limit of increasingly concave functions; because it spends all of the type 1 error rate immediately, the final critical value is ∞ unless it is the only look at the data. At the other extreme is $\alpha^*(t) = \alpha I(t = 1)$, the limit of increasingly convex spending functions. Because none of the type 1 error rate is spent before the last look, all interim boundaries are ∞ and the final boundary is exactly the same as without monitoring.

Table 5.3. Boundaries for the O-Brien-Fleming-like, linear, and Pocock-like spending functions for a one-tailed test at $\alpha = 0.025$ when looks occur at $t_1 = 0.20$, $t_2 = 0.50$, and $t_3 = 1$.

Information time	O'Brien-Fleming-like	Linear	Pocock-like
$t_1 = 0.20$	4.877	2.576	2.438
$t_2 = 0.50$	2.963	2.377	2.333
$t_3 = 1.00$	1.969	2.141	2.225

5.1.1 Using a Different Time Scale for Spending

As we have described the spending function approach, the amount of type 1 error rate to spend at a given interim analysis depends on the information fraction t. In a trial measuring survival or time to failure, the information fraction depends on how many patients will have events by trial's end, a quantity that must be estimated. If the estimate turns out to be too small, then we will reach information fraction 1 and spend all of the α before the end of the trial. To avoid this problem, we can spend α according to a different time scale such as calendar fraction (Lan and DeMets, 1989a [LD89a]).

For example, suppose we expect 100 deaths by the end of a trial with 2 years of recruitment and 4 years minimum follow-up. We monitor using the O'Brien-Fleming-like spending function α_1^*. The first interim analysis after 1 year corresponds to a calendar fraction of $s = 1/6$. Thus, we are allowed to spend $\alpha_1^*(1/6)$, which is 0 to 4 decimal places. The critical value is 5.36. Suppose 25 deaths have occurred. The estimated information fraction at calendar fraction $s = 1/6$ is $t = 25/100$. We stop the trial if $Z(25/100) > 5.36$. Note that the null distribution of $Z(25/100)$ is standard normal whether or not we estimated the number of deaths by trial's end correctly.

Suppose by the second look at 2 years there are 60 deaths. The calendar fraction and estimated information fraction are $s = 2/6$ and $t = 60/100$, respectively. Because we are spending alpha according to calendar fraction, the cumulative type 1 error rate is $\alpha_1^*(2/6) = 0.0001$. Thus, we determine c_2 such that

$$\Pr(Z(25/100) > 5.36 \cup Z(60/100) > c_2) = \alpha_1^*(0.333) = 0.0001.$$

If our initial estimate of 100 deaths by the end of the trial were correct, the null distribution of $(Z(25/100), Z(60/100))$ would be bivariate normal with 0 means, unit variances, and correlation $\{(25/100)/(60/100)\}^{1/2} = (25/60)^{1/2}$, but by now it is clear that we underestimated the final number of deaths. Suppose we now expect 150 deaths by trial's end, so that the actual information fractions at the first and second looks were $25/150$ and $60/150$. The correlation between $Z(25/150)$ and $Z(60/150)$ is $\{(25/150)/(60/150)\}^{1/2} = \{(25/60)^{1/2}\}$. Because the correlation depends on the information fractions only through their ratio, the expected information by trial's end cancels out and the joint distribution of the z-statistics does not depend on the future number of deaths.

We can determine c_2 using the program in the appendix at the end of the chapter, which computes upper boundaries for a one-tailed test. Because we want the one-tailed cumulative type 1 error rate to be 0.0001, we go to the end of the program and change the highlighted portion beginning with "# Input" to:

```
# Input
##################################################################
tcur<-0.60        # Current value of t.
tprev<-c(.25)     # Previous values of t go in parentheses.
cprev<-c(5.36)    # Previous boundary values go in parentheses.
cumulal<-.0001    # Cumulative alpha up to current look,
                  # alpha_*(tcur).
##################################################################
```

This tells the program that our current look is at $t_2 = 0.60$; there was only one previous look, at $t_1 = 0.25$, at which time we used boundary $c_1 = 5.36$; and the cumulative type 1 error rate to spend by the current information time $t_2 = 0.60$ is 0.0001. The program then tells us that $c_2 = 3.72$.

Suppose the next look is at the end of the trial, $t = 1$. We then change the highlighted portion at the end of the program, beginning with "# Input," to

```
# Input
##################################################################
tcur<-1              # Current value of t.
tprev<-c(.25,.60)    # Previous values of t go in parentheses.
cprev<-c(5.36,3.72)  # Previous boundary values go in
                     # parentheses.
cumulal<-.025        # Cumulative alpha up to current look,
                     # alpha_*(tcur).
##################################################################
```

The program then tells us that $c_3 = 1.96$ to two decimal places (the first two looks used such large boundaries that there is essentially no price to pay for monitoring).

This example used calendar fraction as a surrogate for information fraction, but we could have used a different surrogate. For example, suppose all patients are randomized at the beginning of the trial and their survival times have an exponential distribution. Clearly their survival times remain exponentially distributed if we use calendar fraction. The expected number of patients with an event by calendar fraction t is $N\{1-\exp(-\gamma t)\}$. Thus, of the expected $N\{1-\exp(-\gamma)\}$ patients with events by trial's end, the fraction occurring by calendar fraction t is expected to be $\{1-\exp(-\gamma t)\}/\{1-\exp(-\gamma)\}$. Thus, spending linearly with respect to the expected information fraction at calendar fraction t yields the spending function

$$\alpha_4^*(t) = \alpha \left\{ \frac{1-\exp(-\gamma t)}{1-\exp(-\gamma)} \right\}. \tag{5.5}$$

Hwang, Shih, and DeCani (1990) [HSD90] proposed class (5.5), but allowed γ to be negative. Note that $\alpha_4^*(t)$ has limit $\alpha I(t = 1)$ as $\gamma \to -\infty$, αt as $\gamma \to 0$, and $\alpha I(t \neq 0)$ as $\gamma \to \infty$. Thus, considering different values of γ allows consideration of a wide variety of spending functions.

5.1.2 Data-Driven Looks

As described above, the big advantage of spending functions is their flexibility, for they do not require advance specification of the number or timing of looks. On the other hand, the timing of the looks is assumed independent of the B-value process. In practice, the timing of looks might depend on the outcome. If the test statistic is close to a boundary, the Data and Safety Monitoring Board may decide to meet earlier than originally anticipated. Conversely, in a trial where the test statistic is far from the boundary, the board may opt to delay a meeting. Ethics and practicality tend to trump statistical purity. Fortunately, even with data-driven timing and number of looks, the degree of type 1 error rate inflation is relatively small.

Lan and DeMets (1989b) [LD89b] investigated the impact of increased monitoring when the results were close to reaching a boundary. They looked at both the Pocock- and O'Brien-Fleming-like spending functions with a one-tailed test at $\alpha = 0.025$ and originally planned looks at $t = 0.25, 0.5, 0.75$, and 1. If $0.8c(t) < Z(t) < c(t)$, where $c(t)$ is the boundary at information fraction t, they doubled the number of future looks. Thus, if $0.8c(0.5) < Z(0.5) < c(0.5)$, future looks would occur at 0.625, 0.75, 0.875, and 1 instead of just 0.75 and 1. Power and type 1 error rate were virtually unchanged.

Proschan, Follmann, and Waclawiw (1992) [PFW92] considered the impact of a more nefarious attempt to inflate the type 1 error rate. With three looks, they fixed the information fractions of the first and last looks at δ and 1, respectively, and then used a grid search to find the information fraction t at the second look that maximized the conditional probability of rejection at the second or third looks. With more than three looks they used a less computationally intensive method that still went beyond realistic data-driven looks. Even under this "intention to cheat" approach they were unable to cause more than about a 10 percent inflation of the type 1 error rate.

Some members of data monitoring committees express the concern that the boundaries may become unpredictable for look times very close together. For example, let L and c_L be the information fraction and boundary at the last look. Because $\alpha^*(L + \Delta) - \alpha^*(L)$ is very tiny as Δ becomes tiny, it seems the boundary at $L + \Delta$ must be very large if Δ is small. On the other hand, given that no rejection has occurred by L, we know that $Z(L) \leq c_L$. The critical value at $L + \Delta$ may only need to be slightly larger than c_L. Which of these two lines of reasoning is correct?

Result 5.2 *(Proschan, 1999 [P99]). Fix the times of the previous looks* $t_1, \ldots, L$. *Suppose the z-value boundary at the last look L was c_L, and the next look is at information fraction $L + \Delta$ with z-value boundary $c(L + \Delta)$. If $0 < \alpha^{*\prime}(L) < \infty$, then $c_{L+\Delta} \to c_L$ as $\Delta \downarrow 0$.*

Result 5.2 reassures us that the critical value does not become highly unpredictable if the next look time is very close to the last. Table 5.4 illustrates Result 5.2 in a trial whose first three looks occur at information fractions $t_1 = 0.20$, $t_2 = 0.40$ and $t_3 = 0.60$, and whose fourth look occurs at $t_4 = 0.61$, $t_4 = 0.601$, or $t_4 = 0.6001$. For each of the three spending functions, the boundary c_4 at information fraction t_4 is close to the boundary c_3 at the previous look. For example, for the O'Brien-Fleming-like spending function and $t_4 = 0.6001$, the boundary at t_4 is 2.71, virtually the same as $c_3 = 2.68$.

Table 5.4. Boundaries when the first three looks are at $t = 0.20$, 0.40, and 0.60 and the fourth look is very close to the third.

Information Time	O'Brien-Fleming-Like	Linear	Pocock-Like
$t_1 = 0.20$	4.88	2.58	2.44
$t_2 = 0.40$	3.36	2.49	2.43
$t_3 = 0.60$	2.68	2.41	2.41
$t_4 = 0.61$	2.73	2.51	2.52
$t_4 = 0.601$	2.73	2.47	2.47
$t_4 = 0.6001$	2.71	2.44	2.44

5.2 Upper and Lower Boundaries

Most clinical trials aim to show that a new treatment is superior to either a placebo or a standard treatment. It is nonetheless possible that treatment causes harm, as was the case in the Cardiac Arrhythmia Suppression Trial (CAST) (see Chapter 1). Some have interpreted these unexpected findings as mandating two-tailed testing with a fixed overall type 1 error rate. But for a treatment that really has no effect, the two types of errors—concluding the treatment is effective or concluding the treatment is harmful—are quite different. It is more natural to separate the cases, especially if we want to allow different error rates for the two types of errors. The CAST II investigators wanted to make it easier to conclude harm for the remaining antiarrhythmic drug in light of the CAST I evidence of harm for the other two antiarrhythmic drugs. Thus, the investigators set a lower boundary for harm using a spending function with $\alpha = 0.05$ and an autonomous upper boundary for benefit using a spending function with $\alpha = 0.025$. They were not concerned that the overall type 1 error rate exceeded 0.05 because that overall rate mixes apples (benefit) and oranges (harm).

Another reason for separating the two types of error rates is that many trials would stop for futility before crossing a boundary for harm. We ordinarily would not continue a trial to prove that treatment is harmful. The exception would be if the treatment were already in widespread use, in which case it might be important to prove harm to change clinical practice.

A natural question is whether the upper boundary for benefit should account for the fact that we could have stopped for futility, or should the upper and lower boundaries be autonomous? For example, suppose we construct an $\alpha = 0.025$ monitoring boundary for benefit without considering futility monitoring. The actual probability of a false-positive benefit is Pr(cross upper boundary before crossing futility boundary) < 0.025. The problem with accounting for the lower boundary when calculating the upper boundary is that once one incorporates this probability, one can no longer overrule the lower boundary. Thus, crossing the lower futility boundary *requires* stopping the trial and accepting the null hypothesis. If not, then the probability of a false declaration of treatment benefit will exceed 0.025. Our experience is that Data and Safety Monitoring Boards treat futility boundaries as more advisory than upper boundaries. Furthermore, if the results of a trial do not cross the futility boundary, one can never know what the DSMB would have done had the boundary been crossed. Because the calculation of boundary-crossing probability depends on this contrafactual event, we cannot be certain how to calculate the probability. In summary, we strongly prefer to give the DSMB flexibility by not accounting for the lower boundary when constructing the upper boundary.

When it *does* make sense to combine the two types of errors, such as when the two arms are both active treatments and we use symmetric upper and lower boundaries, we can still very closely approximate—unless α is unusually large— the two-tailed boundary at level α by separate one-tailed boundaries at level $\alpha/2$. The "proper" symmetric two-tailed boundary $\pm c_1$, $\pm c_2$, ... at level α satisfies

$$\Pr(|Z(t_1)| > c_1) = \alpha_*(t_1)$$
$$\Pr(|Z(t_1)| > c_1 \cup |Z(t_2)| > c_2) = \alpha_*(t_2)$$
$$\vdots \qquad (5.6)$$

Nonetheless, if we construct upper boundaries c_1', c_2', ... using the same spending function but at level $\alpha/2$, and then use $-c_1'$, $-c_2'$, ... for the lower boundary, then c_i' and c_i will be virtually identical unless α is unusually large (Proschan, 1999 [P99]). The reader may verify this using the software described in Chapter 14 (see Section 14.3.1).

5.3 Summary

The spending function, which specifies the cumulative type 1 error rate to use by information fraction t, allows monitoring without the need to prespecify the number or timing of interim looks. This is important to data monitoring boards, which often try to meet at regular intervals such as every 6 months, but whose actual schedule is dictated by member availability and sometimes by the data themselves. The practical reality is that a board may increase the frequency of monitoring when the data are close to a boundary for efficacy or harm despite protestations from their statisticians about the invalidity of such a procedure.

We can choose a spending function to produce the type of boundary we want. Spending little alpha until near the end gives us O'Brien-Fleming-like boundaries that are very stringent early and close to $z_{\alpha/2}$ at the end. Spending alpha much more rapidly can produce Pocock-like boundaries. Other spending functions lead to intermediate boundaries.

5.4 Appendix

5.4.1 Proof of Result 5.1

First consider $t = 1$. Note that continuously monitoring a trial and stopping as soon as $B(s) > a$ is the same as using a critical value of a at the end and stopping early as soon as conditional power computed under H_0 exceeds $1/2$ (conditional power under H_0 exceeds $1/2$ at time s iff $B(s) > a$). By Result 3.1, the probability that conditional power ever exceeds $1/2$ is twice the probability that $B(1)$ exceeds a. Thus, Result 5.1 holds when $t = 1$.

For $t < 1$, note that

$$\Pr\left\{ \sup_{0 \le s \le t} B(s) > a \right\} = \Pr\left\{ \sup_{0 \le s \le t} B(s)/t^{1/2} > a/t^{1/2} \right\}$$
$$= \Pr\left\{ \sup_{0 \le u \le 1} B(tu)/t^{1/2} > a/t^{1/2} \right\}. \qquad (5.7)$$

It is an elementary exercise to show that if $B(s)$ is a standard Brownian motion, then $B^*(u) = B(tu)/t^{1/2}$ is also a standard Brownian motion for any positive t, so (5.7) equals $\Pr\{\sup_{0 \leq s \leq 1} B(s) > a/t^{1/2}\}$. Because we have already shown that Result 5.1 holds when $t = 1$, this latter probability is $2\Pr\{B(1) > a/t^{1/2}\} = 2\{1 - \Phi(a/t^{1/2})\}$, completing the proof. ‖

5.4.2 Proof of Result 5.2

Suppose first that $c_{L+\Delta}$ converged to a limit $c < c_L$. Then $\alpha^*(L+\Delta) - \alpha^*(L)$ would tend to the nonzero limit $\Pr(B(t_1) \leq c_1, \ldots, c < B(L) \leq c_L)$. Thus, $\alpha^*(t)$ would have to be discontinuous at $t = L$, contradicting the fact that $\alpha^*(t)$ is differentiable at $t = L$. Similarly, if $\alpha^*(t)$ is continuous at $t = L$, there can be no subsequence Δ_i such that $c_{L+\Delta_i} \to c < c_L$.

If we could establish that there cannot be a subsequence Δ_i such that $c_{L+\Delta_i} \to c > c_L$, then clearly $c_{L+\Delta} \to c_L$ as $\Delta \downarrow 0$. The probability of rejecting at time $L + \Delta_i$, given that no rejection has occurred by L, is no larger than

$$\Pr\left\{ B(L + \Delta_i) > \sqrt{L + \Delta_i} c_{L+\Delta_i} \mid B(L) = \sqrt{L} c_L \right\}$$

$$= 1 - \Phi\left\{ \frac{\sqrt{L + \Delta_i} c_{L+\Delta_i} - \sqrt{L} c_L}{\sqrt{\Delta_i}} \right\}$$

$$\leq 1 - \Phi\left\{ \sqrt{L} \left(\frac{c_{L+\Delta_i} - c_L}{\sqrt{\Delta_i}} \right) \right\}.$$

Thus,

$$(1/\Delta_i)\left\{ \frac{\alpha^*(L + \Delta_i) - \alpha^*(L)}{1 - \alpha^*(L)} \right\} \leq (1/\Delta_i)\left[1 - \Phi\left\{ \sqrt{L} \left(\frac{c_{L+\Delta_i} - c_L}{\sqrt{\Delta_i}} \right) \right\} \right]. \tag{5.8}$$

Suppose that $\alpha^*(t)$ has finite, nonzero derivative $\alpha^{*\prime}(L)$ at $t = L$. As $\Delta \downarrow 0$, the left side of (5.8) tends to $\alpha^{*\prime}(L)/\{1 - \alpha^*(L)\}$. Suppose $c_{L+\Delta_i} \to c > c_L$ as $i \to \infty$. Then $x(\Delta_i) = (L/\Delta_i)^{1/2}\{c(L + \Delta_i) - c(L)\} \to \infty$ and the right side of (5.8) tends to 0 because of the well-known inequality $1 - \Phi(x) \leq \phi(x)/x$, whose proof is simple: $\int_x^\infty \phi(u)du = \int_x^\infty (1/u)u\phi(u)du \leq (1/x)\int_x^\infty u\phi(u)du = \phi(x)/x$. Thus, if $c_{L+\Delta_i} \to c > c_L$, then $\alpha^{*\prime}(L) = 0$. We have established that if $0 < \alpha^{*\prime}(L) < \infty$, then for no subsequence $\Delta_i \downarrow 0$ can $\alpha^*(L + \Delta_i)$ have a limit smaller or larger than c_L. In other words, $\alpha^*(L + \Delta) \to c_L$ as $\Delta \downarrow 0$. ‖

5.4.3 An S-Plus or R Program to Compute Boundaries

The following S-Plus or R program, which computes boundary values iteratively, is helpful when using a nonstandard spending function or when using

one time scale for spending and another for computing the joint distribution
of test statistics (see Section 5.1.1).

For given values of the previous boundaries $c_1, \ldots, c_{k-1}$ and time points
$t_1, \ldots, t_{k-1}$, the program finds the current boundary c_k such that the cumulative crossing probability $\Pr(Z(t_1) \geq c_1 \cup \ldots \cup Z(t_k) \geq c_k)$ is a specified value,
"cumulal." To use the program, go to the end and supply the information
highlighted under "Input." Following the program is a short example.

```
simpson<-function(f,dx){
# Approximates integrals using Simpson's rule.
# f is a vector of function values at 2m+1 equally spaced x
# values (comprising 2m intervals of length dx).
    m<-(length(f)-1)/2
    evens<-2*(1:m); odds<-2*(1:m)+1; last<-2*m+1
    int<-(4*sum(f[evens])+2*sum(f[odds])+f[1]-f[last])*(dx/3)
    return(int)
}


updt<-function(datavec){
# updt gives P(Z_1\le c_1,...,ldots,Z_prev\le c_prev,
# Zcur=zcur);
# datavec consists of:
# First dim1 components contain fprev=P(Z_1\le c_1,\ldots,
# Z_{prev-1}\le c_{prev-1},Z_prev=zprev) for a vector
# prevgrid.
# Next dim1 components contain the vector prevgrid.
# Next 2 components contain information times of previous and
# current looks.
# The last component contains zcur.
dimmy<-length(datavec); dim1<-(dimmy-3)/2; dim1p<-dim1+1
dim2<-2*dim1
dim2p<-dim2+1; dim2pp<-dim2+2; dim2ppp<-dim2+3
fprev<-datavec[1:dim1]; prevgrid<-datavec[dim1p:dim2]
tprev<-datavec[dim2p]
tcur<-datavec[dim2pp]; zcur<-datavec[dim2ppp]
temp<-(zcur*sqrt(tcur)-prevgrid*sqrt(tprev))/sqrt(tcur-tprev)
y<-sqrt(tcur/(tcur-tprev))*exp(-temp^2/2)/sqrt(2*pi)*fprev
dx<-prevgrid[2]-prevgrid[1]
return(simpson(y,dx))
}


distrib<-function(tt,cc){
# Gives P(Z(t_1)\le c_1,...Z(t_k)\le c_k), where
# cc=(c_1,\ldots,c_k),
# tt=(t_1,\ldots,t_k)
```

```
if(length(tt)!=length(cc)){return("dimensions of t and c do
not match")}
if(max(tt)>1 | min(tt)<=0){return("t_i not in (0,1] for
all i")}
if(min(cc)< -7){return(0)}
k<-length(tt)
numint<-50
lengthz<-numint+1
if(k==1){return(pnorm(cc[1],0,1))}
zgrid<-seq(-7,cc[1],length=lengthz)
tprev<-tt[1]
fprev<-exp(-zgrid^2/2)/sqrt(2*pi)
for(i in 2:k){
zcur<-seq(-7,cc[i],length=lengthz)
tprev<-tt[i-1]
tcur<-tt[i]
datmat<-matrix(rep(c(fprev,zgrid,tprev,tcur),lengthz),
nrow=lengthz, byrow=T)
datmat<-cbind(datmat,zcur)
ww<-apply(datmat,MARGIN=1,updt)
fprev<-ww
zgrid<-zcur
}
dz<-zcur[2]-zcur[1]
ans<-simpson(ww,dz)
return(ans)
}


##################################################################


rename<-function(cccur,otherstuff){
# Re-parameterizes the distribution function P(Z(t_1)\le c_1,
# \ldots,Z(t_k)\le c_k) so that first variable is c_k and the
# last variable is the cumulative alpha spent.
kminus1<-(length(otherstuff)-2)/2
i1<-kminus1+1; i2<-kminus1+2; i3<--2*kminus1+1; i4<-2*kminus1+2
ttcur<-otherstuff[1]; ttprev<-otherstuff[2:i1]
ccprev<-otherstuff[i2:i3]
alphacum<-otherstuff[i4]
return(distrib(c(ttprev,ttcur),c(ccprev,cccur))-(1-alphacum))
}

findroot<-function(f,low,high,otherstuff){
# Finds root in interval (low,high) for the increasing (in x)
```

```
# function f(x,otherstuff).
lower<-low; higher<-high
if(f(lower,otherstuff)>0 | f(higher,otherstuff)<0){return(
"findroot can't find the root")}
for(i in 1:20){
midpoint<-(lower+higher)/2
if(f(midpoint,otherstuff) > 0){higher<-midpoint}
else{lower<-midpoint}
}
return((lower+higher)/2)
}
```

```
# Input
###################################################################
tcur<-.80                   # Current value of t
tprev<-c(.20,.45,.65)       # Previous values of t go in
                            # parentheses.
cprev<-c(3.5,2.75,2.50)     # Previous boundary values go in
                            # parentheses.
cumulal<-.015               # Cumulative alpha up to current look,
                            # alpha_*(tcur)
###################################################################
```

```
other<-c(tcur,tprev,cprev,cumulal)
answer<-findroot(rename,-7,7,other)
print(round(answer,digits=4))
```

With the "Input" settings shown, the program will compute the upper boundary at the fourth look at information time 0.80 such that the cumulative type 1 error rate is 0.015, given that the previous boundaries were $c_1 = 3.5$, $c_2 = 2.75$, and $c_3 = 2.50$ at information times $t = 0.20$, $t = 0.45$, and $t = 0.65$, respectively. When we run the program, we get $c_4 = 2.26$

If the next look were at the end of the trial ($t = 1$), so we wanted the cumulative type 1 error rate to be 0.05, we would replace the above input values with:

```
# Input
###################################################################
tcur<-1                         # Current value of t
tprev<-c(.20,.45,.65,.80,1)     # Previous values of t go in
                                # parentheses.
```

```
cprev<-c(3.5,2.75,2.50,2.26)  # Previous boundary values go in
                              # parentheses.
cumulal<-.025                 # Cumulative alpha up to current
                              # look, alpha_*(tcur)
##################################################################
```

When we run the program, we find that the final critical value is $c_5 = 2.08$.

6

Practical Survival Monitoring

6.1 Introduction

Methodology for sequential monitoring of survival data and its applications became popular after several seminal publications in the 1980s (see Andersen et al. 1993 [ABG93]). The stochastic process formulation of sequential monitoring of survival data is analogous to that developed through partial sums of i.i.d. random variables and application of the functional central limit theorem (Billingsley, 1968 [B68]). Partial sum processes are special cases of martingales, as are stochastic processes related to survival monitoring. In the 1980s, the theory of counting processes and the martingale central limit theorem provided us with powerful tools to demonstrate that many stochastic processes other than partial sums approach Brownian motion for large sample sizes. These tools provide a unified approach to monitoring interim data from clinical trials, including trials comparing 1) two means or 2) two survival distributions under the proportional hazards assumption. In this chapter we discuss the similarities between comparing means and comparing survival distributions using the logrank statistic under the proportional hazards assumption. We then consider survival monitoring when the proportional hazards assumption does not hold.

6.2 Survival Trials with Staggered Entry

In Chapter 2, we showed that the joint distribution of sequentially-computed logrank statistics was the same as that of sequentially computed t-statistics, but there we assumed all patients were randomized at the beginning of the trial. In most practical situations, patients do not arrive simultaneously. To see the impact of this "staggered entry," suppose a trial randomizes patient P_1 to treatment (T) and P_2 to control (C) at the very beginning of recruitment, and patient P_3 to T 30 days later. Patients P_1 and P_2 die at respective follow-up times 7 and 9, while patient P_3 survives the entire trial. The trial has two different natural time scales: *calendar time* from the beginning of the trial and each patient's *follow-up time* from time of randomization. Suppose the first two looks at the data occur at calendar times 20 and 40 days (Figure 6.1).

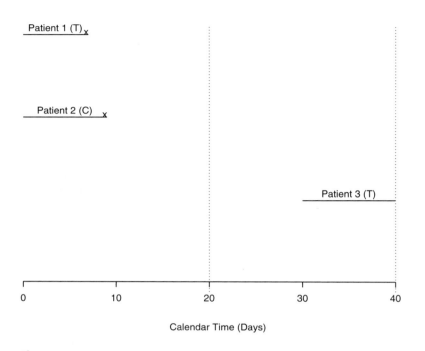

Fig. 6.1. Hypothetical data from a small trial whose first two looks occur at calendar times 20 and 40 days. Each x indicates a death.

By the time of the first interim analysis at calendar time 20 days, patient P_3 has not yet been randomized, so the 2×2 tables at calendar time 20 days are as shown in Table 6.1. The logrank statistic at the first interim analysis is $\{(1 - 1/2) + (0 - 0)\}/\{(1/2)(1 - 1/2) + (0)(1 - 0)\}^{1/2} = 1$. Now suppose the second interim analysis occurs at calendar time $t_c = 40$ days. By that time the third patient has arrived and survived 10 days. Now patient P_3 is included in the risk sets at the first and second death times. The 2×2 tables at the second interim analysis are as shown in Table 6.2.

The logrank statistic is now $\{(1 - 2/3) + (0 - 1/2)\}/\{(2/3)(1 - 2/3) + (1/2)(1 - 1/2)\}^{1/2} = -0.243$. Even though no additional death occurred between the first and second interim analyses, the logrank statistic has changed because the risk sets changed. Thus, to represent the logrank statistic and other survival

Table 6.1. 2×2 tables at interim analysis at calendar time 20 days, follow-up times 7 and 9 days, respectively (first and second death times).

Table 6.2. 2×2 tables at interim analysis at calendar time 40 days, follow-up times 7 and 9 days, respectively (first and second death times).

tests as a stochastic process, we must somehow account for both time scales: calendar time of the entire trial and follow-up time of individual patients.

6.3 Stochastic Process Formulation and Linear Trends

Tsiatis (1982) [T82] accounted for both time scales as follows. Let Y_i denote the calendar time when patient i is randomized; V_i and W_i denote the time from randomization to death and time from randomization to censoring, respectively; and $X_i(t_c)$ denote the follow-up time observed for patient i at calendar time t_c: $X_i(t_c) = \max\{\min(V, W, t_c - Y), 0\}$. For example, at $t_c = 40$ in the small example, $X_i(40)$ is 7, 9, and 10 for $i = 1, 2, 3$. If $\Delta_i(t_c)$ is the indicator that patient i has died (and not been censored) by calendar time t_c, we can write the numerator of the logrank statistic at calendar time t_c as

$$S_n(t_c) = \sum_{i=1}^{n} \Delta_i(t_c) \left\{ Z_i - \sum_{j \in R(t_c, X_i(t_c))} \frac{Z_j}{n(t_c, X_i(t_c))} \right\},$$

where Z_i is the indicator that patient i is assigned to the treatment, and $R(t_c, X_i(t_c))$ and $n(t_c, X_i(t_c))$ are the risk set and its cardinality at calendar time t_c and follow-up time $X_i(t_c)$. The term $\sum_{j \in R(t_c, X_i(t_c))} Z_j / n(t_c, X_i(t_c))$ is analogous to a sample mean; it converges to, and may be replaced by, its expectation for large sample sizes. Replacing $\sum_{j \in R(t_c, X_i(t_c))} Z_j / n(t, X_i(t_c))$ by its expectation allows us to write $S_n(t_c)$ as a sum of i.i.d. stochastic processes. We can then prove that asymptotically, $S(t_c)$ has independent increments and is marginally normal with mean $\{D(t_c)/4\} \ln(r)$ and variance $D(t_c)/4$, where r is the hazard ratio—assumed constant—and $D(t_c)$ is the combined probability of an observed death by calendar time t_c; i.e., $D(t_c)$ is the probability that a randomly selected trial participant will enter the trial and die (without being censored) by calendar time t_c. The denominator of the logrank statistic is approximately $\{D(t_c)/4\}^{1/2}$, so the logrank statistic at calendar time t_c is approximately normally distributed with mean $\{D(t_c)/4\}^{1/2}\ln(r)$ and variance 1. The independent increments property of $S_n(t_c)$ means that we can transform the stochastic process $S_n(t_c)$ to a Brownian motion process by using information time instead of calendar time (see Chapter 2). Define the information time at calendar time t_c to be $t = D(t_c)/D_{\mathrm{end}}$, where D_{end} is the probability of death by trial's end. If $Z(t)$ denotes the logrank statistic at information time t,

$$B(t) = t^{1/2}Z(t)$$

behaves like a Brownian motion with drift $\theta = (D_{\mathrm{end}}/4)^{1/2}\ln(r)$, which is the expected value of the logrank statistic at the end of the trial. We can approximate the information time t by the ratio of the number of deaths observed by calendar time t_c to the number expected by the end of the trial. This is the same result we obtained in Chapter 2 under the much more restrictive condition that everyone was randomized at the very beginning of the trial.

The analogy between monitoring survival and monitoring the t-statistic is striking. Recall that when the treatment and control sample sizes were both n, we wrote the numerator of the t-statistic as S_n, a sum of n i.i.d. differences between treatment and control observations (see Chapter 2); its mean is $n\mu_D$, where $\mu_D = \mu_T - \mu_C$. The mean of S_n is a linear function of the number of observations. Now consider monitoring survival. Recall that under the proportional hazards assumption, the ratio of the treatment to control hazard functions is constant over time. Under proportional hazards, the mean of the numerator $S_n(t_c)$ of the logrank statistic at calendar time t_c is a linear function of the expected number of deaths. The t-statistic and logrank statistic are both approximately normal with variance 1. As the number of observations increases, the expected value and power of the t-statistic increase. As the expected number of expected deaths increases, the expected value and power of the logrank statistic increase, provided that the proportional hazards assumption holds.

6.4 A Real Example

The Beta-Blocker Heart Attack Trial (BHAT) compared survival of patients randomized to the beta-blocker propranolol to that of patients randomized to placebo. The study, begun in 1977, was anticipated to stop in 1982. At the sixth interim look on October 2, 1981, the DSMB recommended termination of BHAT for efficacy, 9 months earlier than scheduled. Many of the calculations for BHAT were made in September 1981. At that time there were 318 deaths, 183 and 135 in the placebo and treatment arms, respectively. Several methods were used to extrapolate the survival curves and estimate the number of deaths by trial's end had it not stopped early; the best estimate was

398 deaths. The information fraction at the sixth look was estimated to be $318/398 = 0.80$. The logrank statistic and B-value were $Z(0.80) = 2.82$ and $B(0.80) = (0.80)^{1/2}(2.82) = 2.52$. Under the proportional hazards assumption and the current trend, the final z-score was expected to be $2.52/0.80 = 3.15$. Conditional power under the current trend was estimated to be

$$CP_{3.15}(0.80) = 1 - \Phi\left(\frac{1.96 - 2.52 - 3.15(1 - 0.80)}{\sqrt{1 - 0.80}}\right)$$
$$= 1 - \Phi(-2.66) > 0.99.$$

Similarly, conditional power assuming the null hypothesis of identical survival curves was

$$CP_0(0.80) = 1 - \Phi\left(\frac{1.96 - 2.52 - 0(1 - 0.80)}{\sqrt{1 - 0.80}}\right)$$
$$= 1 - \Phi(-1.25) \approx 0.89.$$

The first conditional power calculation was predicated on the proportional hazards assumption. The second assumed the null hypothesis, which automatically conforms to the proportional hazards assumption. Sometimes the proportional hazards assumption may not be realistic. For example, a surgical procedure entails certain immediate risks, but the long-term benefit may outweigh those risks.

6.5 Nonlinear Trends of the Statistics: Analogy with Monitoring a t-Test

Consider a t-test comparing two means with equal sample sizes in the two arms. We saw that under the usual assumption of i.i.d. observations across time in a given arm, the expected value of the numerator of the t-statistic is a linear function of the sample size. But suppose that midway through the trial, in response to lagging recruitment, we change the entry criteria to make more patients eligible. If the newly recruited patients differ from those previously recruited, the mean difference $\delta^* = \mu_T^* - \mu_C^*$ of new patients may differ from δ. Consequently, the expected value of the numerator of the t-statistic is no longer linear in the number of patients. Sometimes this effort to increase power by changing the entry criteria and increasing enrollment can actually *decrease* power. For example, with m and $n - m$ patients per arm satisfying the older and newer criteria, respectively, the expected z-score in the known-variance scenario is $\{m\delta + (n-m)\delta^*\}/(2n\sigma^2)^{1/2}$; if $\delta^* < \{(mn)^{1/2} - m\}\delta/(n-m)$, the expected z-score is smaller than if we had only the m original patients!

Now consider the logrank test when the hazard ratio is not constant. Suppose all patients enter at calendar time $t_c = 0$, with half of them assigned to treatment and half control. Suppose that the hazard ratio is greater than 1 during the first 6 months, equal to 1 at 6 months, and less than 1 after

6 months. Then $E(S(t_c))$ increases, reaching its peak at 6 months, and then decreases thereafter. The behavior of $E(S(t_c))$ is similar to that described for the comparison of two means. Add staggered entry. If we do not restrict ourselves to the proportional hazards assumption, the trend of the numerator $S(t_c)$ of the logrank statistic is difficult to describe because of the staggered entry of patients. Analogous to the t-test setting, the expected value of $S(t_c)$, and even of $Z(t_c)$, may not be increasing in t_c. To get an approximate idea of the trend, we can divide the follow-up time into subintervals and estimate the average hazard within each. In other words, we approximate the two survival distributions by two piecewise exponential distributions. Within each subinterval, the hazard ratio is constant and the trend of $S(t_c)$ will be linear. With staggered entry of patients, the trend of $S(t_c)$ is a mixture of trends by different cohorts of patients categorized by entry times. If the hazard ratio were constant over time, even with staggered entry the trend of $S(t_c)$ would be linear.

6.6 Considerations for Early Termination

Suppose a trial is conducted to compare survival for treatments A and B for 4 years. To simplify matters, assume that investigators recruit $2,000$ patients simultaneously into the trial. Imagine that 2 years later, one treatment's survival appears to be so much better than the other's that early termination is considered. What do we lose by stopping the trial early? If we are interested in the comparison of survival curves throughout the interval 0 to 4 years, stopping at 2 years precludes the ability to estimate survival from 2 years to 4 years. If we assume proportional hazards, then the data from years 0 to 2 can be used to estimate the hazard ratio r, and by assumption, this will provide an estimate of the hazard ratio at 3 or 4 years. Continuation of the trial to 4 years will provide a better estimate of r, but if we believe the proportional hazards assumption, a sufficiently large hazard ratio will ethically compel us to stop the trial at year 2. If we do not believe the proportional hazards assumption—because, for example, it does not even appear to hold over the subinterval 0 to 2 years—we may be justified in continuing the trial to compare longer term survival. For instance, as indicated earlier, a surgical treatment may show initial harm because of complications, but longer term benefit. Stopping early would preclude us from seeing that benefit. The second Cardiac Arrhythmia Suppression Trial (CAST-II) was stopped when it became clear that the evidence of harm in the 2-week titration phase was not offset by potential longer term benefit.

In trying to determine whether long-term and short-term treatment effects differ, the DSMB has a difficult task; what may appear to be a long-term effect may actually be a consequence of "survival of the fittest." To understand this, suppose that treatment has no benefit and is actually toxic to some patients. For example, it may kill the sickest 10 percent of patients within 30 days. In the control arm, no one may die within the first 30 days. The patients remaining alive after 30 days in the treatment arm are not comparable to those remaining alive after 30 days in the control arm; the 30-day treatment survivors are the healthiest 90 percent of patients, whereas the 30-day control survivors are all patients. Accordingly, it would not be surprising to see the next death occur in the control arm (assuming patients who do not experience toxicity within 30 days will not experience it later). This "survival of the fittest" phenomenon would tend to bring survival curves back together after initial separation. A similar phenomenon can occur if the treatment is beneficial: the patients remaining alive in the control arm after a specified period of time may have stronger constitutions than those in the treatment arm. A very effective treatment may be able to overcome the unfair advantage afforded control survivors attributable to survival of the fittest. If not, we may erroneously conclude that treatment has long-term harm that offsets initial benefit.

Thus far we have said that we must exercise care in monitoring survival because proportional hazards may not hold, yet we must not overreact in explaining the reason for the appearance of nonproportional hazards. How can we tell whether the appearance of a nonconstant hazard ratio is due to actual short- versus long-term treatment benefit or an artifact caused by survival of the fittest? Statistical techniques can help, but the first and foremost tool is biological judgment. Is there a bonafide biological reason to suspect short-term toxicity or complications but long-term benefit? Conversely, is it reasonable biologically for short-term benefit but toxicity with prolonged use of a drug? Epidemiological and even animal studies might produce corroborative evidence. As far as analyses on data from the trial to try to unveil the mystery, one technique would be to stratify the logrank test by baseline factors such as age or previous heart attack, or to adjust for baseline differences between the arms using a Cox proportional hazards model. The idea is simple: if survivors in one arm are healthier than those in another arm, but that health difference can be explained by differences in baseline factors, we may be able to adjust them away. If, contrary to the logrank analysis, the stratified logrank or Cox model analyses show a consistent treatment effect over time, we would feel more comfortable attributing the apparent diminution of effect over time for the unstratified logrank analysis to survival of the fittest. On the other hand, adjusted analyses that showed a similar diminution of effect over time lend credence to the idea of differential short- and long-term treatment effects.

6.7 The Information Fraction with Survival Data

What determines the power for survival methods such as the logrank test or Cox model is the number of events by trial's end. In fact, many standard methods of calculating sample size actually first calculate the number of events and then, from that, the number of participants required, e.g., George and Desu (1974) [GD74]; Schoenfeld (1981) [S81]; Freedman (1982) [F82]; Lakatos (1988) [L88]. It is therefore appealing to use an *event-driven trial* that continues until a fixed number, d, of events have occurred in the two arms combined. The information fraction at the kth look with d_k events is unambiguously determined as $t_k = d_k/d$ because d is fixed. The EPHESUS trial (Pitt, Remme, Zannad et al., 2003 [PRZ03]) exemplifies this approach. The trial studied a new drug, eplerenone, in patients with heart failure following a myocardial infarction (heart attack). The study had a pair of co-primary endpoints: (1) time to death from any cause with a type 1 error rate of 0.04 and (2) time to death from heart disease or hospitalization for worsening heart failure with a type 1 error rate of 0.01. The statistical monitoring plan called for formal statistical monitoring only for mortality. The trial randomized 6,632 patients, assigning half to eplerenone and half to placebo. Recruitment lasted 24 months. The protocol specified that the trial would end when 1,012 deaths had occurred. The DSMB calculated the information fraction at each of its looks as $d_k/1,012$.

Although event-driven trials are ideal from a statistical standpoint, trials are budgeted for a given number of patients and length of follow-up. Thus, many trials are designed to end at a fixed calendar time irrespective of whether the desired number of events occurred. This makes it hard to determine the information fraction at an interim analysis. For example, suppose that instead of being an event-driven trial, EPHESUS had been designed to enroll 6,632 people and to continue for 32 months. At the kth look, the DSMB would have observed d_k deaths, but it would not have known how many events would occur in the future. The DSMB would have had two choices—it could have projected the number of deaths it expected and used that projected number to calculate the information fraction or it could have based the spending function on the calendar fraction as detailed in Section 5.1.1.

Basing the calculation on events forces the spending function one has chosen to be identical to one's actual spending; basing the calculation on calendar fraction distorts the desired rate of spending. The degree of distortion depends on how closely the timing of deaths approximates a uniform function over time. In a trial with a very low event rate, exponential survival, and rapid enrollment, calendar fraction and event fraction will be very similar; therefore, if calculation of calendar fraction is easy and calculation of event fraction difficult because of the inevitable uncertainty in the number of future events, we recommend calendar fraction. For example, imagine a trial studying mortality in early-stage breast cancer in which all women are randomized within a 4-month period and the trial is planned to continue for 28 months. Suppose reliable previous data indicate an approximate exponential expected survival distribution. The expected proportion of women dying within the study period is small enough that the number of deaths can be assumed nearly uniform. Therefore, calendar fraction provides a reasonable approximation to information fraction.

The most difficult choices in practice arise in trials in which mortality is expected to follow a pattern markedly different from an exponential distribution. Use of calendar fraction in such cases may be quite inefficient, for it may force spending an undesirable amount of the type 1 error rate in periods of time in which few deaths occur, reducing the efficiency of the trial. The Randomized Aldactone Evaluation Study (RALES) [PZW99], a trial of spironolactone (Aldactone) in New York Heart Association (NYHA) class III and IV heart failure patients, was designed to randomize 1,663 patients. The trial was scheduled to end 45 months after the first patient was randomized. The endpoint was all-cause mortality. The death rate in these heart failure patients is very high. Class III patients breathe comfortably only when they are at rest. Class IV patients are confined to a bed or chair and even there do not breathe comfortably. The hazard function was expected to increase rapidly over time. An O'Brien-Fleming-like spending function was specified as the statistical monitoring plan. Basing the spending function on calendar fraction would almost certainly squander type 1 error rate during a period with relatively few deaths. At each of its meetings, the DSMB instead projected the expected number of deaths on the basis of the experience in the trial thus far. Therefore, the expected number of total deaths at the kth look was $D_k + r_k$, the fixed number of deaths d_k that had already occurred plus the variable number r_k expected to occur in the remainder of the study. Clearly, at any of its looks the DSMB might be over- or underestimating the total number of deaths that would occur in the study; however, as time passed and the observed survival curves matured, the DSMB regarded its projections as more and more accurate. At the time of the DSMB's fifth look, 620 participants had died, 269 in the treated group and 351 in the placebo group. The estimated hazard ratio was 0.78 and the logrank z-score was 3.75, giving a nominal two-tailed p-value of $p = .00018$. To determine whether this value crossed the O'Brien-Fleming-like spending function boundary, the DSMB calculated that the expected number of events would be 1,088; therefore, the estimated information fraction was 0.57 and the critical value was $c = 2.79$. Given the uncertainty in the expected number of events, the DSMB also calculated the z-score boundary if calendar fraction had been adopted, as well as the z-score boundary under a variety of reasonable assumptions about the future course of the survival curves. The observed z-score of 3.75 crossed all of these boundaries, assuring the DSMB of the appropriateness of its recommendation to stop the trial and conclude that the data had shown the efficacy of spironolactone in reducing mortality in patients with class III or IV heart failure.

Some caution is in order regarding the updating of information fraction on the basis of new estimates of the number of events by trial's end. First, we must realize that estimates of mortality obtained early in the trial are highly variable, so we should not be concerned if early estimates do not match the originally expected number of deaths. Over-reacting by dramatically changing the expected number of events by trial's end subjects us to the criticism that we deliberately tried to "doctor" the information fraction to stop the trial early. For example, suppose we observed an interim z-score of 2.5 that did not exceed the boundary if we used the originally projected number of events to calculate the current information fraction. By revising the number of events downward, we can increase the current information fraction, changing the current boundary such that 2.5 may now exceed it. To avoid this criticism, we recommend not making dramatic changes in the projected number of events on the basis of early, "noisy" data.

If there are only small differences between originally hypothesized and actual numbers of deaths, we can continue to spend according to the originally projected number of deaths until the very end of the trial, at which time we spend the remainder of the alpha. For example, suppose we used the power spending function $0.025t^{1.5}$ for a one-tailed test at level 0.025, and we initially projected 100 deaths. Suppose that the two interim looks and one final look occurred after 28, 54, and 85 deaths, respectively (in other words, 15 fewer deaths occurred than expected). The information fractions at the first two looks were estimated to be $28/100 = 0.28$ and $54/100 = 0.54$. The boundary at the first look was determined by setting $\Pr(Z_1 > c_1) = 0.025(0.28)^{1.5} = 0.0037$, where Z_1, the logrank statistic after 28 deaths, has a standard normal distribution under the null hypothesis. We find that $c_1 = 2.678$. At the second look, we selected c_2 such that $\Pr(Z_1 > 2.678 \cup Z_2 > c_2) = 0.025(0.54)^{1.5} = 0.0099$. Note that under the null hypothesis, Z_1 and Z_2 are marginally standard normal and have correlation $(t_1/t_2)^{1/2}$, where t_1 and t_2 are the actual information fractions $28/85$ and $54/85$ at the first two looks rather than our initially estimated information fractions $28/100$ and $54/100$. But the joint distribution of Z_1 and Z_2 depends on information fractions only through their ratio/indexinformation fraction/time!invariance to incorrect guess of final information, $28/54$. The number of deaths expected by the end of the trial is completely irrelevant. Thus, inputing information fractions 0.28 and 0.54 will yield the correct value of $c_2 = 2.433$.

At the final look with 85 deaths, we "fix up" the information fraction. That is, we specify information fraction 1. We determine c_3 such that $\Pr(Z_1 > 2.678 \cup Z_2 > 2.433 \cup Z_3 > c_3) = 0.025(1)^{1.5} = 0.025$. Computation of c_3 now becomes tricky. If we specify $t_3 = 1$, the program will compute boundaries assuming that the correlation between Z_1 and Z_3 is $(0.28/1)^{1/2}$ and $(0.54/1)^{1/2}$, whereas the correct correlations should be $(28/85)^{1/2}$ and $(54/85)^{1/2}$. On the other hand, if we tell the program that $t_1 = 28/85$ and $t_2 = 54/85$, it will spend $0.025(28/85)^{1.5}$ at the first look instead of what we actually spent, which was $0.025(0.28)^{1.5}$. We can get around the problem by using the S-Plus or R program in the appendix of Chapter 5, replacing the lines beginning with "# Input" (near the end of the program) with

```
# Input
###############################################################
tcur<-1                    # Current value of t.
```

```
tprev<-c(28/85,54/85)   # Previous values of t go in
                        # parentheses.
cprev<-c(2.678,2.433)   # Previous boundary values go in
                        # parentheses.
cumulal<-.025           # Cumulative alpha up to current look,
                        # alpha_*(tcur).
###################################################################
```

This yields $c_3 = 2.056$.

The problem is more difficult to fix if we have grossly *underestimated* the number of deaths by trial's end. If we continue to spend according to the original projections, we will spend all of the alpha before the trial is completed. Try explaining to a DSMB that any additional events between now and the scheduled end of the trial in one year do not count because we have spent all our alpha already! It is best to avoid this problem by trying to overestimate the number of deaths by trial's end during the design phase. If it becomes clear after the analysis at look i that we have underestimated the number of deaths, we could adopt the following procedure. Let α_i denote the cumulative alpha spent up to and including look i. We now compute the new number of deaths we expect by trial's end, and from it we compute the information fraction t_i at the ith look. For $t \geq t_i$, we modify the spending function as follows. We make the ratio of the incremental alpha spent between now (information fraction t_i) and future information fraction t to the incremental alpha spent between now and the end of the trial $(t = 1)$ the same as for the original spending function. For the original spending function $\alpha_*(\cdot)$, the ratio of these incremental alphas is

$$\frac{\alpha_*(t) - \alpha_*(t_i)}{\alpha - \alpha_*(t_i)}. \tag{6.1}$$

For the new spending function $\alpha'_*(\cdot)$, the ratio of incremental alphas is

$$\frac{\alpha'_*(t) - \alpha_i}{\alpha - \alpha_i}. \tag{6.2}$$

Equating (6.2) to (6.1) results in

$$\alpha'_*(t) = \alpha_i + \left(\frac{\alpha - \alpha_i}{\alpha - \alpha_*(t_i)} \right) \{\alpha_*(t) - \alpha_*(t_i)\}. \tag{6.3}$$

for $t \geq t_i$.

For example, suppose we use the power spending function $0.025t^{1.5}$ for a trial originally expecting 80 deaths and using one-tailed $\alpha = .025$. Suppose the first look occurs after 20 deaths, so the information fraction is estimated to be $20/80 = 0.25$. We spend $0.025(0.25)^{1.5} = 0.003125$, which, using the software at www.medsch.wisc.edu/landemets/, results in a boundary of $c_1 = 2.7344$. At the next look, with 47 deaths, we spend $0.025(47/80)^{1.5} = 0.01126$, yielding boundary $c_2 = 2.3612$. At this point we realize that the final number of deaths is likely to be 95 instead of 80. To be somewhat conservative, we now assume 100 deaths by the end of the trial. In the notation above, $i = 2$ and t_2 is the new estimate of the information fraction at the last look, namely $t_2 = 47/100 = 0.47$. We have already spent $\alpha_2 = 0.01126$, so from now on the spending function is, from (6.3),

$$\alpha'_*(t) = 0.01126 + \left(\frac{0.025 - 0.01126}{0.025 - (0.025)(0.47)^{1.5}} \right) \{ 0.025t^{1.5} - 0.025(0.47)^{1.5} \}$$
$$= 0.0047 + 0.0203t^{1.5}$$

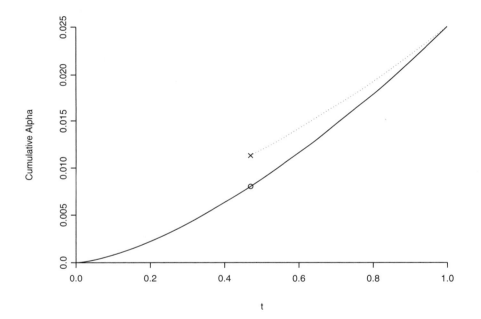

Fig. 6.2. Fixing the spending function when the number of events has been underestimated (we originally estimated 80 deaths, but now we estimate 100 deaths). The actual information fraction at the last look was $t = 0.47$, so instead of spending the amount indicated by the solid curve at $t = 0.47$, we have spent 0.01126 (indicated by the x). The "fixed-up" spending function is the original function before $t = 0.47$, and the dotted line from $t = 0.47$ to $t = 1$.

(see Figure 6.2). If the next look occurs after 71 deaths, the information fraction is $71/100 = 0.71$, so we will choose boundary value c_3 such that

$\Pr(Z_1 \geq 2.7344 \cup Z_2 \geq 2.3612 \cup Z_3 \geq c_3) = 0.0047 + 0.0203(0.71)^{1.5} = 0.0168.$
We use the S-Plus or R computer program in the appendix of Chapter 5, changing the lines beginning with "# Input" to

```
# Input
################################################################
tcur<-.71                  # Current value of t.
tprev<-c(20/100,47/100)    # Previous values of t go in
                           # parentheses.
cprev<-c(2.7344,2.3612)    # Previous boundary values go in
                           # parentheses.
cumulal<-.0168             # Cumulative alpha up to current look,
                           # alpha_*(tcur).
################################################################
```

to find that $c_3 = 2.3549$.

7

Inference Following a Group-Sequential Trial

7.1 Likelihood, Sufficiency, and (Lack of) Completeness

Sequential and group-sequential procedures were designed to test hypotheses. Their adoption in clinical trials for the purpose of speeding drug development (or minimizing the number of patients on the inferior arm of a trial) emphasized their ability to select the better treatment, not their ability to provide a measure of strength of evidence or to produce an estimate of the size of effect. Nonetheless, in a clinical trial, simply concluding that one treatment is better than another as demonstrated by rejecting a hypothesis tested at a type 1 error rate of α leaves the interpretation hanging. Without an estimate of the size of the effect and an assessment of how compelling the conclusion, the interpretation of the results of the trial is incomplete. An article summarizing data on 143 randomized clinical trials that stopped early for benefit between 1990 and 2004 reported that 129 of them did not adjust the treatment effect estimate to account for interim monitoring and truncation. They conclude that many of these trials report implausibly large treatment effects and recommend that "clinicians should view the results of such trials with skepticism" (Montori, Devereaux, Adhikari, et al., 2005 [MDA05]).

In fixed sample size trials, the test statistic, α-level, p-value, and estimated size of effect flow naturally from the same theory. Group-sequential trials cleave these relationships. Generally, as this chapter will show, the p-value and estimated treatment effect reported in the literature from most sequential trials are more extreme than the data support. Experientially, we have attended DSMB meetings where a boundary has been crossed and the committee discusses the p-value. Some statisticians argue, "The p-value is simply the value that would have been calculated had this been a fixed sample size study" (see, for example, Dupont, 1983 [D83]). Others demur, "No, it's different. We need to account for the fact that this was a sequential trial. I don't know what the p-value is, but it is not what it appears." This type of statement is hardly music to the ears of the clinician members who want an unambiguous answer to "what is the p-value?" Unfortunately, there is no unique p-value in the sequential setting; rather, one must decide what criteria to use to define it. Consequently, we urge that in sequential or group-sequential clinical trials—especially phase III trials aimed at regulatory registration—the designers should select not only the sequential boundaries, but also the algorithm by which they intend to calculate their p-values.

Similarly, most statisticians acknowledge that the observed effect from a trial that is stopped early overestimates the true value, but may recommend using the observed estimate for simiplicity (see, for example, Pocock, 2005 [Po05]). This chapter points to methods for unbiased estimation.

Consider a trial with scheduled looks at information fractions $(t_1, \ldots, t_k)$. We observe the summary data $(\tau, Z(t_1), \ldots, Z(\tau))$, where τ is the information fraction when we stop. For example, with scheduled looks at $t = 0.20, 0.50, 0.70$, and 1, stopping at the third look means we observe $(\tau = 0.70, Z(0.20), Z(0.50), Z(0.70))$. Equivalently, we can view the data in terms of increments: $(\tau = 0.70, B(0.20), B(0.50) - B(0.20), B(0.70) - B(0.50))$. If θ denotes the drift parameter, the likelihood of observing $(\tau = t_j, B(t_1) = b_1, B(t_2) - B(t_1) = b_2 - b_1, \ldots, B(t_j) - B(t_{j-1}) = b_j - b_{j-1})$ is

$$L(\theta) = \left[\prod_{i=1}^{j} \{2\pi(t_i - t_{i-1})\}^{-1/2} \right] \exp \left[-\sum_{i=1}^{j} \frac{\{b_i - b_{i-1} - \theta(t_i - t_{i-1})\}^2}{2(t_i - t_{i-1})} \right],$$

where $t_0 = b_0 = 0$. It is slightly easier to work with the likelihood ratio $L(\theta)/L(0)$, which, as a function of θ, is a constant multiple of $L(\theta)$.

$$L(\theta)/L(0) = \exp \left[\sum_{i=1}^{j} \frac{(b_i - b_{i-1})^2 - \{b_i - b_{i-1} - \theta(t_i - t_{i-1})\}^2}{2(t_i - t_{i-1})} \right].$$

Now apply the identity $x^2 - y^2 = (x - y)(x + y)$ to $x = b_i - b_{i-1}$ and $y = b_i - b_{i-1} - \theta(t_i - t_{i-1})$ to deduce that

$$L(\theta)/L(0) = \exp \left\{ \theta \sum_{i=1}^{j} (b_i - b_{i-1}) - (\theta^2/2) \sum_{i=1}^{j} (t_i - t_{i-1}) \right\}$$

$$= \exp\{\theta b_j - (\theta^2/2)t_j\} \quad \text{(because the sums telescope)}$$

$$= \exp\{\theta B(\tau) - (\theta^2/2)\tau\}. \tag{7.1}$$

The factorization theorem implies that $(\tau, B(\tau))$ or, equivalently, $(\tau, Z(\tau))$, is a sufficient statistic; therefore, the search for estimators or tests concerning θ should be confined to those based on $(\tau, Z(\tau))$. One such estimator is the MLE $\hat{\theta}$, obtained by differentiating the logarithm of (7.1) with respect to θ and equating to 0. This results in $\hat{\theta} = B(\tau)/\tau$ (Chang, 1989 [C89]).

Completeness, another important concept in inference, guarantees the uniqueness of certain statistical procedures that are based on the sufficient statistic. Recall from section 2.5.2 that a random vector $\underline{X}$ with distribution function $F(\underline{X}, \theta)$ is said to be *complete* if there is no nontrivial unbiased estimator of 0; i.e., the only function $h(\underline{X})$ such that $\mathrm{E}_\theta\{h(\underline{X})\} = 0$ for all θ is $h(\underline{X}) \equiv 0$ (more precisely, $h(\underline{X}) = 0$ except on a set whose probability is 0 irrespective of θ). Completeness ensures that there cannot be more than one function of $\underline{X}$ that is unbiased for θ because if $h_1(\underline{X})$ and $h_2(\underline{X})$ were unbiased for θ, then $h_1(\underline{X}) - h_2(\underline{X})$ would be an unbiased estimator of 0, so $h_1(\underline{X}) - h_2(\underline{X}) \equiv 0$.

In a nonmonitoring setting, the $N(\theta, 1)$ distribution of the z-score is complete, so the only function of Z that is unbiased for θ is Z. Here we show that $(\tau, Z(\tau))$ is not complete in a group-sequential trial. To demonstrate this, we must consider the distribution function of $(\tau, Z(\tau))$, or equivalently, the distribution function of $(\tau, B(\tau))$. In the following, we define $f_\theta(t, b) = P_\theta(\tau = t, B(\tau) = b)$; that is, $f_\theta(t, b)$ is the density function such that $\Pr(\tau = t, B(\tau) \in A \mid \theta) = \int_A f_\theta(t, b)db$ (note that we assume a finite number of looks at fixed times, so the distribution of τ is discrete). Then

$$
\begin{aligned}
f_\theta(t_j, b_j) &= \int \cdots \int L(\theta; b_1, \ldots, b_j)db_1 \ldots db_{j-1} \\
&= \int \cdots \int \frac{L(\theta; b_1, \ldots, b_j)}{L(0; b_1, \ldots, b_j)} L(0; b_1, \ldots, b_j)db_1 \ldots db_{j-1} \\
&= \exp\{\theta b_j - (\theta^2/2)t_j\} \int \cdots \int L(0; b_1, \ldots, b_j)db_1 \ldots db_{j-1} \\
&= \exp\{\theta b_j - (\theta^2/2)t_j\} \, f_0(t_j, b_j), \tag{7.2}
\end{aligned}
$$

where the range of integration is the continuation region. For example, for a two-tailed, symmetric z-score boundary of $\pm c_i$ at look i, the range of the ith integral of Equation (7.2) is $-c_i$ to c_i.

Equation (7.2) shows the relationship between the density functions for $(\tau, B(\tau))$ for arbitrary θ and for $\theta = 0$. Liu and Hall (1999) [LH99] used representation (7.2) and the theory of Laplace transforms to prove that $(\tau, B(\tau))$ is not complete and to characterize the set of nontrivial functions $h(\tau, B(\tau))$ with zero expectation. We content ourselves with finding a nontrivial unbiased estimator of 0 when $k = 2$ and looks are at $t = t_1$ and $t = 1$.

The simplest function we can try is constant on $t = t_1$; $h(t_1, b_1) = \lambda$ for all b_1. Then

$$
\mathrm{E}_\theta\{h(\tau, B(\tau))\} = \lambda P_\theta(\tau = t_1) + \int_{-\infty}^{\infty} h(1, b)f_\theta(1, b)db. \tag{7.3}
$$

Even though stopping at $t = t_1$ precludes us from seeing $B(1)$, we can still imagine $B(1)$ and the probability density $g_\theta(t_1, b)$ corresponding to $\tau = t_1$ and $B(1) = b$; that is, $\int_A g_\theta(t_1, b)db = P_\theta(\tau = t_1, B(1) \in A)$. If we take $h(1, b) = -\lambda g_\theta(t_1, b)/f_\theta(1, b)$, then the $f_\theta(1, b)$ terms cancel out and

$$
\mathrm{E}_\theta\{h(\tau, B(\tau))\} = \lambda P_\theta(\tau = t_1) - \lambda \int_{-\infty}^{\infty} \{g_\theta(t_1, b)/f_\theta(1, b)\}f_\theta(1, b)db
$$

$$= \lambda P_\theta(\tau = t_1) - \lambda \int_{-\infty}^{\infty} g_\theta(t_1, b)db$$
$$= \lambda P_\theta(\tau = t_1) - \lambda \Pr(\tau = t_1, -\infty < B(1) < \infty)$$
$$= \lambda P_\theta(\tau = t_1) - \lambda P_\theta(\tau = t_1) = 0. \tag{7.4}$$

But $h(\tau, b)$ is supposed to be a statistic; however, $h(1, b) = -\lambda g_\theta(t_1, b)/f_\theta(1, b)$ seems to depend on θ. To see that it does not, write $g_\theta(t_1, b)/f_\theta(1, b)$ as $P_\theta(\tau = t_1 \mid B(1) = b)/P_\theta(\tau = 1 \mid B(1) = b)$. Imagine a trial in which we proceed to the second look regardless of the first stage result; then $B(1)$ is sufficient, so $\Pr(\tau = t_1 \mid B(1) = b)$ and $\Pr(\tau = 1 \mid B(1) = b)$ are both free of θ. Thus, if we define

$$h(t, b) = \begin{cases} \lambda & \text{if } t = t_1 \\ -\lambda g_0(t_1, b)/f_0(1, b) & \text{if } t = 1, \end{cases} \tag{7.5}$$

then

$$\mathrm{E}_\theta\{h(\tau, B(\tau))\} = \lambda P_\theta(\tau = t_1) - \lambda \int_{-\infty}^{\infty} \{g_0(t_1, b)/f_0(1, b)\} f_\theta(1, b)db$$
$$= \lambda P_\theta(\tau = t_1) - \lambda \int_{-\infty}^{\infty} \{g_\theta(t_1, b)/f_\theta(1, b)\} f_\theta(1, b)db$$
$$= \lambda P_\theta(\tau = t_1) - \lambda \int_{-\infty}^{\infty} g_\theta(t_1, b)db = 0$$

by the same arguments leading to (7.4). Because $h(\tau, B(\tau))$ has zero expectation for all θ, $(\tau, B(\tau))$ is not complete. Therefore, there is more than one unbiased function of the sufficent statistic.

7.2 One-Tailed p-Values

7.2.1 Definitions of a p-Value

The fact that unadjusted monitoring causes inflation of the type 1 error rate implies that an unadjusted, or *nominal*, p-value will tend to overstate the evidence against the null hypothesis. The same forces driving us to raise boundaries to account for monitoring also drive us to adjust p-values, though, as described at the beginning of this chapter, not everyone agrees that this is necessary (Dupont, 1983 [D83]).

A trial with no monitoring has two equivalent definitions of a p-value: 1) the smallest α level for which the observed result would be statistically significant, and 2) the null probability of obtaining a test statistic value at least as extreme as that observed. We now try to extend these definitions to group-sequential trials. The first definition requires us to consider a class of similar boundaries with different alpha levels, e.g., O-F$_{k,\alpha}$, the class of O'Brien-Fleming boundaries with k equally spaced looks and type 1 error rate α. On the other hand, the second definition requires us to specify what "at least as extreme" means; i.e., we must specify how to order different outcomes. We shall see that if we order outcomes in a manner consistent with the ordering implied by the class of boundaries specified in definition 1), the two definitions are equivalent.

This section considers one-tailed testing with rejection for large values of the z-statistic. Consider the first definition of p-value, the smallest α level for which the observed result would be statistically significant. The following example illustrates a subtle technical difficulty with what seems like a natural approach.

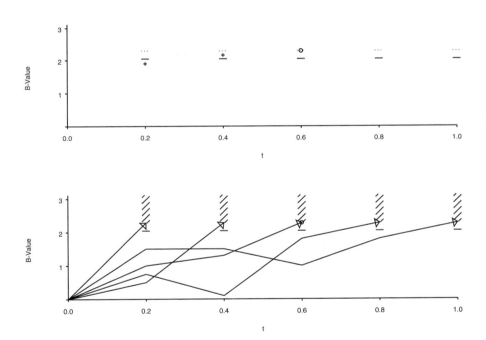

Fig. 7.1. The p-value when ($\tau = 0.6$, $B(0.6) = 2.28$) in a five-look trial with O'Brien-Fleming boundaries. We raise the O'Brien-Fleming boundary until the observed result barely reaches it (dotted line in upper panel); however, the boundary actually used precludes outcomes such as $B(0.2) = 1.90$, $B(0.4) = 2.15$ (pluses in upper panel), which would have caused the trial to stop at $t = 0.4$. Thus, the p-value is the sum of probabilities of paths that remain within the boundary until termination, at which time the B-value equals or exceeds 2.28. Each broken line in the lower panel shows one such outcome with termination at $t = 0.2$, 0.4, 0.6, 0.8, or 1. The p-value is $p = .010$.

Example 7.1. Suppose a five-look trial with the O'Brien-Fleming constant B-value boundary 2.04 terminates at the third look with $B(3/5) = 2.28$. Typically, investigators report the p-value in this case as .002, the nominal p-value corresponding to the associated z-score of $2.28/(3/5)^{1/2} = 2.94$. Clearly, such a calculation overstates the evidence against the null hypothesis. Instead, we ask, "At what level of α would we have just barely rejected the null hypothesis?" We raise the B-value boundary from 2.04 to 2.28, as shown in Figure 7.1. It appears that the smallest α level at which we would reject the null hypothesis is $\alpha = \Pr(\cup_{i=1}^{5} B(i/5) \geq 2.28) = 0.013$, and therefore the p-value appears to be .013. This is not quite correct, however. Using a constant B-value boundary of 2.28 would yield a one-tailed type 1 error rate of 0.013 had all outcomes leading to $B(i/5) \geq 2.28$ for some $1 = 1, \ldots, 5$ been possible, but the boundaries actually used preclude certain outcomes. For example, we cannot observe the outcome $B(1/5) = 1.90$, $B(2/5) = 2.15$ (shown as pluses in the upper panel of Figure 7.1), $B(3/5) = 2.28$ because the trial would have have terminated at the second look. When we add the probabilities of paths remaining within the original boundaries until the trial is stopped and then equaling or exceeding 2.28, we get $p = .010$ (a detailed calculation is provided in Example 7.3). Thus, the actual p-value is .010.

We can do an analogous computation for the class of Pocock boundaries.

Example 7.2. Consider a two-look trial using the Pocock constant z-score boundary of 2.18. The trial continues until the end, with $Z(1) = 2.30$. The one-sided p-value associated with a nonsequential test would have been .011. To obtain the p-value in this sequential setting, we raise the Pocock boundary to 2.30 as shown in Figure 7.2. Once again, the p-value is not $\Pr(Z(1/2) \geq 2.30 \cup Z(1) \geq 2.30)$, but rather $\Pr(Z(1/2) \geq 2.30) + \Pr(Z(1/2) < 2.18 \cap Z(1) \geq 2.30) = .018$.

The reader should, as an exercise, compute the p-value if the observed z-score had instead been $Z(1) = 1.5$. The correct answer is $\Pr(Z(1/2) \geq 2.18) + \Pr(Z(1/2) < 2.18 \cap Z(1) \geq 1.5)$ because we would not have stopped at the first stage unless $Z(1/2) \geq 2.18$.

The second definition of the p-value was the null probability of a result at least as extreme as that observed. But it is not obvious what is more extreme when the outcome is the pair $(\tau, Z(\tau))$. In Example 7.2, would the evidence have been stronger or weaker if the trial had stopped at the first look with $Z(1/2) = 2.40$? Equation (7.1) shows that the log likelihood ratio for testing $\theta = 0$ against $\theta = \theta_1$ is $\theta_1 B(\tau) - (\theta_1^2/2)\tau = \theta_1 \tau^{1/2} Z(\tau) - (\theta_1^2/2)\tau$. Suppose the alternative hypothesis were $\theta_1 = 1$. Then the log likelihood ratio would have been $\tau^{1/2} Z(\tau) - \tau/2$. A z-score of 2.40 at $\tau = 1/2$ yields a log likelihood ratio of $(1/2)^{1/2} 2.40 - (1/2)/2 = 1.447$, whereas a z-score of 2.30 at $\tau = 1$ yields a log likelihood ratio of $1^{1/2} 2.30 - 1/2 = 1.80$. Thus, for deciding whether $\theta = 0$ versus $\theta = 1$, a z-score of 2.30 at $\tau = 1$ is more compelling than a z-score of 2.40 at $\tau = 1/2$. On the other hand, suppose the alternative hypothesis were

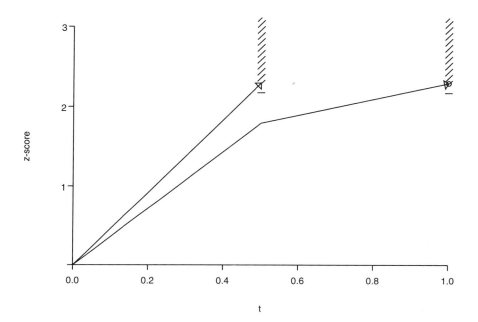

Fig. 7.2. The p-value when $(\tau = 1, Z(1) = 2.30)$ for a two-look trial using the Pocock boundary. We raise the Pocock boundary until the observed result barely reaches it. The p-value is the sum of probabilities of paths remaining within the boundary until termination, at which time the z-score equals or exceeds 2.30. The broken lines show two such outcomes.

$\theta_1 = 3$. Now the log likelihood ratio, $3\tau^{1/2}Z(\tau) - 4.5\tau$, would have been 2.841 for $\tau = 1/2$ and $Z(1/2) = 2.40$, and 2.400 for $\tau = 1$ and $Z(1) = 2.30$. In this case a z-score of 2.40 at $\tau = 1/2$ is more compelling than a z-score of 2.30 at $\tau = 1$. Thus, there is no best way to order the sample outcomes even when there are only two looks (Table 7.1).

It may seem strange to consider likelihood ratio tests when, after all, the boundaries c_i already define an α-level test. Nonetheless, we may think about constructing a test on the sample space $\mathcal{S}$ of possible outcomes for this trial: $\mathcal{S} = \{(t_j, Z(t_j)) : Z(t_1) < c_1, \ldots, Z(t_{j-1}) < c_{j-1}, Z(t_j) \geq c_j\}$. Because the log likelihood ratio

$$\ln\{L(\theta_1)/L(0)\} = \theta_1\{B(\tau) - (\theta_1/2)\tau\} \tag{7.6}$$

is very close to $\theta_1 B(\tau)$ for θ_1 close to 0, the likelihood ratio test, the most powerful test defined on $\mathcal{S}$, of $\theta = 0$ versus $\theta = \theta_1$, orders outcomes essentially

Table 7.1. Likelihood ratio for testing $H_0 : \theta = 0$ against two different alternative hypotheses under two different stopping scenarios. When the alternative hypothesis is $\theta = 1$, stopping when $\tau = 1$ and $Z(1) = 2.30$ is more compelling evidence than stopping when $\tau = 1/2$ and $Z(1/2) = 2.40$, but when the alternative hypothesis is $\theta = 3$, stopping when $\tau = 1/2$ and $Z(1/2) = 2.40$ is more compelling evidence than stopping when $\tau = 1$ and $Z(1) = 2.30$.

	$\tau = 1/2$ $Z(1/2) = 2.40$	$\tau = 1$ $Z(1) = 2.30$
$H_1 : \theta = 1$	1.447	1.800
$H_1 : \theta = 3$	2.841	2.400

by the B-value, $B(\tau)$ for small θ_1. Another way to see that ordering outcomes by their B-values is optimal for small θ_1 is to consider the locally most powerful test, obtained by differentiating (7.6) with respect to θ and evaluating at $\theta = 0$. This yields the score statistic $B(\tau)$ (Rosner and Tsiatis, 1988 [RT88]).

The *B-value (partial) ordering*, also called the *score test ordering*, defines $(\tau_2, Z(\tau_2))$ to be at least as extreme as $(\tau_1, Z(\tau_1))$, written $(\tau_2, Z(\tau_2)) \succeq (\tau_1, Z(\tau_1))$ or $(\tau_1, Z(\tau_1)) \preceq (\tau_2, Z(\tau_2))$, iff the B-value associated with the pair $(\tau_2, Z(\tau_2))$ is at least as large as the B-value associated with the pair $(\tau_1, Z(\tau_1))$. That is, for the B-value ordering,

$$\text{B-value ordering: } (\tau_2, B(\tau_2)) \succeq (\tau_1, B(\tau_1)) \Leftrightarrow \tau_2^{1/2} Z(\tau_2) \geq \tau_1^{1/2} Z(\tau_1).$$

If $b_{\text{obs}} = \tau^{1/2} z_{\text{obs}}$ denotes the observed B-value, the p-value using the B-value ordering is $\Pr(B(\tau) \geq b_{\text{obs}}) = \sum_{i=1}^{k} \Pr(\tau = t_i \cap B(t_i) \geq b_{\text{obs}})$. We saw in Example 7.1 that this p-value arises naturally when the boundaries c_i are those of O'Brien-Fleming, but it can be computed for any boundaries.

We have seen that the B-value ordering arises from consideration of testing $\theta = 0$ against $\theta = \theta_1$ for small θ_1. We could also look at the maximum likelihood ratio test over all alternatives $\theta_1 > 0$ instead of just over small values. Assuming that the data are consistent with $\theta > 0$ (i.e., $Z(\tau) > 0$), the maximum likelihood estimator (MLE) for θ is $\hat{\theta} = B(\tau)/\tau$. Substituting this value into (7.6) gives $(1/2)\{B(\tau)\}^2/\tau = (1/2)\{Z(\tau)\}^2$. In other words, the maximum likelihood ratio test orders nonnegative outcomes by the z-score.

The *z-score (partial) ordering*, also called the *likelihood ratio ordering*, orders by the magnitude of the z-score:

$$\text{z-score ordering: } (\tau_2, Z(\tau_2)) \succeq (\tau_1, Z(\tau_1)) \Leftrightarrow Z(\tau_2) \geq Z(\tau_1).$$

The p-value using the z-score ordering for an observed z-score of z_{obs} is $\Pr(Z(\tau) \geq z_{\text{obs}}) = \sum_{i=1}^{k} \Pr(\tau = t_i \cap Z(t_i) \geq z_{\text{obs}})$. It arose naturally in Example 7.2 with the Pocock boundary, but like the p-value based on the B-value ordering, it can be used with any boundaries (see Example 7.3 below).

Thus, with k equally spaced looks, we can achieve equivalence of the two definitions of the p-value if we use the B-value ordering for the O'Brien-Fleming boundaries and the z-score ordering for Pocock boundaries.

One could also order outcomes in terms of the MLE $\hat{\theta}$ for the drift parameter. The *MLE(partial) ordering* orders by the magnitude of the MLE $B(\tau)/\tau$:

$$\text{MLE ordering: } (\tau_2, Z(\tau_2)) \succeq (\tau_1, Z(\tau_1)) \Leftrightarrow B(\tau_2)/\tau_2 \geq B(\tau_1)/\tau_1,$$

where $B(\tau_i) = \tau_i^{1/2} Z(\tau_i)$. The p-value using the MLE ordering is $\Pr(\hat{\theta} \geq \hat{\theta}_{\text{obs}}) = \sum_{i=1}^{k} \Pr(\tau = t_i \cap \hat{\theta} \geq \hat{\theta}_{\text{obs}})$.

We would like to view $\preceq$ and $\succeq$ the same way we view $\leq$ and $\geq$ for numbers. One important similarity of $\preceq$ and $\succeq$ to $\leq$ and $\geq$ for any of the three (partial) orderings is that any two outcome pairs $(\tau_1, Z(\tau_1))$ and $(\tau_2, Z(\tau_2))$ are comparable in the sense that either $(\tau_1, Z(\tau_1)) \succeq (\tau_2, Z(\tau_2))$ or $(\tau_2, Z(\tau_2)) \succeq (\tau_1, Z(\tau_1))$ or both.

An important difference between $\preceq, \succeq$ and $\leq, \geq$ is that for numbers a and b, if $a \leq b$ and $b \leq a$, then $a = b$. This immediately implies that $\Pr(Z \geq z) = 1 - \Pr(Z \leq z)$ for any number z because $1 = \Pr(Z \leq z \cup Z \geq z) = \Pr(Z \leq z) + \Pr(Z \geq z) - \Pr(Z = z)$, and $\Pr(Z = z) = 0$. But $(\tau, Z(\tau)) \preceq (t, z)$ and $(\tau, Z(\tau)) \succeq (t, z)$ together do not imply that $(\tau, Z(\tau)) = (t, z)$. For example, for the B-value ordering, $(\tau = 0.25, Z(0.25) = 3) \succeq (\tau = 1, Z(1) = 1.5)$ and $(\tau = 1, Z(1) = 1.5) \succeq (\tau = 0.25, Z(0.25) = 3)$; for the z-score ordering, $(\tau = 0.25, Z(0.25) = 3) \succeq (\tau = 1, Z(1) = 3)$ and $(\tau = 1, Z(1) = 3) \succeq (\tau = 0.25, Z(0.25) = 3)$; for the MLE ordering, $(\tau = 0.25, Z(0.25) = 2) \succeq (\tau = 1, Z(1) = 4)$ and $(\tau = 1, Z(1) = 4) \succeq (\tau = 0.25, Z(0.25) = 2)$. Nonetheless, it is clear that for each of these orderings, $\Pr\{(\tau, Z(\tau)) \succeq (t, z) \cap (\tau, Z(\tau)) \preceq (t, z)\} = 0$, and therefore that $\Pr\{(\tau, Z(\tau)) \succeq (t, z)\} = 1 - \Pr\{(\tau, Z(\tau)) \preceq (t, z)\}$.

Example 7.3. We return to Example 7.1 and provide a detailed calculation of the p-values under the B-value, z-score, and MLE orderings. Recall that the trial stopped at the third look with a B-value of 2.28.

For the B-value ordering, the important quantity is the observed B-value $b_{\text{obs}} = 2.28$. The p-value is

$$
\begin{aligned}
p &= \Pr(B(\tau) \geq 2.28) = \Pr\{\cup_{i=1}^{5} \tau = t_i \cap B(t_i) \geq 2.28\} \\
&= \Pr(B(.2) \geq 2.28) \\
&\quad + \Pr(B(.2) < 2.04, B(.4) \geq 2.28) \\
&\quad + \Pr(B(.2) < 2.04, B(.4) < 2.04, B(.6) \geq 2.28) \\
&\quad + \Pr(B(.2) < 2.04, B(.4) < 2.04, B(.6) < 2.04, B(.8) \geq 2.28) \\
&\quad + \Pr(B(.2) < 2.04, B(.4) < 2.04, B(.6) < 2.04, B(.8) < 2.04, B(1) \geq 2.28) \\
&= 0.010.
\end{aligned}
$$

We obtained the final answer by converting each probability involving B-values to a first exit probability involving the z-scores and then using readily available, free software (www.medsch.wisc.edu/landemets/). For example,

$\Pr(B(0.2) < 2.04, B(0.4) \geq 2.28) = \Pr(Z(0.2) < 2.04/(0.2)^{1/2}, Z(0.4) \geq 2.28/(0.4)^{1/2})$.

For the z-score ordering, the important quantity is the z-score $Z(\tau) = 2.28/(0.6)^{1/2} = 2.94$ at the time the trial was stopped. The z-score boundaries for the O'Brien-Fleming procedure with five looks are $2.040/(i/5)^{1/2} = (4.56, 3.23, 2.63, 2.28, 2.04)$. The p-value using the z-score ordering is

$$
\begin{aligned}
p &= \Pr(Z(\tau) \geq 2.94) = \Pr\{\cup_{i=1}^{5}\tau = t_i \cap Z(t_i) \geq 2.94\} \\
&= \Pr(Z(.2) \geq 4.56) \\
&+ \Pr(Z(.2) < 4.56, Z(.4) \geq 3.23) \\
&+ \Pr(Z(.2) < 4.56, Z(.4) < 3.23, Z(.6) \geq 2.94) \\
&+ \Pr(Z(.2) < 4.56, Z(.4) < 3.23, Z(.6) < 2.63, Z(.8) \geq 2.94) \\
&+ \Pr(Z(.2) < 4.56, Z(.4) < 3.23, Z(.6) < 2.63, Z(.8) < 2.28, Z(1) \geq 2.94) \\
&= 0.003.
\end{aligned}
$$

For the MLE ordering, the important quantity is the MLE at the time the trial was stopped, $\hat{\theta} = B(0.6)/(0.6) = Z(0.6)/(0.6)^{1/2} = 2.94/(0.6)^{1/2} = 3.80$. We first convert the z-score boundaries to boundaries for the MLE $\hat{\theta}(t) = B(t)/t = Z(t)/t^{1/2}$. The MLE boundaries are $(10.20, 5.10, 3.40, 2.55, 2.04)$.
The p-value using the MLE ordering is

$$
\begin{aligned}
p &= \Pr(\hat{\theta}(\tau) \geq 3.80) = \Pr\{\cup_{i=1}^{5}\tau = t_i \cap \hat{\theta}(t_i) \geq 3.80\} \\
&= \Pr(\hat{\theta}(.2) \geq 10.20) \\
&+ \Pr(\hat{\theta}(.2) < 10.20, \hat{\theta}(.4) \geq 5.10) \\
&+ \Pr(\hat{\theta}(.2) < 10.20, \hat{\theta}(.4) < 5.10, \hat{\theta}(.6) \geq 3.80) \\
&+ \Pr(\hat{\theta}(.2) < 10.20, \hat{\theta}(.4) < 5.10, \hat{\theta}(.6) < 3.40, \hat{\theta}(.8) \geq 3.80) \\
&+ \Pr(\hat{\theta}(.2) < 10.20, \hat{\theta}(.4) < 5.10, \hat{\theta}(.6) < 3.40, \hat{\theta}(.8) < 2.55, \hat{\theta}(1) \geq 3.80) \\
&= 0.002
\end{aligned}
$$

We obtained the final answer by converting each probability involving $\hat{\theta}(t)$ to a first exit probability involving the z-scores. For example, because $\hat{\theta}(t) = B(t)/t = Z(t)/t^{1/2}$, $\Pr(\hat{\theta}(0.2) < 10.20, \hat{\theta}(0.4) \geq 5.10) = \Pr(Z(0.2) < 10.20(0.2)^{1/2}, Z(0.4) \geq 5.10(0.4)^{1/2})$.

7.2.2 Stagewise Ordering

The calculations in Example 7.3 clearly show that the p-values for the z-score, B-value, and MLE orderings depend not only on the data observed thus far, but also on future plans. Even though we stopped at the third look, we needed to know the boundaries at the fourth and fifth looks. But future look times may be unpredictable. Why should the degree of evidence observed thus far depend on the number and times of looks in the future? This violates the likelihood principle.

A way to avoid this drawback is to order outcomes in terms of the stage at which the trial was stopped, with earlier stopping providing more compelling

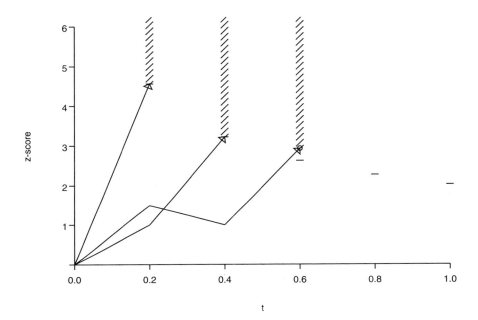

Fig. 7.3. The stagewise p-value for observed outcome $(\tau = 0.6, Z(0.6) = 2.94)$ is the probability of either stopping earlier than $t = 0.6$ or stopping at $t = 0.6$ with a z-score of 2.94 or more. The paths shown correspond to $(\tau = 0.2)$, $(\tau = 0.4)$, and $(\tau = 0.6, Z(0.6) \geq 2.94)$, respectively.

evidence of treatment differences than later stopping. For two trials stopping at the same time t, the one with the larger z-score is more extreme. Thus, $(\tau_2, Z(\tau_2))$ is at least as extreme as $(\tau_1, Z(\tau_1))$ in the *stagewise ordering* iff $\tau_2 < \tau_1$ or $\tau_2 = \tau_1$ and $Z(\tau_2) \geq Z(\tau_1)$. The so-called *stagewise ordering* assigns to the outcome $(\tau = t_j, Z(t_j) = z)$ the p-value

$$p = \Pr(\cup_{i=1}^{j-1} Z(t_i) \geq c_i) + \Pr(\cap_{i=1}^{j-1} Z(t_i) < c_i, Z(t_j) \geq z_j)$$

$$= \Pr(\cup_{i=1}^{j-1} Z(t_i) \geq c_i \cup Z(t_j) \geq z_j).$$

It is easy to compute the stagewise p-value in a one-tailed setting using software that computes cumulative crossing probabilities. We simply compute the cumulative crossing probability using boundaries $c_1, \ldots, c_{j-1}$ at looks $1, \ldots, j-1$ and z_j at the jth look.

For the trial of Example 7.1, the z-score boundaries are 4.56, 3.23, 2.63, 2.28, and 2.04. The p-value using the stagewise ordering after observing $\tau =$

0.6 and $Z(0.6) = 2.94$ is $\Pr(Z(0.2) \geq 4.56 \cup Z(0.4) \geq 3.23 \cup Z(0.6) \geq 2.94) = 0.002$ (Figure 7.3).

Table 7.2 summarizes the p-values calculated for this example. In this particular case, the p-value for the B-value ordering differs markedly from the other four, which are quite similar.

Table 7.2. p-values using different approaches.

Method	p-value
Unadjusted $\Pr(Z(3/5) \geq 2.94)$	0.002
B-value ordering	0.010
z-score ordering	0.003
MLE ordering	0.002
Stagewise ordering	0.002

Example 7.4. Suppose a trial with unpredictable look times uses the O'Brien-Fleming-like spending function. The z-score at the first look at information fraction 0.15 is $Z(0.15) = 1.5$, well below the boundary of 5.67. The second look at information fraction 0.37 produces a z-score of $Z(0.37) = 3.60$, which exceeds the boundary of 3.50. The one-tailed p-value using the stagewise ordering is $\Pr(Z(0.15) \geq 5.67 \cup Z(0.37) \geq 3.60) = 0.00016$, which is virtually the same as the unadjusted value. The p-value for the other three orderings cannot even be computed without knowing the number of future looks and their information fractions.

Unlike the previous three orderings, the stagewise ordering is a linear ordering, meaning that if $(\tau_1, Z(\tau_1)) \succeq (\tau_2, Z(\tau_2))$ and $(\tau_2, Z(\tau_2)) \preceq (\tau_1, Z(\tau_1))$, then $(\tau_1, Z(\tau_1)) = (\tau_2, Z(\tau_2))$.

7.2.3 Two-Tailed p-Values

We can extend the definition of p-values to two-tailed testing with arbitrary upper and lower z-score boundaries U_i and L_i, respectively. Again let τ be the first exit time, $\tau = \min\{t_i : Z(t_i) \geq U_i$ or $Z(t_i) \leq L_i\}$. We modify the stagewise ordering to account for the fact that either the upper or lower boundary may be crossed: (τ_2, z_2) is more extreme than (τ_1, z_1) iff either 1) $\tau_1 = \tau_2$ and $z_1 \leq z_2$, or 2) $\tau_1 < \tau_2$ and z_1 crossed the lower boundary, or 3) $\tau_1 > \tau_2$ and z_2 crossed the upper boundary. The other orderings require no modification. For observed result $(\tau_{\text{obs}}, z_{\text{obs}})$ we compute upper and lower p-values $p_U = P_0\{(\tau, Z(\tau)) \succeq (\tau_{\text{obs}}, z_{\text{obs}})\}$ and $p_L = P_0\{(\tau, Z(\tau)) \preceq (\tau_{\text{obs}}, z_{\text{obs}})\}$. The two-tailed p-value is $2\min(p_L, p_U)$.

It is easy to see that when the upper and lower boundaries are symmetric about 0, the two-tailed p-value is the one-tailed p-value of the previous section applied to $|Z_i|$. For example, the two-tailed p-value for the stagewise ordering with upper and lower z-score boundaries c_i and $-c_i$ is

$$p = \Pr(\cup_{i=1}^{j-1}|Z(t_i)| \geq c_i) + \Pr(\cap_{i=1}^{j-1}|Z(t_i)| < c_i, |Z(t_j)| \geq z_j)$$

$$= \Pr(\cup_{i=1}^{j-1}|Z(t_i)| \geq c_i \cup |Z(t_j)| \geq z_j)$$

A word of caution is in order about upper and lower boundaries. As mentioned in Chapter 1 and Section 5.2, lower boundaries are sometimes regarded as more advisory than binding. This is particularly true if they are futility boundaries. One may include futility boundaries for, say, 10 percent conditional power and 20 percent conditional power, but the trial might continue even if one or both of these boundaries are crossed. In other cases, the lower boundary might be considered more binding. One should carefully consider which of these situations applies to the current trial. If the lower boundary is advisory, it may be best to ignore it and compute a one-tailed p-value. If it is considered binding, one may wish to compute a two-tailed p-value as outlined in this section.

7.3 Properties of p-Values

The stagewise one-and two-tailed p-values have desirable properties. For example, suppose that the stagewise p-value is less than α. Then we must have either crossed the boundary before the scheduled end of the trial or continued to the end and crossed it. If not, then $Z(t_1) < c_1, \ldots, Z(1) < c_k$ in a one-tailed testing setting, so the p-value would have been $p = \Pr(\cup_{i=1}^{j-1}Z(t_i) \geq c_i \cup Z(t_j) \geq z_j) > \Pr(\cup_{i=1}^{j}Z(t_i) \geq c_i) = \alpha$. Thus, if the p-value is less than α, the boundary was crossed. Similarly, if we cross the boundary, the stagewise p-value must be α or less. In other words, the group-sequential boundary is crossed if and only if the stagewise p-value is α or less. The other orderings sometimes lack this property.

Example 7.5. Consider a one-tailed, two-look trial with a z-score boundary of 1.9600 at $t = 0.5$ and, say, 10 at $t = 1$. The trial is stopped at $t = 0.5$ because $Z(0.5) = 1.9601$. With the z-score ordering, the p-value is $\Pr(Z(\tau) \geq 1.9601) = \Pr(Z(0.5) \geq 1.9601) + \Pr(Z(0.5) < 1.9600, Z(1) \geq 1.9601) \approx \Pr(Z(0.5) \geq 1.96 \cup Z(1) \geq 1.96) = .042$. Although we crossed the $\alpha = .025$ boundary, the p-value using the z-score ordering is greater than .025.

Although Example 7.5 was extreme in the sense that the final boundary was huge, it illustrates the possibility of inconsistent results between the boundaries and p-value when the stagewise ordering is not used.

In a nonmonitoring setting, the p-value has a uniform distribution when the test statistic has a continuous distribution. Is this true under monitoring? Consider the one-tailed p-value using the B-value ordering: $\Pr\{B(\tau) \geq b_{\text{obs}}\}$, where b_{obs} is the observed B-value. As b increases from $-\infty$ to ∞, $\Pr(B(\tau) > b)$ decreases from 1 to 0, attaining every value in between. It follows that for any $u \in (0,1)$, there exists a b_u with $\Pr(B(\tau) \geq b_u) = u$. The p-value associated with the observed outcome $(\tau_{\text{obs}}, z_{\text{obs}})$ is u or less if and only if $b_{\text{obs}} \geq b_u$. The null probability of this event is $\Pr(B(\tau) \geq b_u) = u$. Thus, the p-value is uniformly distributed. A similar argument works for the z-score and MLE orderings. For the stagewise ordering, a similar argument works, where for each u we find an outcome (t_u, z_u) such that $\Pr(\tau, Z(\tau)) \succeq (t_u, z_u)) = u$. Two-tailed p-values are also uniformly distributed.

Desirable p-value properties are:

1. The p-value is uniformly distributed.
2. The p-value is consistent with the boundaries (i.e., the p-value is α or less iff the boundary is crossed).
3. The p-value does not depend on the number or timing of future looks.
4. If the trial is stopped at the first look, the p-value is the same as for a trial with no monitoring.

All four orderings have the first property; the stagewise ordering has each of the other three, whereas the other orderings have none of the other three. The stagewise ordering is therefore our ordering of choice. Unless otherwise stated, we confine attention to the stagewise ordering for the remainder of the book.

With no monitoring, if the z-score barely exceeds the critical value, the p-value will be close to α. This need not hold with monitoring, as illustrated with the stagewise ordering in a five-look trial using the O'Brien-Fleming boundary; $Z(0.2) = 4.57$ barely crosses the boundary at the first look, yet the one-tailed p-value using the stagewise ordering is $\Pr(Z(0.2) \geq 4.57) \leq .0001$.

7.4 Confidence Intervals

One way to obtain a confidence interval in a nonmonitoring situation is as follows. Having observed $Z = z_{\text{obs}}$, we determine the value θ_L such that $P_{\theta_L}(Z \geq z_{\text{obs}}) = \alpha/2$, where Z is the z-score for testing whether $\theta = 0$ (Figure 7.4). This leads to $(\hat{\theta} - \theta_L)/\{\text{var}(\hat{\theta})\}^{1/2} = z_{\alpha/2}$. The resulting value for θ_L is $\hat{\theta} - z_{\alpha/2}\{\text{var}(\hat{\theta})\}^{1/2}$. Similarly, we determine θ_U such that $P_{\theta_U}(Z < z_{\text{obs}}) = \alpha/2$ (Figure 7.4). Then $(\hat{\theta} - \theta_U)/\{\text{var}(\hat{\theta})\}^{1/2} = -z_{\alpha/2}$. The resulting value of θ_U is $\hat{\theta} + z_{\alpha/2}\{\text{var}(\hat{\theta})\}^{1/2}$. The confidence interval is (θ_L, θ_U). The rationale behind this method is depicted in Figure 7.5.

The monitoring analog of the above method is as follows. Having observed $(\tau_{\text{obs}}, z_{\text{obs}})$, we choose the value θ_L such that $P_{\theta_L}\{(\tau, Z(\tau)) \succeq (\tau_{\text{obs}}, z_{\text{obs}})\} = \alpha/2$, where $\succeq$ is with respect to the stagewise ordering. Similarly, we choose θ_U such that $P_{\theta_U}\{(\tau, Z(\tau)) \preceq (\tau_{\text{obs}}, z_{\text{obs}})\} = \alpha/2$. Equivalently, θ_U satisfies $P_{\theta_U}\{(\tau, Z(\tau)) \succeq (\tau_{\text{obs}}, z_{\text{obs}})\} = 1 - \alpha/2$. We emphasize that $(\tau, Z(\tau))$ represent the z-statistic and stopping time associated with the test of $\theta = 0$.

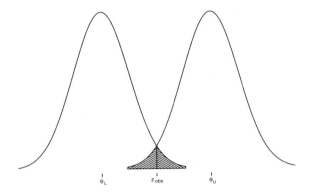

Fig. 7.4. Method of constructing confidence intervals in the nonmonitoring setting: Find θ_L and θ_U such that $P_{\theta_L}(Z > z_{\text{obs}}) = \alpha/2$ and $P_{\theta_U}(Z \leq z_{\text{obs}}) = \alpha/2$.

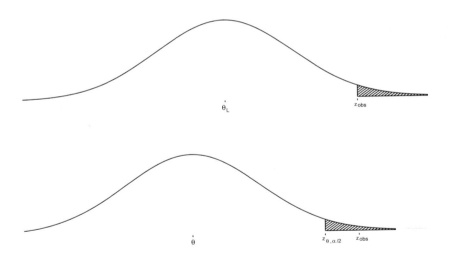

Fig. 7.5. Why the method of Figure 7.4 works. We chose θ_L such that the area to the right of z_{obs} is $\alpha/2$ (top panel). The bottom panel shows $\theta < \theta_L$. Note that $\{\theta < \theta_L\} \Leftrightarrow P_\theta(Z \geq z_{\text{obs}}) < \alpha/2 \Leftrightarrow z_{\text{obs}} > z_{\theta,\alpha/2}$, where $z_{\theta,\alpha/2}$ is the $1 - \alpha/2$th percentile of a normal distribution with mean θ and variance 1. Thus, $P_\theta(\theta < \theta_L) = P_\theta(Z_{\text{obs}} \geq z_{\theta,\alpha/2}) = \alpha/2$. Similarly, $P_\theta(\theta > \theta_U) = \alpha/2$, so $P_\theta(\theta_L < \theta < \theta_U) = 1 - \alpha$.

Implicit in the above formulation is that $\Pr(\tau, Z(\tau) \succeq (t, z))$ is an increasing function of θ for the stagewise ordering. This *monotonicity property* clearly holds for the stagewise ordering because we can obtain a Brownian motion with drift θ_2 from one with drift $\theta_1 < \theta_2$ by adding the nonnegative quantity $(\theta_2 - \theta_1)t$; $B_{\theta_2}(t) = B_{\theta_1}(t) + (\theta_2 - \theta_1)t$. If $(\tau, Z(\tau)) \succeq (t, z)$ for the Brownian motion with drift θ_1, then the same must hold for $B(t) + (\theta_2 - \theta_1)t$.

An equivalent way to obtain a confidence interval in the nonmonitoring setting is to invert a test of $\theta = \theta_L$ versus $\theta > \theta_L$ and similarly for θ_U. That is, we could have started by forming the test statistic $Z(\theta_L) = (\hat{\theta} - \theta_L)/\hat{\sigma}_{\hat{\theta}_L}$. The z-score at which we would have just rejected the null hypothesis is $z_{\alpha/2}$. Setting $(\hat{\theta} - \theta_L)/\hat{\sigma}_{\hat{\theta}_L} = z_{\alpha/2}$ and solving for θ_L gives $\theta_L = \hat{\theta} - z_{\alpha/2}\{\mathrm{var}(\hat{\theta})\}^{1/2}$. Similarly, setting $Z(\theta_U) = -z_{\alpha/2}$ and solving for θ_U gives $\theta_U = \hat{\theta} + z_{\alpha/2}\{\mathrm{var}(\hat{\theta})\}^{1/2}$. This confidence interval coincides with that of the first method.

Although not obvious, this alternative method of constructing confidence intervals, when extended to monitoring, is equivalent to the first. When we extend the second method to monitoring, the outcome is a pair $(\tau, Z(\tau))$. If we had been testing $\theta = \theta_L$ from the beginning, the boundaries would have been different from those of testing $\theta = 0$, and therefore the stopping time τ may have been different. Nonetheless, the monotonicity property of the stagewise ordering means we can regard the boundaries actually used as a test of $\theta = \theta_L$ versus $\theta > \theta_L$ and $\theta = \theta_U$ versus $\theta < \theta_U$. Thus, we can also regard the first method of constructing confidence intervals as inverting tests ot $\theta = \theta_L$ versus $\theta > \theta_L$ and $\theta = \theta_U$ versus $\theta < \theta_U$.

Example 7.6. In a cancer trial we wish to compare a new treatment with an active control with respect to the proportion of patients whose tumors show substantial regression from baseline to 30 days after randomization. The plan is to examine the data after approximately 60, 120, and 180 patients per arm have been evaluated using the O'Brien-Fleming-like spending function for a two-tailed test at $\alpha = 0.05$.

As it turns out, the first analysis takes place with 62 control and 64 treatment participants evaluated, the second analysis with 111 control and 115 treatment patients evaluated, and the third with 173 control and 176 treatment patients evaluated. If we had been clairvoyant, we would have known that the information fractions at the first two looks were really $t_1 = (1/62 + 1/64)^{-1}/(1/173 + 1/176)^{-1} = 0.361$ and $t_2 = (1/111 + 1/115)^{-1}/(1/173 + 1/176)^{-1} = 0.647$. Because we thought there would be 180 patients per arm at the end, we thought the information fractions were $t_1 = (1/62 + 1/64)^{-1}/(2/180)^{-1} = 0.350$ and $t_2 = (1/111 + 1/115)^{-1}/(2/180)^{-1} = 0.628$. Remember that the null joint distribution of $(Z(t_1), Z(t_2))$ depends only on the ratio t_1/t_2, which is invariant to misspecification of the information at the end of the trial. Thus, the boundaries are exactly the same whether or not we correctly specify the total information. For the purpose of p-values and confidence intervals, we can pretend the total sample sizes 173 and 176 had been fixed in advance. We can treat the information fractions and drift parameter as $t_1 = 0.361$, $t_2 = 0.647$, $t_3 = 1$ and

$$\theta = \frac{\delta}{\sqrt{p_C(1-p_C)/173 + p_T(1-p_T)/176}}, \qquad (7.7)$$

where $\delta = p_T - p_C$. Note that just as in the nonmonitoring case, we do not assume that $p_T = p_C$ when we construct confidence intervals; we do so only when we test whether $p_C = p_T = 0$. The boundaries using the O'Brien-Fleming-like spending function are $c_1 = 3.552$, $c_2 = 2.558$, $c_3 = 1.989$. No z-score was close to reaching statistical significance. At the end of the trial, the proportions of patients with substantial tumor regression in the control and treatment arms are $\hat{p}_C = 41/173$ and $\hat{p}_T = 45/176$. The final z-score is $Z(1) = 0.405$. The sufficient statistic is $(\tau = 1, Z(\tau) = 0.405)$; the interim z-scores are no longer important. The set of outcomes at least as extreme as the observed outcome $(\tau = 1, Z(\tau) = 0.405)$ is

$$A = \{\tau = .361, Z(.361) \geq 3.552\} \cup \{\tau = .647, Z(.647) \geq 2.558\}$$
$$\cup \{\tau = 1, Z(1) \geq .405\}$$

We can express this set in terms of events involving the three z-scores. For example, the event $\{\tau = 1, Z(1) \geq 0.405\}$ may be written as $\{|Z(0.361)| < 3.552, |Z(0.647)| < 2.558, Z(1) \geq 0.405\}$. The two-tailed p-value is twice the null probability of A. Because the boundaries are symmetric about 0, the p-value is equivalent to $P_0(|Z(0.361)| \geq 3.552 \cup |Z(0.647)| \geq 2.558 \cup |Z(1)| \geq 0.405) = 0.69$.

For the confidence interval, we determine through numerical integration and a grid search the values θ_L and θ_U such that $P_{\theta_L}(A) = 0.025$ and $P_{\theta_U}(A) = 0.975$. This yields $\theta_L = -1.555$, $\theta_U = 2.366$. We translate this interval into one for the natural parameter $\delta = p_T - p_C$. The denominator of (7.7) is 0.046, so the confidence interval for the difference in proportions, δ, is $(-1.555(0.046), 2.366(0.046)) = (-0.072, 0.109)$. Thus, we are 95 percent confident that $p_T - p_C$ is between -0.072 and 0.109.

Example 7.7. A trial comparing two diets with respect to weight change over 3 months in 200 participants per arm uses the O'Brien-Fleming-like spending function with four planned looks after roughly equal increments of information. At the third look, the mean weight loss is 8.1 kg among the 152 active diet participants compared to 6.0 kg among the 144 control participants. The current information fraction is $(1/152 + 1/144)^{-1}/(2/200)^{-1} = 0.74$. The pooled standard deviation estimate is 4.8 kg, so the t-statistic is $(8.1 - 6.0)/\{4.8^2(1/152 + 1/144)\}^{1/2} = 3.76$ with 294 degrees of freedom. We can treat it as a z-statistic because of the large number of degrees of freedom. Because the first two looks were at estimated information fractions $t_1 = 0.22$ and $t_2 = 0.55$, the z-score boundary at the third look at information fraction $t_3 = 0.74$ is 2.39. Thus, the outcome for this trial is $(\tau = 0.74, Z(0.74) = 3.76)$.

For the stagewise ordering, the set of outcomes at least as extreme as that observed is

$$A = \{\tau = .22, Z(.22) \geq 4.64\} \cup \{\tau = .55, Z(.55) \geq 2.81\}$$

$$\cup \{\tau = .74, Z(.74) \geq 3.76\}$$

The two-tailed p-value is twice the probability of A, which is equivalent to $P_0(|Z(0.22)| \geq 4.64 \cup |Z(0.55)| > 2.81 \cup |Z(0.74)| \geq 3.76) = 0.005$. Note that the p-value calculated without accounting for the sequential nature of the trial would have been .0002.

We obtain the confidence interval by determining through numerical integration the values θ_L and θ_U such that $P_{\theta_L}(A) = 0.025$ and $P_{\theta_U}(A) = 0.975$. The resulting values are $\theta_L = 1.134$ and $\theta_U = 6.211$. We translate this into a confidence interval for the natural parameter $\delta = \mu_T - \mu_C$. The drift and natural parameters are related by

$$\theta = \frac{\delta}{\sqrt{2\sigma^2/200}}, \qquad \delta = \theta\{2\sigma^2/200\}^{1/2}.$$

Substituting the current pooled standard deviation estimate, 4.8, for σ yields $\delta = 0.48\theta$. Multiplying the lower and upper limits of the confidence interval for θ by 0.48 yields the confidence interval $(0.544, 2.981)$. Thus, the new diet reduces weight by between roughly half a kilogram to almost 3 kilograms.

One quirk of confidence intervals using the stagewise ordering is that the confidence interval could exclude the MLE $B(\tau)/\tau$ in certain extreme settings (Rosner and Tsiatis, 1988 [RT88]), as we see in the following example.

Example 7.8. Suppose a two-look trial with one-tailed $\alpha = 0.025$ uses the Pocock z-score boundary $c = 2.18$ for its planned looks at $t = 0.5$ and $t = 1$. The trial is stopped at the second look with a very large z-score, z_{obs}. The set of outcomes at least as extreme as the observed outcome, $(\tau = 1, Z(1) = z_{\text{obs}})$, is $\{\tau = 0.5\} \cup \{\tau = 1, Z(1) \geq z_{\text{obs}}\} = \{Z(1/2) \geq 2.18\} \cup \{\tau = 1, Z(1) \geq z_{\text{obs}}\}$. The upper limit θ_U of the 95 percent confidence interval, obtained by setting

$$P_\theta(Z(1/2) \geq 2.18) + P_\theta(\tau = 1 \cap Z(1) \geq z_{\text{obs}}) = 0.975 \qquad (7.8)$$

and solving for θ, requires numerical integration. We can get an upper bound on θ_U without numerical integration by solving the simpler equation $P_\theta(Z(1/2) \geq 2.18) = 0.975$:

$$0.975 = P_\theta(Z(1/2) \geq 2.18) = P_\theta\left(B(1/2) \geq 2.18\sqrt{1/2}\right)$$
$$= 1 - \Phi\left(\frac{2.18\sqrt{1/2} - (1/2)\theta}{\sqrt{1/2}}\right) = 1 - \Phi\left(2.18 - \sqrt{1/2}\,\theta\right)$$

so

$$\Phi\left(2.18 - \sqrt{1/2}\,\theta\right) = 0.025$$
$$2.18 - \sqrt{1/2}\,\theta = \Phi^{-1}(0.025) = -1.96$$
$$(2.18 + 1.96)\sqrt{2} = \theta = 5.855.$$

Thus, the upper limit of the confidence interval can be no greater than 5.855 irrespective of the observed z-score at the final look. Because the MLE is $B(1)/1 = Z(1) = z_{obs}$, if $z_{obs} > 5.855$, the confidence interval will exclude the MLE.

Though we showed that $\theta_U < 5.885$, θ_U is actually quite close to 5.885 for very large values of z_{obs}. For example, when $z_{obs} = 6$, the confidence interval for θ is $(0.311, 5.850)$. The reason that θ_U is so close to our upper bound is that θ_U satisfies (7.8), and $P_\theta(\tau = 1 \cap Z(1) \geq z_{obs}) \leq \Pr(Z(1) \geq z_{obs}) \approx 0$ for very large z_{obs}.

Example 7.8 was extreme; the first stage z-score had to fall within its boundary of 2.18, but the second stage z-score had to be close to 6. Such an outcome has microscopically low probability. If we lower the confidence level, then less extreme z-scores could produce confidence intervals that exclude the MLE. For example, Rosner and Tsiatis (1988) [RT88] give an example based on a 90 percent confidence interval and the Pocock boundary with five looks and two-tailed $\alpha = 0.05$. The 90 percent confidence interval excluded the MLE when the z-score at the fifth look was 2.

7.5 Estimation

Estimation of the drift parameter θ following a group-sequential trial is problematic because of the possibility of stopping on a random high. For example, consider one-tailed testing with two looks. We know that if we agreed to continue to the end of the trial regardless of the interim results, both $\hat{\theta}(t_1) = B(t_1)/t_1$ and $\hat{\theta}(1) = B(1)/1$ would be unbiased estimates of θ. With monitoring, however, we will stop early if $\hat{\theta}(t_1)$ is large enough. Clearly $\hat{\theta}(t_1)$ will tend to overestimate θ (see Section 7.7 for a proof for an arbitrary number of looks).

How can we adjust the MLE to make it unbiased? Suppose we knew, for each value of θ, the bias $\beta(\theta)$ of the MLE when the true value of the drift is θ. Note that

$$\mathrm{E}(\hat{\theta}) = \theta + \beta(\theta). \tag{7.9}$$

A method of moments approach is to substitute $\hat{\theta}$ for its expectation on the left side of (7.9) and determine $\tilde{\theta}$ such that

$$\hat{\theta} = \tilde{\theta} + \beta(\tilde{\theta}) \tag{7.10}$$

(Whitehead, 1997 [W97]). We iterate to solve (7.10) for $\tilde{\theta}$, beginning by estimating $\tilde{\theta}$ by the MLE

$$\tilde{\theta}_0 = B(\tau)/\tau.$$

We adjust $\tilde{\theta}_0$ by subtracting its bias $\beta(\tilde{\theta}_0)$:

$$\tilde{\theta}_1 = \tilde{\theta}_0 - \beta(\tilde{\theta}_0).$$

We now treat the revised estimate $\tilde{\theta}_1$ as the true θ for the purpose of re-evaluating the bias of the MLE. We compute

$$\tilde{\theta}_2 = \tilde{\theta}_0 - \beta(\tilde{\theta}_1).$$

Continuing in this fashion, we find at the $i + 1$st step

$$\tilde{\theta}_{i+1} = \tilde{\theta}_0 - \beta(\tilde{\theta}_i). \tag{7.11}$$

Suppose $\tilde{\theta}_i$ converges to some number θ_* as $i \to \infty$. Then from 7.11, $\theta_* = \tilde{\theta}_0 - \beta(\theta_*)$, so

$$\tilde{\theta}_0 = \theta_* = \tilde{\theta}_0 + \beta(\theta_*). \tag{7.12}$$

In other words, θ_* is the solution to (7.10). In practice, we might have to estimate $\beta(\theta)$, as in the following example.

Example 7.9. A trial comparing two diets with respect to change in diastolic blood pressure (DBP) from baseline to the end of the study uses a t-test with planned looks after $30, 50, 80, 140$, and 200 participants per arm are evaluated. Thus, the information fractions are $t_1 = 0.15, t_2 = 0.25, t_3 = 0.40, t_4 = 0.70$, and $t_5 = 1$. Applying the O'Brien-Fleming-like spending function yields the B-value and z-score boundaries in Table 7.3.

Table 7.3. Boundaries a_i and c_i for $B(t_i)$ and $Z(t_i)$, respectively.

t_i	a_i	c_i
0.15	2.20	5.67
0.25	2.17	4.33
0.40	2.13	3.36
0.70	2.04	2.44
1.00	2.00	2.00

Suppose we observe B-values of $1.00, 1.40$, and 2.20 at the first three looks. At the third look, the boundary is crossed and the MLE for θ is $B(0.40)/0.40 = 2.2/0.40 = 5.50$. The drift parameter θ is related to the natural parameter $\delta = \mu_T - \mu_C$ through

$$\theta = \frac{\delta}{\sqrt{2\sigma^2/N}}, \quad \delta = \theta\sqrt{2\sigma^2/N},$$

where $N = 200$. Substituting the pooled standard deviation estimate $\hat{\sigma} = 5.00$ produces an estimated δ of 2.75 mm Hg.

To estimate the bias of the MLE, we generate 10,000 five-dimensional vectors $\{B_*(t_1), \ldots B_*(t_5)\}_1, \ldots, \{B_*(t_1), \ldots, B_*(t_5)\}_{10,000}$ with drift 0, each representing a single clinical trial generated under the null hypothesis. We add

$5.5(t_1, t_2, t_3, t_4, t_5)$ to each five-vector to simulate a trial under drift 5.5 corresponding to the MLE. For the ith simulated trial we use the same boundaries as for the actual trial, and we compute: (τ_{*i}, B_{*i}); $\theta_{*i} = B_{*i}/\tau_{*i}$; and estimated bias $\theta_{*i} - \tilde{\theta}_0$, where $\tilde{\theta}_0 = 5.5$ The average of these $10,000$ biases gives our estimate of the bias function, $\hat{\beta}(5.5)$, evaluated at the MLE 5.5. Suppose that $\hat{\beta}(5.5) = 0.3$.

The next step is to calculate a new drift parameter estimate $\tilde{\theta}_1 = 5.5 - \hat{\beta}(5.5) = 5.5 - 0.3 = 5.2$ and generate $10,000$ trials with drift 5.2. No new random number generation is needed; we use the original $10,000$ trials generated under the null hypothesis but this time add $5.2(t_1, \ldots, t_5)$. We use the same stopping boundaries, compute the MLE and bias estimate for each simulated trial, and average the biases to get the best estimate, $\hat{\beta}(5.2)$, of the bias evaluated at $\tilde{\theta}_1 = 5.2$. Suppose $\hat{\beta}(5.2) = 0.2$.

We next compute $\tilde{\theta}_2 = 5.5 - 0.2$ and continue in this way until the estimated drift changes very little from one iteration to the next. The resulting drift parameter and natural parameter estimates were 5.17 and 2.59 mm Hg (recall that the MLE for the natural parameter was 2.75 mm Hg).

Of course there is no reason to assume that this bias-corrected estimate based on the MLE is necessarily the optimal estimator. Kim's (Kim, 1989 [K89]) *median unbiased estimator* is more directly tied to p-values and confidence intervals; one determines the value $\theta_{0.50}$ such that the one-tailed p-value for testing $\theta = \theta_{0.50}$ versus $\theta > \theta_{0.50}$ is .50. Interestingly, the median unbiased estimate for θ in Example 7.9 is the MLE value, 5.5.

We close this section by searching for the minimum variance unbiased estimate of θ. We could improve any unbiased estimator $\hat{\theta}$ (not necessarily based on the sufficient statistic) by computing its conditional expectation given the sufficient statistic $(\tau, B(\tau))$. The new estimator $\tilde{\theta} = \mathrm{E}\{\hat{\theta} \mid (\tau, B(\tau))\}$ is an unbiased function of the sufficient statistic having variance no greater than that of $\hat{\theta}$ because of the familiar argument

$$
\begin{aligned}
\mathrm{var}(\hat{\theta}) &= \mathrm{E}(\hat{\theta} - \tilde{\theta} + \tilde{\theta} - \theta)^2 \\
&= \mathrm{E}(\hat{\theta} - \tilde{\theta})^2 + \mathrm{E}(\tilde{\theta} - \theta)^2 + 2\mathrm{E}\{(\hat{\theta} - \tilde{\theta})(\tilde{\theta} - \theta)\} \\
&= \mathrm{E}(\hat{\theta} - \tilde{\theta})^2 + \mathrm{var}(\tilde{\theta}) \\
&\geq \mathrm{var}(\tilde{\theta}).
\end{aligned}
$$

Line 3 follows from line 2 because $\mathrm{E}\{(\hat{\theta} - \tilde{\theta})(\tilde{\theta} - \theta)\} = 0$ by the following argument: first compute the conditional expectation of $(\hat{\theta} - \tilde{\theta})(\tilde{\theta} - \theta)$ given $(\tau, B(\tau))$; the term $(\tilde{\theta} - \theta)$ is already a function of $(\tau, B(\tau))$ and may be pulled out of the conditional expectation, while $\mathrm{E}\{\hat{\theta} - \tilde{\theta} \mid (\tau, B(\tau))\} = \tilde{\theta} - \tilde{\theta} = 0$.

Emerson and Fleming used this tack (Emerson and Fleming, 1990 [EF90]) to improve the first stage MLE $\hat{\theta}(t_1)$ by $\tilde{\theta} = \mathrm{E}\{\hat{\theta}_1 \mid (\tau, B(\tau))\}$; however, they mistakenly claimed that $\tilde{\theta}$ is the minimum variance unbiased estimator for θ. This would be true if $(\tau, B(\tau))$ were complete; in that case there would be only one function of the sufficient statistic that was unbiased for θ. But as we saw in Section 7.1, $(\tau, B(\tau))$ is not complete. In fact, Liu and Hall (1999) [LH99] showed that there is no minimum variance unbiased estimator.

Even though it is not a minimum variance unbiased estimator—because there is none in the group-sequential setting—Emerson and Fleming's estimator is appealing. Only the first stage data is guaranteed to be observed, and the best estimator for a one-stage design is the MLE $\hat{\theta}_1 = B(t_1)/t_1$. Thus, $\tilde{\theta} = \mathrm{E}\{\hat{\theta}_1 \mid (\tau, B(\tau))\}$ seems as if it should be optimal in some sense. Liu and Hall (1999) [LH99] formalized this idea by considering the class of *truncation-adaptive unbiased estimators*, unbiased estimators whose value given $(\tau = t_j, B(\tau) = b)$ does not depend on the number or timing of future looks. They showed that only one unbiased function of the sufficient statistic $(\tau, B(\tau))$ is truncation-adaptive, so there is a unique minimum variance truncation-adaptive unbiased estimator—Emerson and Fleming's $\tilde{\theta} = \mathrm{E}\{B(t_1)/t_1 \mid (\tau, B(\tau))\}$. Because $(\tau, B(\tau))$ is sufficient, this conditional expectation does not depend on θ. Thus, we can compute it assuming $\theta = 0$.

For example, suppose a trial terminates at the second look with a B-value of b_2. To compute the Emerson-Fleming estimator $\mathrm{E}\{B(t_1)/t_1 \mid (\tau = t_2, B(t_2) = b_2)\}$, we need the conditional distribution of $B(t_1)$ given $(\tau = t_2, B(t_2) = b_2)$. Because $(\tau, B(\tau))$ is sufficient, this conditional distribution is the same for all θ, so we can assume $\theta = 0$. In the following, $P_0(B(t_1) = b_1 \mid \tau = t_2, B(t_2) = b_2)$ denotes the conditional density of $B(t_1)$ (evaluated at b_1) given $\tau = t_2, B(t_2) = b_2$, and similarly for the other expressions.

$$P_0(B(t_1) = b_1 \mid \tau = t_2, B(t_2) = b_2)$$
$$= \frac{P_0(B(t_1) = b_1, B(t_2) - B(t_1) = b_2 - b_1, \tau = t_2)}{P_0(\tau = t_2, B(t_2) = b_2)}$$
$$= \frac{\phi_{t_1}(b_1)\phi_{t_2-t_1}(b_2 - b_1)}{f_0(t_2, b_2)},$$

for $b_1 < c_1 t_1^{1/2}$ (boundary for the B-value), where $\phi_t(x)$ denotes the normal density with mean 0 and variance t evaluated at x while $f_0(t_2, b_2)$ denotes $P_0(\tau = t_2, B(t_2) = b_2)$. Thus, the expectation of $B(t_1)/t_1$ given $(\tau = t_2, B(t_2) = b_2)$ is

$$\psi(t_2, b_2) = \frac{\int_{-\infty}^{c_1}(b_1/t_1)\phi_{t_1}(b_1)\phi_{t_2-t_1}(b_2 - b_1)}{f_0(t_2, b_2)}.$$

After considerable simplification,

$$\psi(t_2, b_2) = \frac{\exp\left(\frac{-b^2}{2t_2}\right)}{2\pi t_1 t_2^{1/2} f_0(t_2, b_2)}\left[\frac{t_1 b_2 \sqrt{2\pi}}{t_2}\Phi\left(\frac{c_1 - \frac{t_1 b_2}{t_2}}{\sqrt{\frac{t_1}{t_2}(t_2 - t_1)}}\right)\right.$$
$$\left. - \sqrt{t_1(t_2 - t_1)/t_2}\exp\left\{\frac{-(c_1 - t_1 b_2/t_2)^2}{2(t_1/t_2)(t_2 - t_1)}\right\}\right].$$

7.6 Summary

Inference following a group-sequential trial is problematic because p-values, confidence intervals, and point estimates are biased if monitoring is not taken into account. The p-values cited in the medical literature when a trial stops early often fail to account for the sequential monitoring that took place. Often the corrected and uncorrected p-values are nearly the same, but sometimes the difference can be large enough so that the uncorrected value produces an overly optimistic view of the strength of the evidence for a treatment effect. The magnitude of the difference between the two p-values depends on the nature of the monitoring boundary and the look at which the trial is stopped. The fact that the sufficient statistic is the pair $(\tau, Z(\tau))$ causes problems because the likelihood ratio cannot be written as a monotone function of a statistic as it can in the nonmonitoring setting. Each way (B-value, z-score, MLE, or stagewise ordering) to order outcomes yields a different p-value. We strongly recommend the stagewise ordering because its p-value depends only on what has happened thus far, not on future plans. The stagewise ordering is also consistent in the sense that the p-value is α or less iff the boundary was crossed.

A confidence interval for the drift parameter θ may be constructed using the stagewise ordering by finding θ_L and θ_U such that $P_{\theta_L}\{(\tau, Z(\tau)) \succeq (\tau_{\text{obs}}, z_{\text{obs}})\} = \alpha/2$ and $P_{\theta_U}\{(\tau, Z(\tau)) \preceq (\tau_{\text{obs}}, z_{\text{obs}})\} = \alpha/2$. This method's only drawback is that in some cases the confidence interval can exclude the MLE $\hat{\theta} = B(t)/t$; however, this potential is less disconcerting than it sounds because the MLE produces a biased estimator of the drift parameter.

Whitehead (1997) [W97] proposed a method of correcting for the bias, while others have searched for the minimum variance unbiased estimate of θ. Emerson and Fleming [EF90] proposed starting with the best first-stage estimate (the first stage is the only one guaranteed to occur) $B(t_1)/t_1$ and computing its conditional expectation given the sufficient statistic $(\tau, Z(\tau))$. Although $(\tau, Z(\tau))$ is not complete and no minimum variance unbiased estimate exists, Emerson and Fleming's estimator is the best among those estimators that do not depend on future monitoring plans (Liu and Hall, 1999) [LH99].

7.7 Appendix: Proof that $B(\tau)/\tau$ Overestimates θ in the One-Tailed Setting

Note that

$$B(\tau)/\tau - \theta = \sum_{i=1}^{k} (1/\tau)\{B(t_i) - B(t_{i-1}) - \theta(t_i - t_{i-1})\} I(\tau \geq i)$$

$$= \sum_{i=1}^{k} (1/\tau) Y_i I(\tau \geq i), \tag{7.13}$$

where $Y_i = B(t_i) - B(t_{i-1}) - \theta(t_i - t_{i-1})$. The bias is the expectation of (7.13). To find the expectation of the ith term of the sum on the right side of (7.13), we first compute its conditional expectation given $\mathcal{F}_{-i}$ where $\mathcal{F}_{-i} = B(t_1) - B(t_0), \ldots, B(t_{i-1}) - B(t_{i-2}), B(t_{i+1}) - B(t_i), \ldots, B(t_k) - B(t_{k-1})$ includes all but the ith increment. Note that $I(\tau \geq i)$, being a function of the first $i - 1$ increments, becomes constant once we condition on $\mathcal{F}_{-i}$. Pulling $I(\tau \geq i)$ out of the conditional expectation, we get $I(\tau \geq i)\mathrm{E}\{(1/\tau)Y_i \,|\, \mathcal{F}_{-i}\}$.

We claim that $\mathrm{E}\{(1/\tau)Y_i \,|\, \mathcal{F}_{-i}\} = \mathrm{cov}(1/\tau, Y_i \,|\, \mathcal{F}_{-i})$. To see this, note first that the independent increments property of Brownian motion ensures the independence of Y_i and $\mathcal{F}_{-i}$, so $\mathrm{E}\{Y_i \,|\, \mathcal{F}_{-i}\} = \mathrm{E}(Y_i) = 0$. This means that

$$\mathrm{E}\{(1/\tau)Y_i \,|\, \mathcal{F}_{-i}\} = \mathrm{E}\{(1/\tau)Y_i \,|\, \mathcal{F}_{-i}\} - \mathrm{E}(1/\tau \,|\, \mathcal{F}_{-i})\mathrm{E}(Y_i \,|\, \mathcal{F}_{-i})$$
$$= \mathrm{cov}\{1/\tau, Y_i \,|\, \mathcal{F}_{-i}\}.$$

The conditional expectation of the ith term of (7.13) given $\mathcal{F}_{-i}$ is therefore

$$I(\tau \geq i)\mathrm{cov}\{1/\tau, Y_i \,|\, \mathcal{F}_{-i}\}. \tag{7.14}$$

Note that $1/\tau$ and Y_i are both increasing functions of $B(t_i) - B(t_{i-1})$ for fixed values of the other increments. Thus, $\mathrm{cov}(1/\tau, Y_i \,|\, \mathcal{F}_{-i})$ is nonnegative with probability 1. That means $\mathrm{E}\{(1/\tau)Y_iI(\tau \geq i)\} = \mathrm{E}[\mathrm{E}\{(1/\tau)Y_iI(\tau \geq i) \,|\, \mathcal{F}_{i-1}\}] \geq 0$. Because every term of the right side of (7.13) has nonnegative expectation, $\mathrm{E}\{B(\tau)/\tau - \theta\} \geq 0$, so $\mathrm{E}\{B(\tau)/\tau\} \geq \theta$.

8

Options When Brownian Motion Does Not Hold

Thus far we have considered trials we can monitor using Brownian motion. Brownian motion breaks down if 1) the sample size is so small that the variance is estimated very poorly; 2) the test statistic is not normally distributed; or 3) the increments are not independent. In this chapter, we explore options for dealing with these scenarios.

With normally distributed data, failure to account for the fact that we have estimated the variance inflates the type 1 error rate in a monitoring context, just as using the standard normal distribution to approximate the t-distribution does in a nonmonitoring context. We demonstrate how large the sample size must be to produce negligible inflation. We also present one approximate and two exact solutions to the problem of type 1 error rate inflation when the sample size is small.

When the data are not normally distributed and the sample size is small, a permutation test provides an attractive alternative, yielding a valid p-value in diverse settings. We demonstrate how to apply a permutation test with continuous or dichotomous outcomes. With dichotomous outcomes, the permutation approach amounts to combining 2×2 tables using Fisher's exact test.

When the increments are not independent and we opt not to use a permutation test, we can combine the Bonferroni inequality with a spending function to obtain a conservative test irrespective of the true joint distribution of the test statistic over information time. We show through examples that the degree of conservatism increases with the number of looks and is more pronounced with Pocock than with O'Brien-Fleming boundaries.

8.1 Small Sample Sizes

In either a monitoring or nonmonitoring situation, the accuracy of treating t-statistics as if they were standard normal depends on whether the sample size is large enough. We assess the accuracy of the Brownian motion approximation assuming the underlying observations are normally distributed. Without loss of generality, we take $\sigma^2 = 1$.

The appendix details a parsimonious method for simulating repeated t-statistics. Because the method considers the joint distribution of the sufficient statistics $\sum X_i$ and $\sum X_i^2$ rather than the individual observations, simulations need only generate two statistics in each arm for each of the k looks, irrespective of the sample sizes.

Table 8.1. Simulated type 1 error rate and power applying the six-look, one-tailed $\alpha = 0.025$ O'Brien-Fleming and Pocock boundaries to t-statistics with m observations per arm between successive looks. The noncentrality parameter selected yields 90 percent power when the variance is known. For each m, we simulated 1/2 million clinical trials.

	O-F		Pocock	
m	Type 1 Error Rate	Power	Type 1 Error Rate	Power
2	.057	.905	.098	.913
3	.037	.901	.062	.906
4	.033	.900	.049	.904
5	.030	.900	.043	.902
10	.027	.900	.033	.902
20	.026	.900	.028	.900
50	.025	.900	.026	.900

Table 8.1 shows the type 1 error rate and power applying the O'Brien-Fleming and Pocock six-look, one-tailed $\alpha = 0.025$ boundaries to repeatedly computed t-statistics. As we might expect, the type 1 error rate is unacceptably high when the sample sizes are very small. For example, the type 1 error rate with two participants per arm between successive looks (a total of $2 \times 2 \times 6 = 24$ participants) is 0.057 and 0.098 for the O'Brien-Fleming and Pocock $\alpha = 0.025$ boundaries. The Pocock boundary leads to high type 1 error rate inflation because early stopping is more likely than with the O'Brien-Fleming boundary, and approximating the t-distribution by a standard normal is particularly inaccurate with few degrees of freedom. The inflation remains high for the Pocock boundary until each arm has about 20 observations between successive looks (a total sample size of $2 \times 20 \times 6 = 240$), whereas the inflation for the O'Brien-Fleming boundary becomes acceptable with only about 10 per arm between successive looks.

Interestingly, power remains close to 0.90 even with only two observations per arm between successive looks.

Fortunately, there is a very simple method that largely fixes the problem of inflation of the type 1 error rate. We illustrate the approach using the two-tailed O'Brien-Fleming boundary with $\alpha = 0.05$ and m observations per arm between each of six looks. The upper z-score boundaries are $c_i = 5.029$, 3.556, 2.903, 2.514, 2.249, and 2.053 with corresponding nominal two-tailed p-values $2\{1 - \Phi(c_i)\} = 5.0 \times 10^{-7}$, .0004, .0037, .0119, .0245, and .0401 (but remember from Chapter 7 that we should not cite these p-values if we cross the boundary). At the first look, we compute the two-tailed p-value using the t-distribution with $2(m - 1)$ degrees of freedom, and we reject if that p-value is 5×10^{-7} or less. At looks $i = 2, 3, 4, 5$ and 6, we reject the null hypothesis if the two-tailed p-value based on the t-distribution with $2(im - 1)$ degrees of freedom is less than or equal to .0004, .0037, .0119, .0245, and .0401, respectively. This process of converting z-score boundaries to p-value boundaries and applying them to p-values from the t-distribution is called the *nominal p-value approach.*

Equivalently, we can convert the z-score boundaries to two-tailed p-values as above, and then convert to t-score boundaries. For example, with a six-look trial and three observations per arm between looks, there are $2(3 - 1) = 4$ degrees of freedom at the first look; $\Pr(|T_4| > 59.035) = 5 \times 10^{-7}$, so the first t-score boundary is 59.035. At the second look, there are $2(6 - 1) = 10$ degrees of freedom; $\Pr(|T_{10}| \geq 5.244) = 0.0004$, so the second t-score boundary is 5.244. The degrees of freedom and the t-score boundaries at the six looks are $(4, 10, 16, 22, 28, 34)$ and $(59.035, 5.244, 3.395, 2.741, 2.377, 2.135)$, respectively.

Reformulating the nominal p-value approach to t-score boundaries facilitates calculation of approximate power. Recall that although the type 1 error rate could be profoundly affected by treating the standard deviation as known for small sample sizes per arm between successive looks, power was not. Thus, a good method of approximating power under drift θ is to compute $P_\theta(Z(t_1) > c'_1, \ldots, Z(t_k) > c'_k)$, where $(c'_1, \ldots, c'_k)$ are the t-score boundaries and $Z(t) = B(t)/t_1^{1/2}$, where $B(t)$ is Brownian motion with drift θ. This probability can be computed using standard group-sequential software.

For example, in the six-look example with three observations per arm between successive looks, assume the true treatment difference and standard deviation are $\delta = 2$ and $\sigma = 1.8$. The drift parameter is the expected z-score at the end, $\theta = \delta/\{2\sigma^2/18\}^{1/2} = 3.333$. Using the Windows version (winld.exe) of the free software available at www.medsch.wisc.edu/landemets/, we enter the "Compute" menu and select "Probability." From "**Analysis Parameters**" we type 6 in the "Interim Analyses" box. When we press enter, the six equally spaced times appear in the "Time" portion of the table at the upper right. We then go to "Determine bounds" under "**Probability Parameters**" and select "User input." We type the upper bounds 9.9, 5.244, 3.395, 2.741, 2.377, 2.135 in the "Upper" portion of the table at the top right. Note that we replaced the first boundary, 59.035, with the smaller but still practically unreachable value 9.9 to prevent the program from bogging down. We then move to the "Drift" box under "**Probability Parameters**" and type 3.333. Clicking on "Calculate" and hitting the enter button gives the cumulative exit probability 0.89060 at the final look, meaning that power is approximately 0.89.

Table 8.2 illustrates the remarkable accuracy of the nominal p-value approach for a six-look trial using the O'Brien-Fleming or Pocock one-tailed $\alpha = 0.025$ boundaries with m observations per arm between successive looks. The simulated type 1 error rate for O'Brien-Fleming was 0.025 or 0.026 irrespective of the number of looks, while for Pocock it was at most 0.028, occurring when $m = 2$. Power in all cases is extremely close to 0.90.

Table 8.2. Simulated type 1 error rate and power for the nominal p-value approach for the O'Brien-Fleming and Pocock boundaries with six looks and m observations per arm between successive looks. We simulated 1/2 million trials for each scenario.

	m	Type 1 Error Rate	Power, drift θ
	2	.026	.898
O-F	3	.026	.898
	4	.025	.899
	5	.025	.900
	2	.028	.900
Pocock	3	.027	.902
	4	.026	.902
	5	.026	.902

Jennison and Turnbull (1991) [JT91] used numerical integration to fix the nominal p-value approach so it has type 1 error rate exactly α. They considered the one-sample problem with r observations between looks, which translates to degrees of freedom $r - 1, 2(r - 1), \ldots, k(r - 1)$ at looks $(1, \ldots, k)$. But in the two-sample setting with m per arm between successive looks, the degrees of freedom for the pooled variance are $2(m - 1), 2(2m - 1), \ldots, 2(km - 1)$, so the tables of Jennison and Turnbull do not strictly apply. Fortunately, as can be deduced from Table 8.2, the nominal p-value approach needs very little adjustment to make it exact.

Another way to make the Brownian motion approximation exact when the data are normally distributed with unknown variance is to apply the *inverse normal method*, first proposed by Stouffer et al. (1949) [SSD49] and used in other contexts such as meta-analysis (pages 39-40 of Hedges and Olkin, 1985 [HO85]) and adaptive sample size estimation (Lehmacher and Wassmer, 1999 [LW99]). The idea is simple: the t-statistics $T_{i-1,i}$ computed on the incremental data between looks $i - 1$ and i are independent t-deviates, so their associated one-tailed p-values $p_{i-1,i}$ are independent uniforms under H_0. The transformation $Y_i = \Phi^{-1}(1 - p_{i-1,i})$ converts these p-values to i.i.d. standard normals under the null hypothesis. If the incremental sample sizes between successive looks are equal, we take simple averages of the Ys to form our cumulative z-statistics: $Z_1 = Y_1, Z_2 = (Y_1 + Y_2)/2^{1/2}, \ldots, Z_k = (Y_1 + \ldots + Y_k)/k^{1/2}$. For unequal incremental sample sizes, a weighted combination (Mosteller and Bush, 1954 [MB54]) can be used. Let $V_{i-1,i}$ be the variance of the treatment effect estimator $\hat{\delta}_{i-1,i}$ based on the incremental data between looks $i - 1$ and i, and let $I_{i-1,i} = 1/V_{i-1,i}$ be the information associated with $\hat{\delta}_{i-1,i}$. At look j, we form the cumulative z-score

$$Z(t_j) = \sum_{r=1}^{j} \sqrt{I_{r-1,r}/I_j}\, Y_r, \qquad (8.1)$$

where $I_j = \sum_{r=1}^{j} I_{r-1,r}$ and $t_j = I_j/I_k$. The unknown variance σ^2 cancels out in the numerator and denominator of (8.1) and in the definition of t_j. It is easy to see that $Z(t_1), \ldots, Z(t_k)$ have a multivariate normal distribution with zero means under the null hypothesis, unit variances, and covariances

$$\begin{aligned}
\text{cov}\{Z(t_i), Z(t_j)\} &= I_i^{-1/2} I_j^{-1/2} \sum_{r=1}^{i} I_{r-1,r} \\
&= I_i^{-1/2} I_j^{-1/2} I_i \\
&= (I_i/I_j)^{1/2} = (t_i/t_j)^{1/2}
\end{aligned}$$

for $i \le j$. Thus, $t_j^{1/2} Z(t_j)$ behaves like Brownian motion. Therefore, we can apply standard z-score boundaries to the z-statistics (8.1).

To illustrate the inverse normal method, consider a three-look, continuous endpoint trial using a two-tailed test with the linear spending function $\alpha_*(t) = 0.05t$ and 19 observations per arm at the end of the trial. Suppose there are five control and six treatment observations at the first look, so the variance of the treatment effect estimate is $V_{0,1} = \sigma^2(1/5 + 1/6) = 11\sigma^2/30$. The information is $I_1 = I_{0,1} = 30/(11\sigma^2)$. Note that the treatment and control sample sizes differed slightly so that the information at the end of the trial, $I_{0,1} + I_{1,2} + I_{2,3}$, is slightly less than $(2\sigma^2/19)^{-1}$ because we lose information when the sample sizes are unequal. Without knowing the sample sizes at future looks we cannot know $I_3 = I_{0,1} + I_{1,2} + I_{2,3}$, and therefore we cannot know the current information fraction precisely. Still, $(2\sigma^2/19)^{-1}$ is a good estimate (if the incremental data between successive looks were balanced across arms, it would be exact). Furthermore, we only need to estimate I_3 to determine how much type 1 error rate to spend at each of the three looks; as in the discussion of spending functions, the joint distribution of $Z(t_1)$, $Z(t_2)$, $Z(t_3)$ depends only on ratios of information fractions and is therefore invariant to erroneous guesses of I_3. The estimated current information fraction is $t_1 = \{30/(11\sigma^2)\}/\{2\sigma^2/19\}^{-1} = 0.287$. We are allowed to spend $\alpha_*(0.287) = (0.05)(0.287) = 0.0144$, which from a standard normal table corresponds to a two-tailed z-score boundary of ±2.447.

We compute the z-score at look 1 by converting the one-tailed p-value based on the t-distribution to a z-score. Suppose the observed one-tailed p-value at the first look is 0.14. The $1 - 0.14$th percentile of the standard normal distribution is $Y_1 = 1.080$, which is within the z-score boundaries ± 2.447. Therefore, we continue to the second look.

Suppose there are six observations per arm between the first and second looks, so $V_{1,2} = 2\sigma^2/6$, $I_{1,2} = 6/(2\sigma^2) = 3/\sigma^2$, $I_2 = I_{0,1} + I_{1,2} = 30/(11\sigma^2) + 3/\sigma^2$, $I_{0,1}/I_2 = (30/11)/(30/11 + 3) = 0.4762$, and $I_{1,2}/I_2 = 3/(30/11 + 3) = 0.5238$. The information fraction is $I_2/(2\sigma^2/19)^{-1} = 0.603$. The cumulative type 1 error rate we are allowed to spend is $\alpha_*(0.603) = (0.05)(0.603) = 0.030$. Using the program winld.exe at www.medsch.wisc.edu/landemets/, we enter the "Compute" menu and choose "Bounds." Under "**Analysis Parameters**, Interim Analyses," we type 3 and hit the enter button. From the "Information times" box under "**Analysis Parameters**" we select "User Input" and hit enter. Moving to the "Time" column of the table at the upper right we enter 0.287, 0.603, and 1, making sure to hit enter after each. We then enter the "**Spending Function**" area, select "Power Family," and then type 1 under the "Phi" box to indicate that we want the linear spending function. Clicking on "Calculate" makes the z-score boundaries appear. The boundary at the second look is ± 2.33.

We next compute Y_2, the z-score on the 12 incremental observations between the first and second looks. If the one-tailed p-value for those 12 observations (using the t-distribution) is $p_{1,2} = 0.05$, we compute the $1 - 0.05 = 0.95$ quantile of a standard normal distribution: $Y_2 = 1.645$. From (8.1), the cumulative z-score at the second look is $Z(t_2) = (0.4762)^{1/2}(1.080) + (0.5238)^{1/2}(1.645) = 1.936$. Because $-2.33 \le 1.936 \le 2.33$, we continue to the last look.

Between the second and third look, there are seven control and eight treatment observations, so $I_{2,3} = \{\sigma^2(1/7 + 1/8)\}^{-1} = 56/(15\sigma^2)$, $I_3 = (30/11 + 6/2 + 56/15)/\sigma^2$, $I_{0,1}/I_3 = 0.2883$, $I_{1,2}/I_3 = 0.3171$, $I_{2,3}/I_3 = 0.3946$. The program winld.exe gives the z-score boundary of 2.18 at the final look.

We next compute Y_3, the z-score associated with the 15 incremental observations between the second and third looks. Suppose the observed one-tailed p-value (using the t-distribution) applied to these 15 observations is $p_{2,3} = .002$. The $1 - 0.002 = 0.998$ quantile of the standard normal distribution is 2.878. Thus, (8.1) becomes $(0.2883)^{1/2}(1.080) + (0.3171)^{1/2}(1.645) + (0.3946)^{1/2}(2.878) = 3.314$. Because $3.314 \ge 2.18$, we reject the null hypothesis.

The inverse normal method is not attractive when the sample size is small because it is less powerful than the nominal p-value approach. As seen in Table 8.3, the nominal p-value method has substantially higher power than the inverse normal method when m is small. This comparison is slightly unfair because the inverse normal method has type 1 error rate exactly α whereas the nominal p-value method does not. Still, even if we correct the nominal

p-value approach to yield type 1 error rate exactly α, its power is superior to that of the inverse normal method.

Table 8.3. Simulated power for the inverse normal approach compared to the nominal p-value approach for the O'Brien-Fleming and Pocock boundaries with six looks and m observations per arm between successive looks. The noncentrality parameter was selected to give 90 percent power if the variance were known.

| | O-F | | Pocock | |
m	Inverse Normal	Nominal p	Inverse Normal	Nominal p
2	.789	.870	.740	.850
3	.843	.882	.822	.868
4	.863	.887	.850	.878
5	.873	.889	.862	.883

8.2 Permutation Tests

We now address the problem of nonnormally distributed data. Even in the nonmonitoring setting, strikingly non-normal data can invalidate the t-test unless the sample size is large. A permutation test provides one solution. In a nonmonitoring setting, a permutation test treats the aggregate data as fixed; the only stochastic component is the random reordering of the treatment labels. A similar idea can be applied in a monitoring setting. This time we consider the aggregate data at each look fixed so that the random relabeling of treatments induces a joint distribution of the treatment effect estimate over time. We illustrate with two small examples, one from a continuous outcome and one from a binary outcome.

8.2.1 Continuous Outcomes

Consider a continuous outcome trial designed to have 12 observations per arm at the end and a single interim look at roughly the halfway point. We use the spending function $\alpha_*(t) = 0.05t^3$ and a two-tailed test at $\alpha = 0.05$. At the interim analysis there are five treatment and six control observations, so the information fraction is $\{\sigma^2(1/5 + 1/6)\}^{-1}/(2\sigma^2/12)^{-1} = 0.455$. Thus, we can spend a type 1 error rate of $0.05(0.455)^3 = 0.0047$.

The interim data are as follows: Control: $-6, -3, -1, -1, 0, 1$; Treatment: $-10, -8, -4, -4, -2$. First we combine and order the treatment and control data: $-10, -8, -6, -4, -4, -3, -2, -1, -1, 0, 1$. We treat the data as fixed but the treatment labels as random, with each of the $\binom{11}{5} = 462$ ways of selecting five people to label as treatment observations being equally likely. For each such labeling, we compute the sum S_{T1} of the treatment observations, generating the permutation distribution of S_{T1} (Table 8.4), which can be converted to a permutation distribution for the mean difference $\hat{\delta}_1 = \bar{x}_{T1} - \bar{x}_{C1} = S_{T1}/5 - (-38 - S_{T1})/6 = 11S_{T1}/30 + 38/6$ (Figure 8.1).

Table 8.4. Permutations of first-stage data. Treatment numbers in bold.

Permutation	S_{T1}	Probability
-10,-8,-6,-4,-4,-3,-2,-1,-1,0,1	-32	1/462
⋮	⋮	⋮
⋮	⋮	⋮
-10,-8,-6,-4,-4,-3,**-2,-1,-1,0,1**	-3	1/462

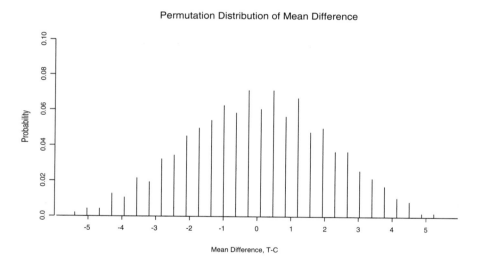

Permutation Distribution of Mean Difference

Fig. 8.1. The permutation distribution of $\bar{x}_T - \bar{x}_C$ at the interim analysis with five treatment and six control observations.

The most extreme permutations in which the largest five or smallest five observations all occur in the treatment arm each have probability $1/\binom{11}{5} = 1/462$, so $\Pr(S_{T1} = -32 \text{ or } S_{T1} = -3) = 2/462 = 0.0043$. Because 0.0043 is barely smaller than the spending allotment of $\alpha_*(0.455) = 0.0047$, we reject at the first interim analysis only if either $S_{T1} = -32$ or $S_{T1} = -3$.

The actual result was $S_{T1} = -28$, so we proceed to the end of the trial and observe the following second-stage data: Control: $-7, -6, -4, -1, 0, 3$; Treatment: $-9, -7, -6, -3, 0, 1, 3$. Consider the joint permutation distribution of $(S_{T1}, S_{T1} + S_{T2})$, where S_{T2} is the sum of the seven treatment observations among the 13 total observations in stage 2. The total number of ways to select five of 11 in the first-stage data and seven of 13 in the second stage to label as treatment observations is $\binom{11}{5}\binom{13}{7} = 792,792$. The probability of rejecting at the first stage was $\Pr(S_{T1} = -3 \text{ or } -32) = 0.0043$ (recall we could not achieve 0.0047), and we want the cumulative probability of rejecting by the end of the study to be 0.05. Thus, we want $\Pr(\text{do not reject at stage 1, reject at stage 2})$ to be $0.05 - 0.0043 = 0.0457$. In other words, we want $\Pr(-32 < S_{T1} < -3, \text{reject at stage 2}) = 0.0457$. Enumerating all the possibilities yields

$$\Pr(-32 < S_{T1} < -3, S_{T1} + S_{T2} \leq -55) = 0.0251$$
$$\Pr(-32 < S_{T1} < -3, S_{T1} + S_{T2} \geq -18) = 0.0225.$$

Thus, if we set rejection region $\{S_{T1} + S_{T2} \leq -55\} \cup \{S_{T1} + S_{T2} \geq -18\}$, the incremental type 1 error rate spent will be $0.0251 + 0.0225 = 0.0476$. This slightly exceeds the allotment of $0.05 - 0.0043 = 0.0457$, and yields a total type 1 error rate of $0.0043 + 0.0476 = 0.0519$. Because this exceeds 0.05 (albeit slightly), we choose the lower boundary -56 instead of -55. In that case

$$\Pr(-32 < S_{T1} < -3, S_{T1} + S_{T2} \leq -56) = 0.0190$$
$$\Pr(-32 < S_{T1} < -3, S_{T1} + S_{T2} \geq -18) = 0.0225,$$

so the incremental and total type 1 error rates are $0.0190 + 0.0225 = 0.0415$ and $0.0043 + 0.0415 = 0.0458$, respectively.

Suppose the observed data produced $S_{T1} + S_{T2} = -28 + -21 = -49$. Because $-56 < -49 < -18$, we do not reject the null hypothesis. We obtain the two-tailed p-value by doubling the smaller of the one-tailed p-values. For the stagewise ordering, the smaller of the one-tailed p-values is the probability of stopping earlier with a smaller value of S_{T1} or not stopping at the first look but seeing a smaller value of $S_{T1} + S_{T2}$. Thus, the p-value is

$$2\{\Pr(S_{T1} = -32) + \Pr(-32 < S_{T1} < -3, S_{T1} + S_{T2} \leq -49)\} = 0.20.$$

8.2.2 Binary Outcomes

Consider next the application of permutation testing in the binary outcome setting. We illustrate with a small example. This time we use the O'Brien-Fleming spending function with looks at the data after each of the first 3

Table 8.5. Data at the first interim analysis in a binary outcome trial.

	Event Yes	No	
Control	5	8	13
Treatment	1	14	15
	6	22	28

years and a one-tailed test at $\alpha = 0.025$. We spend according to calendar time. Suppose the data at the first look are as shown in Table 8.5.

At year 1, we are allowed to spend $\alpha_*(0.33) = 0.0001$. We consider all possible ways to select 15 of the 28 participants to label as treatment observations. For each such relabeling, the total number of events remains 6. Furthermore, each 2×2 table with a fixed total number of events corresponds to one or more relabelings of the treatment assignments. Thus, the permutation distribution of X_1, the number of control events, is the hypergeometric distribution

$$\Pr(X_1 = i) = \frac{\binom{13}{i}\binom{15}{6-i}}{\binom{28}{6}}.$$

We must determine c_1 such that $\Pr(X_1 \geq c_1) \leq 0.0001$. Table 8.6 shows the most extreme result possible. The null probability for this table is $\binom{13}{6}\binom{15}{0}/\binom{28}{6} = 0.005$. Because this probability exceeds the O'Brien-Fleming limit of 0.0001, $c_1 = \infty$. Thus, there is no way to stop at the first analysis and we spend no alpha.

Table 8.6. The only table more extreme than that observed.

	Event Yes	No	
Control	6	7	13
Treatment	0	15	15
	6	22	28

The additional data from the first to second analyses are presented in Table 8.7.

We must now determine c_2 such that $\Pr\{(X_1 \geq \infty) \cup (X_1 + X_2 \geq c_2)\} = \alpha_*(0.67) = 0.006$. Thus, we determine c_2 that makes

$$\sum_{i=0}^{6}\sum_{j=0}^{6} \Pr(X_1 = i)\Pr(X_2 = j)I(X_1 + X_2 \geq c_2) \qquad (8.2)$$

Table 8.7. Incremental data between the first and second analyses.

	Event Yes	No	
Control	5	14	19
Treatment	1	16	17
	6	30	36

equal to 0.006, where $\Pr(X_2 = j) = \binom{19}{j}\binom{17}{6-j}/\binom{36}{6}$. We find that with $c_2 = 11$, (8.2) is 0.0012, whereas with $c_2 = 10$, (8.2) is 0.0104. Because the cumulative type 1 error rate is less than 0.006 for $c_2 = 11$ and greater than 0.006 for $c_2 = 10$, we select $c_2 = 11$. That is, we stop at the second look if the cumulative number of control events is 11 or more. Because the actual number (Tables 8.5 and 8.7) was $5 + 5 = 10$, we continue to the final look at the data.

The data accruing between the second and third interim analyses are presented in Table 8.8.

Table 8.8. Incremental data between the second and third looks.

	Event Yes	No	
Control	4	11	15
Treatment	0	15	15
	4	26	30

We must now determine c_3 such that $\Pr\{(X_1 \geq \infty) \cup (X_1 + X_2 \geq 11) \cup (X_1 + X_2 + X_3 > c_3)\} = 0.025$. We must therefore find c_3 making

$$\sum_{i=0}^{6}\sum_{j=0}^{6}\sum_{k=0}^{4}[\ \Pr(X_1 = i)\Pr(X_2 = j)\Pr(X_3 = k)$$
$$\times I\{(X_1 + X_2 \geq 11) \cup (X_1 + X_2 + X_3 \geq c_3)\}] \qquad (8.3)$$

equal to 0.025. Critical values $c_3 = 12$ and $c_3 = 13$ make (8.3) equal to 0.0253 and 0.006, respectively. Although $c_3 = 12$ results in a type 1 error rate slightly exceeding the desired 0.025, $c_3 = 13$ results in a very conservative procedure with type 1 error rate 0.006, so we select $c_3 = 12$. The actual number of control events is $x_1 + x_2 + x_3 = 5 + 5 + 4 = 14$, which is at least as large as c_3, so we reject the null hypothesis and declare the treatment beneficial.

We next compute the one-tailed p-value using the stagewise ordering. Outcomes at least as extreme as observed are those for which we would have stopped earlier, or those for which we would not have stopped earlier but would have seen $X_1 + X_2 + X_3 \geq 14$, the observed value. Remember we had no chance of stopping at the first look, so the null probability of stopping earlier is

$$\Pr(X_1+X_2 \geq 11) = \sum_{i=0}^{6} \sum_{j=0}^{6} \Pr(X_1 = i)\Pr(X_2 = j)I(X_1+X_2 \geq 11) = 0.0012.$$

The probability of not stopping earlier but having $X_1 + X_2 + X_3 \geq 14$ is

$$\sum_{i=0}^{6} \sum_{j=0}^{6} \sum_{k=0}^{4} \Pr(X_1 = i)\Pr(X_2 = j)\Pr(X_3 = k)I(X_1 + X_2 \leq 10,$$
$$X_1 + X_2 + X_3 \geq 14) = 0.0005,$$

so the p-value is $.0012 + .0005 = .0017$.

We can obtain a one-sided confidence interval as follows. At look 1, the distribution of X_1 under the alternative hypothesis that the control-to-treatment odds ratio $\{p_C/(1 - p_C)\}/\{p_T/(1 - p_T)\}$ is λ can be obtained from the noncentral hypergeometric distribution (see appendix to this chapter):

$$P_\lambda(X_1 = i) = \frac{\binom{13}{i}\binom{15}{6-i}\lambda^i}{\sum_{j=0}^{6} \binom{13}{j}\binom{15}{6-j}\lambda^j},$$

and similarly for the second and third looks. Thus, the probability under the alternative of obtaining a result at least as extreme as that observed is

$$\sum_{i=0}^{6} \sum_{j=0}^{6} P_\lambda(X_1 = i)P_\lambda(X_2 = j)I(X_1 + X_2 \geq 11)+$$
$$\sum_{i=0}^{6} \sum_{j=0}^{6} \sum_{k=0}^{4} \{ P_\lambda(X_1 = i)P_\lambda(X_2 = j)P_\lambda(X_3 = k)$$
$$\times \ I(X_1 + X_2 \leq 10, X_1 + X_2 + X_3 \geq 14)\}. \tag{8.4}$$

Equating (8.4) to 0.025 and solving for λ yields $\lambda = 1.79$. Thus, we can be 97.5 percent confident that the control-to-treatment odds ratio is at least 1.79.

The above examples demonstrated the use of the permutation approach in both continuous and binary data. It is applicable in more complicated settings as well. Pawitan and Hallstrom (1990) [PH90] used it in a survival setting with the Cardiac Arrhythmia Suppression Trial. The examples we gave were sufficiently tractable that we could enumerate the outcomes and compute the exact permutation distribution. When this is not possible, one can simulate by generating a huge number of permutations and obtaining the empirical distribution of the treatment effect estimate.

A disadvantage of the permutation approach is that, technically speaking, the conclusions apply only to the participants of the trial. Conditioning on the aggregate data answers the question of whether the observed results demonstrate conclusively that treatment is effective in these specific patients. Generalization to a broader population is, to some degree, speculative. We contend that such generalization is always somewhat difficult in clinical trials. Clinical trial participants never really comprise a random sample from the patients about whom we intend to generalize. People who agree to participate in a clinical trial often differ considerably from those who do not, making generalization always somewhat speculative.

8.3 The Bonferroni Method

The Bonferroni method is another choice when we do not trust the Brownian motion approximation because of small sample sizes, nonindependence of increments—as with some survival statistics such as the Gehan (see Chapter 13)— or other reasons. All we need is the null marginal distribution of the test statistic at each look; nothing is assumed about the joint distribution over time.

We have already seen an example of the Bonferroni method, namely the Haybittle-Peto boundary, one variant of which rejects at the ith look if the p-value is less than .001 for $i < k$, and rejects at the end if the p-value is less than $\alpha - (k-1)(.001)$. By the Bonferroni inequality, the total type 1 error rate is no greater than $(k-1)(.001) + \{\alpha - (k-1)(.001)\} = \alpha$.

To apply the Bonferroni method in conjunction with a spending function $\alpha_*(t)$, assume that the marginal distribution of the test statistic at any look is continuous, so its p-value has a uniform distribution under the null hypothesis. At the first look at information fraction t_1, the trial is stopped if the p-value is less than $\alpha_*(t_1)$. Denote the p-value based on the cumulative data up to the second look by p_2. We reject the null hypothesis at the second look if $p_2 \leq \alpha_*(t_2) - \alpha_*(t_1)$. By the Bonferroni inequality, the cumulative probability of rejecting by the second analysis is no greater than $\Pr(\text{reject at } t_1) + \Pr(\text{reject at } t_2) = \alpha_*(t_1) + \alpha_*(t_2) - \alpha_*(t_1) = \alpha_*(t_2)$. Similarly, we reject at look j if $p_j \leq \alpha_*(t_j) - \alpha_*(t_{j-1})$. Again the Bonferroni inequality implies that the cumulative type 1 error rate used by look j is no greater than $\sum_{i=1}^{j}\{\alpha_*(t_i) - \alpha_*(t_{i-1})\} = \alpha_*(t_j)$, $j = 1, \ldots, k$. In particular, the type 1 error rate used by the end of the trial is no greater than α irrespective of the true null joint distribution of the test statistics over (information) time.

The degree of conservatism of the Bonferroni method depends on the number of looks and how rapidly alpha is spent. For example, with the Haybittle-Peto method and five looks, the final test statistic requires a nominal p-value of .045 instead of .05. The difference in power between not monitoring at all and monitoring using the Haybittle-Peto boundary will be small. Similarly, with the O'Brien-Fleming-like spending function and not too many looks, the Bonferroni method will not be overly conservative. It is more conservative for the Pocock-like spending function and other methods that spend alpha more rapidly. For any spending function, the degree of conservatism increases with the number of looks.

Table 8.9 shows the actual type 1 error rate used by the Bonferroni method in conjunction with the Pocock and O'Brien-Fleming boundaries with equally spaced looks when the data are normally distributed with known variance. We see that with only two or three looks, we lose very little power compared to using Brownian motion to compute boundaries with the O'Brien-Fleming-like spending function. The loss in power becomes more pronounced with a larger number of looks. On the other hand, for the Pocock-like spending function, the loss in power using the Bonferroni boundary instead of the one based on Brownian motion is noticeable even with only two or three looks.

Table 8.9. The conservatism of the Bonferroni inequality used in conjunction with the O'Brien-Fleming-like and Pocock-like spending functions when the Brownian motion paradigm holds and looks are equally spaced. The null hypothesis is rejected at look j if the p-value is less than $\alpha_*(j/k) - \alpha_*\{(j-1)/k\}$. Shown are the actual type 1 error rate and power. The noncentrality parameter was selected to yield 90 percent power under Brownian motion.

Number of Looks	O-F		Pocock	
	Type 1 Error Rate	Power	Type 1 Error Rate	Power
2	.024	.897	.022	.877
3	.021	.886	.020	.862
4	.019	.874	.018	.850
5	.017	.864	.017	.839
6	.015	.854	.016	.831
7	.014	.845	.015	.822
8	.013	.838	.015	.815
9	.012	.830	.014	.808
10	.012	.823	.014	.802

8.4 Summary

Appealing to Brownian motion may be inappropriate if the sample size is too small, the test statistic is not normally distributed, or the increments are not independent. Of these problems, a small sample size is the least troubling because sample sizes in clinical trials are usually large enough for Brownian motion to be a good approximation, and there is a relatively easy fix if the sample size is too small. The problem of nonindependent increments is more difficult. It can arise with certain survival statistics like the Gehan statistic, or when the short-term outcome of interest differs from the long-term outcome. For example, even though ultimate interest might be in comparing time to fatal/nonfatal stroke using the logrank test, if one treatment is a risky surgery, at an interim analysis we might want to monitor 30-day mortality using a test of proportions. We cannot assume independent increments if a different outcome and test statistic are used at different monitoring times.

If the sample size is too small for Brownian motion to hold, the nominal p-value approach converting z-score boundaries to p-value boundaries and applying them to p-values computed using the t-distribution is highly accurate, yielding type 1 error rate and power very close to the desired levels. The inverse normal method preserves the type 1 error rate exactly, but loses considerable power.

When the test statistic is not normally distributed and the sample size is small, a permutation test can be applied. Permutation tests, which are applicable in continuous, binary, or other outcome trials, provide valid inference under minimal assumptions. They may be computationally intensive, however.

When only the marginal distribution of the test statistic is known, a conservative approach is to use the Bonferroni inequality in conjuction with a spending function. The overall type 1 error rate will be α or less irrespective of the true null joint distribution of the test statistic over time; however, if the number of looks is large, the method entails a noticeable loss in power.

8.5 Appendix

8.5.1 Simulating the Distribution of t-Statistics Over Information Time

Without loss of generality, assume that $\sigma^2 = 1$, and consider the joint distribution of $(U_j, V_j)_{j=1}^k$, where $U_j = \sum_{i=1}^{n_j} X_i$ and $V_j = \sum_{i=1}^{n_j} X_i^2$ are the sums of the n_j control observations and their squares, respectively, accumulated by look j. Observe that

$$
\begin{aligned}
\{U_j, V_j\} &= \left\{ U_{j-1} + \sum X_i; \; V_{j-1} + \sum X_i^2 \right\} \\
&= \left\{ U_{j-1} + \sum X_i; \; V_{j-1} + \sum X_i^2 - \frac{(\sum X_i)^2}{n_j - n_{j-1}} + \frac{(\sum X_i)^2}{n_j - n_{j-1}} \right\} \\
&= \left\{ U_{j-1} + \sum X_i; \; V_{j-1} + \sum (X_i - \bar{X}_{j-1,j})^2 + \frac{(\sum X_i)^2}{n_j - n_{j-1}} \right\} \\
&= \left\{ U_{j-1} + (n_j - n_{j-1})^{1/2} Z_{j-1,j}; \; V_{j-1} + \chi^2_{j-1,j} + Z^2_{j-1,j} \right\}, \quad (8.5)
\end{aligned}
$$

where

$$
Z_{j-1,j} = (n_j - n_{j-1})^{-1/2} \sum X_i \qquad (8.6)
$$

$$
\chi^2_{j-1,j} = \sum (X_i - \bar{X}_{j-1,j})^2, \qquad (8.7)
$$

$\bar{X}_{j-1,j}$ is the mean of the $n_j - n_{j-1}$ observations between looks $j-1$ and j, and the range of the sums of (8.5), (8.6), and (8.7) is from $n_{j-1}+1$ to n_j. Note that $Z_{j-1,j}$ has a standard normal distribution. Because $Z_{j-1,j}/(n_j - n_{j-1})^{1/2}$ and $\chi^2_{j-1,j}/(n_j - n_{j-1} - 1)$ are the sample mean and variance of $X_{n_{j-1}+1}, \ldots, X_{n_j}$, $\chi^2_{j-1,j}$ has a chi-squared distribution with $n_j - n_{j-1} - 1$ degrees of freedom and is independent of Z.

The sample variance of all n_j control observations by look j is

$$\hat{\sigma}^2_j = \frac{V_j - U_j^2/n_j}{n_j - 1}. \tag{8.8}$$

A similar decomposition holds in the treatment arm, the only difference being the mean of $Z_{j-1,j}$ of (8.6). The control and treatment observations have mean 0 and μ_T, respectively, so the mean of the Z-score comparing the two treatments at the end of the trial is $\theta = (\mu_T - 0)/\sqrt{2/n_k}$. It follows that $\mu_T = \theta\sqrt{2/n_k}$. Thus, in the treatment arm, (8.6) has mean

$$\mathrm{E}\left\{ (n_j - n_{j-1})^{-1/2} \sum_{i=n_{j-1}+1}^{n_j} X_i \right\} = (n_j - n_{j-1})^{-1/2}(n_j - n_{j-1})\mu_T$$

$$= \{2(n_j - n_{j-1})/n_k\}^{1/2}\theta.$$

The pooled variance, assuming equal sample sizes in the two arms, is just the average of the two sample variances.

In summary, we 1) simulate (U_j, V_j) using (8.5), (8.6), (8.7), 2) form the sample variances using (8.8), and 3) form the t-statistics

$$T_j = \frac{U_{jT} - U_{jC}}{\sqrt{n_j\{\hat{\sigma}^2_{jC} + \hat{\sigma}^2_{jT}\}}}.$$

8.5.2 The Noncentral Hypergeometric Distribution

In a trial with an immediate-response outcome, we are sometimes interested in the conditional distribution of X, the number of control events, given the number m and n of treatment and control patients and the total number of events k (Table 8.10).

Table 8.10. Data from an immediate-response outcome trial with m control patients, n treatment patients, and a total of k patients with events across both arms.

	Event Yes	No	
Control	X		m
Treatment	Y		n
	k		

Unconditionally, X and Y are independent binomials with parameters (m, p_C) and (n, p_T), respectively. Thus,

$$\Pr(X = x, Y = y) = \binom{m}{x} p_C^x (1 - p_C)^{m-x} \binom{n}{y} p_T^y (1 - p_T)^{n-y}.$$

The conditional probability that $X = x$ given $X + Y = k$ is

$$\Pr(X = x \mid X + Y = k) = \Pr(X = x, Y = k - x)/\Pr(X + Y = k)$$

$$= \frac{\binom{m}{x}\binom{n}{k-x} p_C^x (1 - p_C)^{m-x} p_T^{k-x}(1 - p_T)^{n-(k-x)}}{\sum_{j=0}^{k} \Pr(X = j, Y = k - j)}$$

$$= \frac{\binom{m}{x}\binom{n}{k-x} p_C^x (1 - p_C)^{m-x} p_T^{k-x}(1 - p_T)^{n-(k-x)}}{\sum_{j=0}^{k} \binom{m}{j}\binom{n}{k-j} p_C^j (1 - p_C)^{m-j} p_T^{k-j}(1 - p_T)^{n-(k-j)}}$$

$$= \frac{(1 - p_C)^m p_T^k (1 - p_T)^{n-k} \binom{m}{x}\binom{n}{k-x} \lambda^x}{(1 - p_C)^m p_T^k (1 - p_T)^{n-k} \sum_{j=0}^{k} \binom{m}{j}\binom{n}{k-j} \lambda^j}$$

$$= \frac{\binom{m}{x}\binom{n}{k-x} \lambda^x}{\sum_{j=0}^{k} \binom{m}{j}\binom{n}{k-j} \lambda^j}, \tag{8.9}$$

where λ is the control-to-treatment odds ratio $\{p_C/(1 - p_C)\}/\{p_T/(1 - p_T)\}$. This is the noncentral hypergeometric distribution with parameter λ. If $p_C = p_T$, then $\lambda = 1$ and (8.9) reduces to the central hypergeometric distribution

$$\frac{\binom{m}{x}\binom{n}{k-x}}{\binom{m+n}{k}}.$$

9

Monitoring for Safety

9.1 Example: Inference from a Sample Size of One

On June 4, 1998, the National Institute of Diabetes and Digestive and Kidney Diseases (NIDDK) announced the discontinuation of the troglitazone (Rezulin) arm of its four-arm Diabetes Prevention Program (DPP). The press release explained:

> One of the 585 recipients of troglitazone in the DPP, a multi-center controlled clinical trial, died on May 17 following liver failure and a liver transplant. The clinical course and ultimate death of the patient were complex. However, a three member panel of experts concluded that drug-induced liver toxicity was probably the cause of liver failure. Largely in view of this report and because the DPP is a prevention study, the [Data Safety Monitoring] Board recommended to the Institute discontinuation of the troglitazone arm of the study.

From a purely statistical point of view, the action may appear to have been premature. After all, conditional on the occurrence of this single event, the p-value for the tragedy is identically one—the event, having happened, had to have occurred in one of the four arms. Even if one defines a one-sided p-value as the probability that the event would have occurred in the troglitazone arm, the p-value value would be .25, hardly a surprising happening. Obviously, the internal statistical data alone could not have provided the basis for the decision to stop; instead, the action was based on data external to the trial as well as the experts' judgment of the causal linkage of troglitazone usage to fatal liver failure in this specific case.

The study had begun randomizing participants in 1997. On November 19, 1997, the Food and Drug Administration (FDA) added a new warning to its label for troglitazone, "Rare cases of severe idiosyncratic hepatocellular [liver] injury have been reported during marketed use. The hepatic injury is usually reversible, but very rare cases of hepatic failure, including death, have been reported. Injury has occurred after both short- and long-term troglitazone treatment" (www.fda.gov/medwatch/SAFETY/1997/nov97.htm). Thus, the decision to stop the study arm was governed by extra-statistical thinking.

9.2 Example: Inference from Multiple Endpoints

Cyclooxygenase-2 (Cox-2) inhibitors relieve the pain of arthritis with theoretical reasons to believe, supported by some data from clinical trials, that they cause less gastric disturbance than does aspirin. Moreover, some members of this class of drug have shown promise in prevention of cancer and other diseases. At the end of September 2004, however, the manufacturer of one drug in the class removed its drug rofecoxib (Vioxx) from the market because a randomized trial had shown more serious cardiovascular events in patients on rofecoxib than on placebo (Bresalier, 2005 [B05]). In the wake of that recall, the DSMB for a trial of celecoxib (Celebrex), another member of the class, asked for a special review of cardiovascular events that had occurred in the trial it was monitoring. The trial was designed to show whether prophylactic treatment with celecoxib for people with adenomatous colon polyps—which sometimes become malignant—could prevent the growth of further polyps. The study randomized participants into one of three groups: low- or high-dose celecoxib, or placebo.

The DSMB established a committee consisting of a blinded Endpoints Review Subcommittee that classified each serious adverse event as cardiovascular or not and, if cardiovascular, categorized it into one of several specific diagnoses (myocardial infarction, stroke, congestive heart failure, etc.). The DSMB also convened an unblinded Safety Subcommittee to interpret the data. The committee established a hierarchical classification of events such that each successive event added to the hierarchy was considered less clearly in the putative pathophysiologic pathway: 1) cardiovascular (CV) death; 2) CV death or myocardial infarction (MI); 3) CV death or MI or stroke;... 6) CV death or MI or stroke or heart failure or angina or CV procedure. The committee hypothesized that if celecoxib truly adversely affected the cardiovascular system, the hazard ratio of celecoxib to placebo, as estimated in a Cox model, would decrease monotonically over this classification. They did not expect the statistical significance of the results to reflect this monotonicity because statistical significance is a function both of effect size and of sample size. They predicted that the most statistically significant of the endpoints would be one of the composites in the middle of the hierarchy. The results were consistent with the prior hypotheses. For both the high- and the low-dose celecoxib groups, the relative risks showed a clear trend—the relative risk was elevated for each endpoint in the hierarchy, with the level of relative risk highest at the top of the classification and lowest at the bottom. The most statistically significant composite was the endpoint CV death, MI, stroke, or congestive heart failure. Table 9.1 shows the data for the high-dose celecoxib and placebo groups (Solomon, 2005 [SMP05]).

Table 9.1. Hierarchical classification of safety endpoints for a study of celecoxib. The data shown come from the high dose and placebo groups as reported by Solomon (2005) [SMP05]. CHF is congestive heart failure and MI is myocardial infarction.

Endpoint	Number of Events Placebo	Number of Events Celecoxib	Hazard Ratio	95% CI	p-value
Cardiovascular (CV) death	1	6	6.1	(0.7, 50.3)	.10
CV death or MI	4	15	3.8	(1.3, 11.5)	.015
CV death, MI, or stroke	6	20	3.4	(1.4, 8.5)	.007
CV death, MI, stroke, or CHF	7	23	3.4	(1.4, 7.8)	.006
CV death, MI, stroke, CHF, or angina	11	25	2.3	(1.1, 4.7)	.027
CV death, MI, stroke, CHF, angina, or CV procedure	17	31	1.9	(1.0, 3.3)	.05

In light of this analysis and other data from the trial, the DSMB recommended stopping the trial.

In contrast to the troglitazone example, the inference about safety in this trial relied heavily on statistical thinking.

9.3 General Considerations

While earlier chapters have presented a unified approach to monitoring data for efficacy, this chapter presents some nonunified stances for safety. The purpose of most clinical trials is to show efficacy, or at least non-inferiority, of a new treatment or to demonstrate that a treatment already in use provides benefit for a new indication. Only under unusual circumstances will patients enroll in a trial to show that an experimental treatment is harmful; rather, rational participants who understand the informed consent document they have signed trust that the investigator will inform them if the ongoing data show more risks than anticipated at the time they agreed to enter the study. In trials during which the investigators are blinded to the ongoing data and therefore remain ignorant of emerging risks, the DSMB must evaluate the risks and benefits on an ongoing basis with the view toward informing the participants, or even stopping the trial, should the balance between risk and benefit change materially.

A well-designed protocol specifies the endpoints measuring efficacy; in safety monitoring, on the other hand, often the most important endpoints are still unknown. A taxonomy of safety endpoints provides a structure for thinking about how to monitor for safety. A drug or other intervention has some risks that are known, some that are unexpected but nonserious, others that are unexpected but serious, some that are unexpected and life-threatening, and some that, though not biologically credible, are frightening if true. A physician friend of ours once pointed out, only somewhat facetiously, that a drug without adverse effects is probably inert (J. Cedarbaum; personal communication). This section introduces some general considerations related to safety; later sections parse the above taxonomy addressing each type of safety signal in turn.

Monitoring for safety presents statistically difficult problems. In looking for safety signals, the DSMB searches for the unknown, the rare unexpected event. Problems of multiplicity abound, for many endpoints and many looks conspire to muddle the sample space and therefore make probabilities ill-defined. While one can, and should, specify precisely the number of endpoints to be evaluated for efficacy, by definition, one cannot specify the number of hypotheses relevant to safety. Instead, the DSMB must remain alert to react to surprises, turning a fundamentally hypothesis-generating ("data-dredging") exercise into somewhat of a hypothesis-testing framework. Taking as our marching order Good's aphorism, "I make no mockery of honest ad hockery" (Good, 1965 [Go65]), we now suggest approaches for a DSMB when it monitors safety.

Complicating the decisions of the DSMB is the fact that data on safety frequently arrive at different times than do data on efficacy. In many cases, safety data appear earlier than efficacy data. In a trial studying the long-term effects of a new therapy for diabetes, the adverse experiences are likely to emerge long before the data can show a decreased probability of occurrence of the long-term sequelae of the disease. Similarly, cancer chemotherapeutic agents will declare their toxicity before data have accrued that can address whether the treatment is beneficial (Wittes, 1996 [W96]). On the other hand, in some cases the adverse effects become manifest late. For example, development of gastric ulcers in trials of analgesia may occur only after relatively long-term use of the drug when benefit on pain is already clear to the DSMB.

The DSMB has several tools for monitoring safety. For adverse events that the drug under study is known to cause, the DMSB can use the emerging data to estimate the rates with the purpose of ensuring that the rate is not unacceptably higher than previously thought. For example, tetrabenazine, a drug used in Europe for the treatment of chorea, is known to cause drowsiness in some patients (Jankovic and Beach, 1997 [JB97]). In a randomized, blinded study comparing tetrabenazine to placebo for the treatment of the chorea of Huntington's disease, therefore, one expects some participants to complain of drowsiness. The appropriate statistical assessment is not a test of the null hypothesis of no effect; rather, the DSMB should be estimating the incidence rate of drowsiness. For an event whose relationship to the drug is unknown but hypothesized, the DSMB can operate under the unified structure described in the earlier chapters. By analogy with the approach it takes for efficacy, it can set a statistical boundary for safety. Crossing the boundary means that, with respect to this endpoint, the data have shown convincing evidence of harm, or convincing evidence of an incidence rate higher than expected. Under this situation, the safety endpoint would be as clearly defined, standardized, and well-documented as the efficacy endpoint. Later in this chapter we shall discuss how to select such boundaries.

DSMBs take a variety of stances with respect to safety. Some DSMBs use futility bounds for efficacy as ersatz safety bounds. Other DSMBs adopt a bound that is symmetric with respect to the efficacy bounds; that is, one declares excess risk if the evidence for harm is as strong as the evidence for benefit would have been. Another approach used by some DSMBs is to establish a boundary more extreme than futility but less extreme than the symmetric bound. Still another approach is to define an a priori balance of risk and benefit; if the ongoing data show that the balance has changed importantly in the direction of excess risk, the DSMB may recommend stopping the trial for lack of safety (Freedman, Anderson, and Kipnis, 1996 [FAK96]). If the event had previously been unreported in connection with the drug under study, the DSMB may formulate an hypothesis of excess risk and use the remainder of the trial to test whether the excess is real (Lachenbruch and Wittes, 2005 [LW05]).

To fix ideas, consider a two-armed trial in which the treatment group is showing a slight excess in pulmonary emboli, a blood clot that enters the lung. This extremely dangerous condition is sometimes fatal. If the excess is real, then at the very least the DSMB should inform the investigators of the excess risk; if it is not real, then a warning sends an unnecessarily worrisome message. The difference between type 1 and type 2 errors emerges starkly in the decision-making process. Committing a type 1 error—declaring an adverse event so bad that the study should stop when in fact the excess occurred by chance—can destroy a promising drug. On the other hand, a DSMB that commits a type 2 error—failing to react to a serious adverse event—can harm the participants in the trial.

Confronted with what seems like a signal—in this case an excess rate of pulmonary embolism—the DSMB should first take measures to enhance that signal. Summarizing all thrombotic (clotting) events would increase the number of events; observing more total thrombotic events in the treated group provides biological evidence that the observed excess in pulmonary embolism reflects a real effect. On the other hand, if biologically related events occurred more frequently in the control group, then the increase in pulmonary emboli might be simply noise. Next, any laboratory data—for instance, clotting time—that provide insight into the causal mechanism of the event should be examined. Think of the observation as a mystery that the DSMB must solve in real time. The board should identify an adverse event if it is real but not point to one if that is not real. Before discussing some methods for distinguishing these two types of events, we first discuss some practical considerations in dealing with data on safety.

9.4 What Safety Data Look Like

Most information on safety in clinical trials arrives as spontaneous reports. Such unstructured data are notoriously ambiguous. The investigator writes a description of the event on a case report form (Figure 9.1). The form arrives at the data center where a person or a computer algorithm codes the events using a standard dictionary of adverse events. [The system currently accepted by drug regulatory authorities, the MedDRA dictionary (Brown, 2004 [B04]), has thousands of unique terms.]

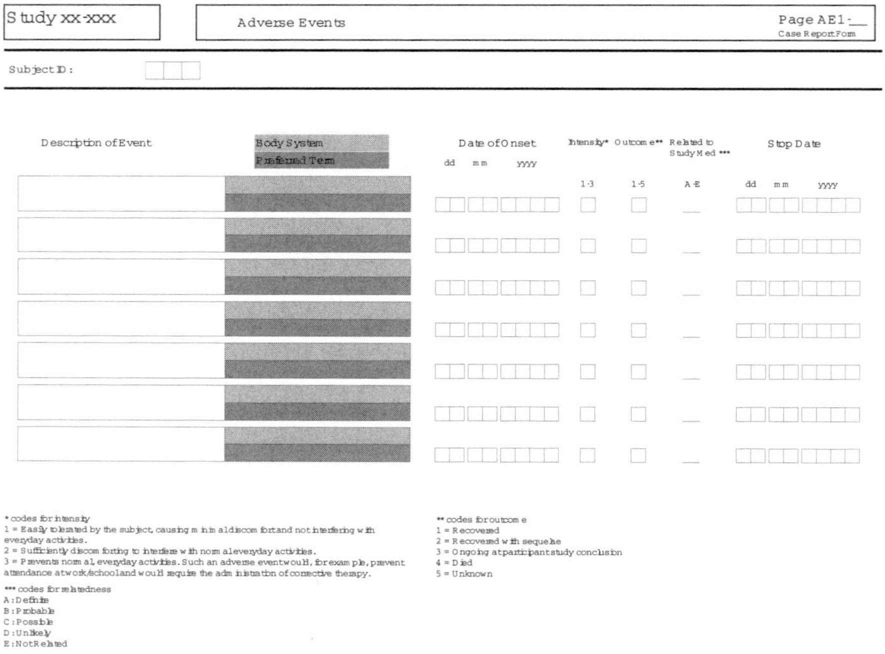

Fig. 9.1. Case report form for adverse events

These individual reports become the basis for a summary table showing the number of adverse events by body system in the study groups (Table 9.2). Typically, the table does not summarize the data by time of exposure; it simply lists the events and their frequency. The table may extend for many pages. Closely related events of interest may be distributed within a body system using different names (e.g., angina pectoris, angina pectoris aggravated, and unstable angina) or even across body systems (e.g., strokes are listed in the nervous system as cerebral vascular accident, hemorrhagic stroke, and stroke; in this example, one is listed in the vascular system termed "cerebral infarction.") During the course of the study, the DSMB is responsible for looking at such tables and identifying potential problems the drug may be causing. Clearly, if the DSMB is to perform its task adequately, the statistician preparing the safety report should work closely with a physician to reclassify events in a way that is more useful to interpret.

One cannot expect classification systems for events as complicated, varied, and idiosyncratic as the possible collective of adverse events to be ideal, but some methods can enhance the quality of these data. For certain events, diaries provide a systematic approach to collection. In many randomized trials that study vaccines, the participant fills out a daily diary card with a list of expected adverse events that occur in the immediate days after immunization.

More generally, the study team may develop specialized case report forms to collect data on known or suspected risks. Codifying the collection can increase the accuracy and completeness of the data. For example, early studies of bevacizumab, a monoclonal antibody against vascular endothelial growth factor, showed evidence of hypertension, thrombosis, serious bleeding, and severe diarrhea. During the course of a study of bevacizumab in metastatic colorectal cancer, Genentech, the sponsor, collected data on specially designed case report forms for each of these events. The DSMB reviewed summaries of these data every 2 weeks during the course of the trial (Hurwitz et al., 2004 [HFN04]). Such a systematic approach to data collection enhances the reliability and interpretability of the data.

For specified serious adverse events of special interest, a blinded endpoint committee may review the investigators' reports. If, for instance, the drug under study is suspected of causing thrombotic events, an endpoint committee can review spontaneously reported events that could potentially be thrombotic.

A DSMB should not rely solely on coding systems; rather, it should feel free to classify and reclassify to identify clusters of similar events. Conventional categorization by body system may underemphasize certain events that occur across systems, for example bleeding or thrombotic events or pain. Further, some events, like stroke, have many synonyms. The problem is even more serious in multinational trials where differences in language and medical terminology can have a large impact on the reporting and coding of adverse events. Listing them as separate types of events makes them appear less frequent than they really are. In Section 9.5, we discuss methods for looking at a single type (or cluster) of adverse events, and in Section 9.6 we discuss approaches for evaluating the collective set of events.

Table 9.2. A typical table of serious adverse events from a randomized clinical trial—number of events by body system.

Preferred term	Treated N=576	Control N=582
Blood and lymph system	*5*	*3*
Anemia NOS[1]	4	1
Iron deficiency anemia	1	2
Cardiac	*45*	*28*
angina pectoris	4	1
angina pectoris aggravated	1	2
arrhythmia NOS	1	0
atrial flutter	2	1
cardiac failure	9	6
cardiac failure left	8	2
cardiac failure right	3	0
.		
.		
.		
unstable angina	6	3
ventricular tachycardia	4	2
.		
.		
.		
Infections and infestations	*6*	*8*
abscess NOS	1	0
cellulitis	0	2
.		
.		
.		
Nervous system disorders	*8*	*1*
Cerebral vascular accident	2	0
.		
.		
.		
hemorrhagic stroke	1	0
.		
.		
.		
stroke	3	1
.		
.		
.		
Vascular disorders	*8*	*6*
.		
.		
.		
cerebral infarction	2	0
.		
.		
.		

[1] NOS, not otherwise specified.

9.5 Looking for a Single Adverse Event

Suppose a DSMB sets out to determine whether a single type of adverse event E (e.g., itchiness) or a prespecified cluster of events (e.g., bleeding) is occurring at a higher rate in the treated than in the control group. How does the DSMB decide that it is interested in E and, once it becomes interested, how does it decide whether the rate of occurrence of E is higher in the treated than in the control group? Finally, having established that the rate in the treated group is indeed higher—or at least probably higher—than in the control group, what action does the DSMB take?

Now obviously, not all Es are equal; as George Orwell said in another context, "Some are more equal than others" [O45]. A minor irritant (drowsiness or itchiness) is less important than death or than a life-threatening event like major bleeding or stroke. Moreover, the importance of a specific event E depends not only on the severity of E itself but also on the disease under study. Healthy people in a study of a drug to alleviate minor muscle aches might be unwilling to tolerate drowsiness because it would interfere with their daily lives, but patients hospitalized with metastatic cancer may willingly accept considerable drowsiness if the treatment has the potential to prolong life. Even life-threatening adverse events weigh differently depending on the disease being studied. A small, but real, increase in the risk of breast cancer may be unacceptable to a patient with coronary heart disease whose life expectancy is measured in decades, but it may be irrelevant to someone with class IV heart failure who is unlikely to survive another year. In the example of troglitazone that began this chapter, one important factor leading to stopping the study arm was the fact that the participants in the trial were reasonably healthy— the purpose of the study was to identify an intervention to prevent or delay the onset of diabetes, not to treat existing disease. The threshold for harm in a prevention study is much lower than in a trial studying people with a disease. Thus, as we consider statistical approaches to monitoring a specific event E, we need to bear in mind not only what we know a priori about the causal relationship of the drug under study to E, but we need to weigh the seriousness of E in the context of the disease under study.

In considering how to monitor a single event (or a single cluster of events like bleeding), we distinguish three situations. In the first case, the event signaling a problem with safety is the same as the event showing efficacy. The CAST study that began this book is an example of such a situation— the study was designed to show that suppressing arrhythmias reduced sudden deaths/cardiac arrests in patients with cardiac arrhythmias and a prior heart attack; the study showed that the drugs used actually *increased* sudden deaths/cardiac arrests. Section 9.5.1 below describes methods for monitoring this type of event, which we term the flip-side of the efficacy endpoint. Obviously, if the data show a real increase in the event rate, then the study should be stopped, for the drug has not achieved its aim.

In the second case, the safety endpoint is serious or frequent enough to warrant stopping the study even if the experimental therapy is showing benefit. The troglitazone study that began this chapter is an extreme example of such a situation. Often, as discussed in Section 9.5.2, the balance between efficacy and safety in this situation is more difficult to weigh.

The third situation is more difficult—the DSMB becomes aware of an event not already known to be caused by the drug (or not sufficiently described in the informed consent document), but it judges the event to be not serious enough to stop the study. In such a case, as described in Section 9.5.3, the DSMB may inform the investigators of the new adverse event.

These three types of examples are statistically very different—the first is amenable to the methods of this book; the second often requires nonstatistical judgment; the third involves statistical thinking different from that related to monitoring for efficacy.

9.5.1 Monitoring for the Flip-Side of the Efficacy Endpoint

The conceptually easiest type of event to consider is the negative of the efficacy endpoint. Consider a study that aims to show that the test drug prevents or cures E. For safety, a reasonable approach is to assume pessimistically that the drug may cause or worsen E. If the endpoint is a major event (e.g., death, kidney failure, heart attack, stroke) or even a very bothersome symptom (e.g., pain or joint immobility), a DSMB may establish two one-sided boundaries. It sets the upper, or efficacy, boundary according to the principles enunciated in earlier chapters; generally, it sets the safety boundary to be less extreme than the efficacy boundary.

As an example, consider a clinical trial studying sepsis. The standard endpoint in sepsis is 28-day mortality. Suppose the study drug is anticipated to reduce mortality by 25 percent; specifically, suppose the anticipated percent mortality is 24 percent and 18 percent in the treated and control groups, respectively. A trial with a one-sided type 1 error rate of 0.025 and a power of 0.90 requires approximately 1000 patients per group. Imagine that the DSMB plans to meet four times over the course of the trial leading to a total of five looks at the data—four during the course of the trial and one at the end. For simplicity, suppose the looks are to occur 28 days after each successive group of 400 patients is randomized. (Of course, in practice, one cannot look so soon after the 400th person's 28th day, for the data are highly likely to lag considerably.) The DSMB plans to monitor efficacy with an O'Brien-Fleming-like spending function (see the upper bound in Figure 9.2). In such a design, the study would stop at the first look for efficacy if the z-value were at least 4.88. If the observed event rate in the control group were 0.20, the mortality rate in the treated group would have to be no greater than 0.041 to exceed this boundary. If the boundary were not crossed at any of the first four looks and the observed event rate in the control group remained at 0.20, the event rate

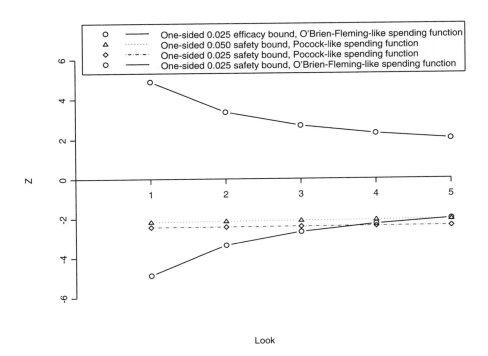

Fig. 9.2. Examples of safety bounds.

would have to be 0.165 in the treated group at the end of the study to show statistically significant benefit.

While in the past we have sometimes advocated not establishing a safety boundary, we have come to believe that a prespecified safety boundary helps a DSMB make judgments about the endpoint of interest when the data are showing harm. So let us consider some safety bounds. Suppose the safety bound were symmetric with respect to the efficacy bound. Then at the first look if the observed mortality rate in the control arm were 0.20, the boundary would not be crossed unless the observed event rate in the treated group were over 0.426 (Figure 9.3). In other words, a DSMB that acted symmetrically with respect to the upper and lower bounds would not stop the trial for safety concerns at the first look unless the event rate in the treated group were at least double that in the control (again, assuming an observed proportion of 0.20 in the control group). We believe few DSMBs would stomach such a large increase in mortality.

Some DSMBs use a less extreme O'Brien-Fleming-like spending function boundary for safety, say a one-sided 0.05 rather than a one-sided 0.025. Many

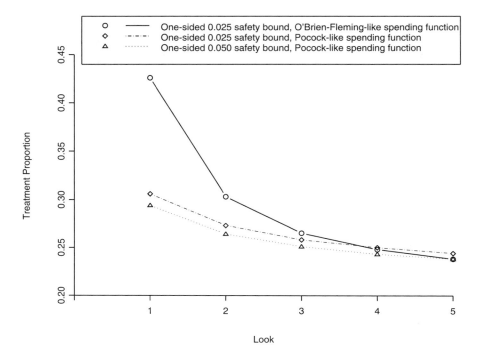

Fig. 9.3. Safety boundaries expressed in terms of the observed treatment proportion if the observed control proportion is 0.20.

use instead a Pocock-like spending function boundary. The advantage of such a boundary in the setting of safety is that it allows earlier termination of the study with a statistically based conclusion of harm. At the first look, an observed rate of 0.306 or 0.294 in the treated group would cross the Pocock 0.025 or 0.05, respectively, one-sided boundary if the observed control rate were 0.20 (Figure 9.3). We believe that a DSMB could feel ethically comfortable with such a boundary early in the study. What leaves us uncomfortable with the Pocock boundary is its persistence at high values toward the end of the study; however, in reality, a DSMB would probably recommend stopping a trial if the z were more than two standard deviations below zero late in the trial.

If an O'Brien-Fleming-like spending function boundary for an adverse event that is life threatening is too conservative early in the trial while a Pocock-like spending function boundary is too conservative late, a boundary that preserves alpha but is somewhat between the two is one that employs a spending function proportional to $t^{1.5}$. For a one-sided 0.05 alpha-level test, the five successive points on the boundary are 2.61, 2.33, 2.14, 1.99, and 1.85 (Figure 9.4).

Because no alpha-preserving boundary has an ideal shape for safety, the sponsor and investigators must be aware that whatever boundary the DSMB agrees to, it may ask the study to pause, it may recommend a change in the informed consent document, or it may recommend stopping the study for harm before the data cross the boundary.

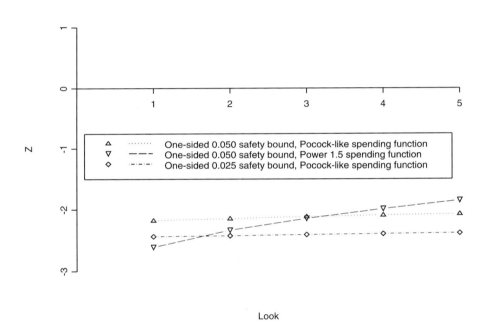

Fig. 9.4. The power spending function $0.05t^{1.5}$ safety boundary compared to the Pocock 0.025 and Pocock 0.05 safety boundaries.

9.5.2 Monitoring for Unexpected Serious Adverse Events that Would Stop a Study

Unknown, but serious, risks that emerge during the course of a study may lead to anxious discussion within the DSMB. If the signal is real, does the possible—as yet undemonstrated—benefit outweigh the risks? Even more troubling are unexpected serious adverse events with dire consequences. For example, in a trial studying a drug to prevent myocardial infarction, a DSMB that observes a small excess of stroke in the treated arm may take immediate action. It may ask for an expert on stroke to join the committee; it may ask for a special data collection instrument to enhance the accuracy of spontaneously reported stroke. Or, if the risk seems unacceptably high compared to the benefit seen or hypothesized in myocardial infarction, it may recommend stopping the trial.

Perhaps the most vexing problem for a DSMB is the observation of an excess rate of an unexpected life-threatening event. Sometimes an event of this type occurs where the relationship to the drug under study is medically not credible, but, if true, devastating. Even a very low rate (a single event, perhaps) of fatal liver failure may lead to stopping the trial. Here judgment of the clinician members of the board often guides decision-making.

Two examples, both somewhat modified from their respective actual trials, point to the problem and provide some suggestions of approaches to dealing with such data. The first comes from an unblinded trial on heart failure testing whether the new treatment decreased mortality relative to standard therapy. Early in the trial, the DSMB observed excess mortality in the treated group. The board, although scheduled to meet every 6 months, asked for a safety update 3 months after its first meeting. At that time, the excess mortality in the treated group had become even more pronounced. Worried lest the unblinded nature of the study might have led the investigators to follow the treated group more intensively and therefore be more quickly aware of the deaths in the treated group, the board asked the investigators to determine the vital status of each participant on a specific date. To preserve the integrity of the study, the board did not describe why it wanted the data—it simply said that responsible monitoring required timely and accurate information on mortality. The investigators then reported many more deaths; in fact, more deaths overall had already occurred in the control than in the treated group. The DSMB, reassured about safety, recommended continuation of the trial. This DSMB had reacted quickly to an apparent risk but it recognized the potential for biased reporting arising from the unblinded nature of the trial. Rather than stop the trial prematurely, it asked for rapid collection of relevant data.

In another example, a DSMB was monitoring a study on quality of life in patients with breast cancer. The treatment was showing clear benefit on symptoms but excess early mortality in the treated group (20 deaths in the treated group and eight in the control group; nominal p-value: .025). The DSMB, recognizing that this difference in mortality could have occurred by chance, asked for more information to help explain the excess mortality. Because the sponsor was unable to give the DSMB the rapid accurate information it required, the DSMB felt it had no choice but to recommend stopping the study.

9.5.3 Monitoring for Adverse Events that the DSMB Should Report

One important role of the DSMB is to report its ongoing findings when the data are strong enough to warrant a change in protocol or a modification in the informed consent document. The threshold differs depending on whether the adverse event is already known and the data suggest that the rate is higher than previously thought or whether the event represents a newly identified risk.

For known risks, the role of safety monitoring is to ensure that during the course of the trial the balance of risk and benefit continues to favor benefit. Even if the known risks are quite serious, the DSMB may recommend continuation of the trial if it is convinced that the participants are being well cared for and that they have been adequately informed of the risks they are incurring. For example, in a trial of cardiovascular disease where the drug under study causes serious bleeding, the DSMB may examine the data to see whether mortality is higher in the treated or the control group and whether the physicians treated the serious bleeds effectively. As long as the excess bleeding does not translate into excess mortality, the DSMB may not ask for any change in protocol or any modification to the process of informed consent. Appealing to statistical significance in this type of situation is rather silly, for the treatment is *known* to cause the events. We have been involved in trials studying drugs with known risk and seen DSMBs not worry about an emerging risk because it was not "statistically significant." Remember that statistical significance is the probability, under the *null* hypothesis, that the observed result or something more extreme would have occurred by chance. If we already know that a treatment causes some adverse event, we do not need to accumulate data to reject an artificial null hypothesis. The reason that statistical thinking was unnecessary in the troglitazone case was that the relationship between the drug and liver failure had already been established in diabetic populations. A single event with laboratory evidence relating the event to the drug confirmed that the event could also occur in individuals at high risk for diabetes.

Lack of statistical evidence of effect within a particular trial in the case of an adverse event known to be related to the activity of the drug is not convincing evidence of no effect; it may simply be the consequence of testing the wrong hypothesis (the null) with inadequate power. We have seen many DSMBs lull themselves into complacency by improperly monitoring against a null hypothesis. The danger is especially important when the event is rare, but serious. Suppose one is studying a drug known to increase the probability of developing a clot and imagine that after 2000 patients have been followed for 3 months, five strokes have occurred in the treatment arm and none in the control. We have seen DSMBs argue as follows: "The two-sided probability of a five to zero split is .06, not even reaching the conventional level of statistical significance. Because we are observing the data on multiple occasions, a difference this large may well occur by chance. Therefore, while we shall continue to monitor stroke, this finding has not raised our level of concern." Instead, we believe that a five to zero split in the situation of a drug *known* to cause clots is strong evidence of harm. Whether the harm is sufficient to lead to action is a different question.

An important role for the statistician on a DSMB is to point to areas where statistical arguments are irrelevant or not particularly useful. For example, heparin is known to cause bleeding. The probability of a major bleed depends on the dose, the medical indication, the individual's condition, and the definition of "major bleed." If a DSMB is monitoring data from a study that is testing heparin, it should start with the knowledge that heparin causes bleeding; the DSMB's goal is not to test that hypothesis, but to estimate the proportion of major bleeds and to establish whether specific subgroups of the population are at unacceptable risk. If the physicians discount data on known adverse events because the excess in the treated group has not yet reached statistical significance, the statistician needs to remind the rest of the board that its role is not to establish whether bleeding is a risk of therapy, but to provide an estimated rate. If that rate is too high, then the board may recommend stopping the study or modifying the protocol.

Boards often find themselves faced with the question of deciding what rate is unacceptably high. If the ongoing data reject the hypothesis that the difference between treated and control is above some "too high" level, then the board may recommend stopping the trial or informing the study leadership of the risk. The methods of this book can apply when the null hypothesis is that the difference between the two groups is Δ; in this case, we reject the hypothesis if the data show a statistically significant difference above Δ. To fix ideas, suppose a study of emergency balloon angioplasty (a method that breaks clots in an artery supplying blood to the heart) is comparing heparin to placebo; the endpoint is the number of meters walked on a treadmill at 6 months (dead people scored as zero). Clinically, the investigators would be comfortable using heparin if the excess number of people experiencing serious bleeds were below, say, 15 percent. The board may establish for itself a guideline that would reject the hypothesis if the data crossed the boundary defined by a null hypothesis of 15 percent. Note that the threshold for an acceptable Δ depends on the efficacy endpoint of the study. If the study were designed to show a decrease in mortality, the investigators might well allow a larger Δ. On the other hand, if the study were to prevent events in a healthy population, the DSMB might select a small Δ.

While arguments from biological plausibility aid in the interpretation of known risks and of risks associated with known mechanisms of action of the drug, observed unexpected events in the treated arm are more difficult to interpret. From a regulatory standpoint, in the United States a sponsor of a clinical trial is required by law to report quickly to the FDA every adverse event that has the three attributes of "serious," "related," and "unanticipated."

"Serious" in the regulatory context usually means that the event led to hospitalization or to an increased length of hospital stay, or that the event was life-threatening or caused death.

"Related" means that the investigator deemed the drug at least probably related to the event (in some settings, the definition is "at least possibly"; sometimes the event must be "definitely" related). While each trial has its own definition of "possibly," "probably," and "definitely" related to study drug, much of the decision is up to the judgment of the investigator. Often, the placebo group has as many "related" events as does the treated group. Investigators tend to classify as "related" an event that is known to be associated with use of the drug. Thus, if a drug is known to cause headache, the investigator will often check "related." On the other hand, if the event is not known to be associated with the use of the drug and it occurs after many months of use, the investigator is unlikely to declare it related. It will appear to the investigator as part of the underlying medical condition of the patient. In particular, heart attacks, strokes, and other major events are often not attributed to the drug, especially in studies that include many elderly participants. For these reasons, in randomized trials, DSMBs usually disregard the attribution of relatedness and consider, instead, the totality of all reported events. It relies on randomization to produce treatment groups at equivalent risk. Therefore, an excess of a particular type of event in the treated arm—whether or not the investigators attributed the event to the treatment—becomes evidence that the treatment is leading to the occurrence of the event.

An "unanticipated" event is one not known to be related either to the process of the disease or to the therapy under study. It is these latter events that the DSMB regards with particular scrutiny because they may lead to a change in protocol or in the informed consent document.

Unanticipated but not serious risks pose uncomfortable questions to the DSMB, but usually a DSMB assumes that the benefits of the drug, while perhaps not yet manifest, will outweigh these risks. Often nonserious adverse events emerge early in the treatment while evidence for benefit occurs later. Suppose, for example, a drug is anticipated to reduce the incidence of myocardial infarction. When patients start taking the drug, many experience some gastrointestinal discomfort. The DSMB may rationally judge that the potential benefit on reduction of risk of heart attack is worth some mild nausea. It may recommend continuing the trial with no change in protocol or it may report nausea as a new adverse event.

In studies of an injected vaccine, adverse events like soreness, headache, sniffles, and fever may frequently occur within a few days of immunization. The effect of the vaccine on preventing disease will not be known for months or even years. The DSMB must make a judgment about the acceptibility of the adverse events under an assumption of the degree of efficacy of the vaccine.

In some special cases a DSMB may recommend early stopping because of an increase in nonserious events. An example, slightly modified from an actual trial, comes from a study of a rapidly fatal neurologic disease that used mortality as its primary endpoint. The DSMB's charter unambiguously specified that it should recommend stopping only for excess mortality in the treated group. After all patients had enrolled and two-thirds of the data were available, the board saw an almost identical proportion of deaths in the two groups (28 percent in the treated group; 29 percent in control). On the other hand, the data were showing an increase in nonserious but bothersome events like "agitation" and "confusion." The board, judging that the balance of risk and benefit no longer favored benefit, recommended stopping the trial. Its thinking stemmed partly from its opinion that the patients did not have long to live. The board could not justify increasing the participants' discomfort in the absence of evidence of benefit. This example points to the inappropriateness of limiting a board's flexibility—if the data are inconsistent with the anticipated scenarios, the board may well ignore its charter, substituting its own judgment to make recommendations.

We have punted the question of what constitutes "statistical significance" in the case of these unanticipated events. Some people use naive uncorrected p-values; some use z-scores; some choose an arbitrary, but low, value (say $p=.01$) as an informal correction for multiplicity. The actual decisions often must rely on medical judgment enhanced by statistical thinking. Lachenbruch and Wittes (2005) [LW05] suggest sentinel event methods for identifying statistical analysis of unexpected adverse events. For individual unexpected serious adverse events, we may consider a) the number of nonevents until the kth event or b) the time until the next (or kth event). For groups of patients in whom the sentinel "event" is an unexpectedly high rate, we can use c) the event rate in the future patients. Various statistical models suggest themselves: for individual events the negative binomial model or a binomial sequential probability ratio test is natural for problem a), while the exponential or gamma distribution is appropriate for problem b). Normal models lend themselves to problem c).

9.6 Looking for Multiple Adverse Events

Sometimes a drug causes not a single adverse event but many. All in all, the patients in the treated group seem to be doing worse than the patients in the control group. Such a finding is hardly surprising, for a drug may have effects on many organs. In a trial of prevention of renal failure in type 2 diabetics, no particular adverse event occurred statistically significantly more frequently in the treated than in the control group, but overall, participants in the treated group experienced more pulmonary, renal, hepatic, and coronary adverse events than did those in the control group. The DSMB informally weighed the overall adverse impact of the drug against the potential gain and, after several years of monitoring, recommended stopping the trial because it judged that a drug that led to so many adverse events would not be useful.

If the adverse events are related to each other, a more formal approach useful in large trials is the method described in the celecoxib example of Section 9.2. Having noted a sentinel event, the DSMB concentrates not on the conventionally presented tables of adverse events, but rather it may create a special targeted hierarchical classification. The pinnacle of the hierarchy is the most specific event, where specificity is defined in terms of biological pathway, seriousness of the event, and low likelihood of misclassification. For the Cox-2 example, cardiovascular death sat at the pinnacle; for thromboembolic events, pulmonary embolism might constitute the pinnacle; for chemotherapy-induced febrile neutropenia, sepsis might serve that role. Let E_1 denote the pinnacle event and suppose there are k events ($A_1 = E_1$, A_2, A_3, ... A_k) within the pathway of interest. Define $E_2 = E_1 \cup A_2$ and, successively, $E_j = E_{j-1} \cup A_j$ ($j = 3, 4, ... k$). Thus each person with a cardiovascular event within the hierarchy enters the pyramid at the highest level consistent with that person's events. Often, the frequency of the event A_j increases as we move down the hierarchy but the relative risk decreases. Thus, in the Cox-2 example where $k = 6$, only six cardiovascular deaths (A_1) occurred, but 12 people had a cardiovascular procedure (A6) as their only cardiovascular event. As one moves down the hierarchy, one adds events that are successively less likely to be related to the putative mechanism of action or that by their nature include events that are likely to be misclassified in a clinical trial. Thus, as one moves down the hierarchy, the power may first increase but then decrease with the addition of more noisy events.

9.7 Summary

The statistical issues posed by monitoring for safety differ considerably from the issues posed by monitoring for efficacy. In the latter case, prior hypotheses govern both the design of the study and the consequent boundaries for monitoring data. For safety monitoring, however, the hypotheses are often data-driven. For anticipated adverse events, the DSMB's role should be to estimate the rates of events with the view to taking some action if they become unacceptably high. For unanticipated events, a DSMB risks reacting to a falsely "discovered" endpoint [MH4], for the event may have occurred in the treatment arm purely by chance. Therefore, DSMBs typically wish to dampen a rush to judgment about the product or intervention. In prevention trials among healthy volunteers or in trials of diseases or conditions not usually accompanied by many types of serious adverse events (e.g., relief of minor headache pain), one analysis might compare the total number of adverse events to a standard rate known from historical data or to the control. Identification of sentinel events during the course of the trial coupled with nimble statistical guidelines for subsequent monitoring afford a DSMB the opportunity to react to unanticipated events at the same time as protecting against overzealous worry.

Especially for safety, purely statistical considerations should not unduly constrain a DSMB. It should not fear what our friend Dr. Rick Ferris terms the "alpha-police." It may recommend termination of a study when no statistical difference in safety can be shown because of the medical implications of an adverse event. On the other hand, it may recommend continuation of a study, even when it is reasonably sure that the experimental treatment is causing serious adverse events, if it believes the benefit outweighs the risk.

10

Bayesian Monitoring

10.1 Introduction

Classical procedures that focus on the type 1 error rate necessarily punish us for taking interim looks at the data; the more we look, the higher the boundaries become. Meier (1975) [M75] puzzled over this: "...it seems hard indeed to accept the notion that I should be influenced in my judgment by how frequently he peeked at the data while he was collecting it." It also seems strange that conclusions should depend on how the data were collected; for example, different p-values will obtain for the same trial results depending on whether the trial was designed for a specified number of patients or a specified number of events. This led Berger and Berry (1988) [BB88] to quip, "Indeed, if the investigator died after reporting the data but before reporting the design of the experiment, it would be impossible to calculate the p-value or other standard measures of evidence." Also, frequentists do not have a universally accepted method of incorporating unplanned data, such as would occur if investigators decided to extend a trial on the basis of promising but not statistically significant results.

Bayesian methodology offers a way of overcoming these obstacles by focusing not on controlling the error rate under a single point null hypothesis $\theta = 0$, but on the trade-off between type 1 and type 2 errors, using prior opinion to help decide how likely each is. A major advantage is that Bayesian monitoring boundaries do not depend at all on how many looks have been taken or how the data were sampled (e.g., whether the trial continued until a fixed number of patients was reached or until a fixed number of events occurred). Bayesian methods also offer a formal way of incorporating information from outside the trial. Their major disadvantage is that they require us to formalize our prior opinion of the treatment effect through a prior distribution, and different priors lead to different conclusions for the same data.

10.2 The Bayesian Paradigm Applied to B-Values

Recall that for many testing scenarios, the B-value $B(t)$ is approximately normally distributed with mean θt and variance t. That is, the conditional distribution of $B(t)$ given the drift parameter θ is normal with mean θt and variance t. We may regard θ as the treatment effect expressed in standardized form.

If we acted like a Bayesian, we would quantify our uncertainty about θ through a probability distribution, the *prior distribution*. We would still regard the treatment effect as a fixed constant; the prior distribution reflects our uncertainty about that fixed constant. Having specified a prior distribution, we update it after observing data. Specifically, we compute the conditional distribution of θ given the observed data, which is called the *posterior distribution* of θ.

The most critical aspect of Bayesian methods is specification of the prior distribution for θ. One mathematically convenient method is to specify a conjugate prior, i.e., a prior distribution resulting in a posterior distribution in the same family. The conjugate family for normally distributed B-values are normal with mean θ_0 and variance σ_0^2. Mathematical convenience is not a compelling reason for choosing a prior, but we shall see that the class of normal priors is sufficiently rich to include a wide spectrum of prior opinion ranging from absolute certainty ($\sigma_0^2 = 0$) to absolute uncertainty ($\sigma_0^2 = \infty$).

As outlined in the discussion of predictive power in Chapter 3, the posterior distribution of θ given the data observed thus far depends only on the current B-value $B(t) = b$. $B(t)$ is normal with posterior mean a weighted combination of the prior estimate θ_0 and the empirical estimate $B(t)/t$:

$$
\begin{aligned}
\mathrm{E}\{\theta \mid B(t) = b\} &= \frac{(1/\sigma_0^2)\theta_0 + [1/\mathrm{var}\{B(t)/t\}](b/t)}{1/\sigma_0^2 + 1/\mathrm{var}\{B(t)/t\}} \\
&= \frac{(1/\sigma_0^2)\theta_0 + t(b/t)}{1/\sigma_0^2 + t} \\
&= \frac{\theta_0 + b\sigma_0^2}{1 + t\sigma_0^2}.
\end{aligned}
\tag{10.1}
$$

The variance of the posterior distribution is

$$
\mathrm{var}\{\theta \mid B(t) = b\} = \frac{\sigma_0^2}{1 + t\sigma_0^2}.
\tag{10.2}
$$

Note that the posterior distribution does not depend on the number or timing of previous looks at the data.

Bayesians tend to emphasize estimation rather than testing a single point null hypothesis $\theta = 0$. They use the posterior distribution to compute a credibility interval for θ. For example, the posterior probability is $1 - \alpha$ that θ lies in the interval

$$\left(\frac{\theta_0 + b\sigma_0^2}{1 + t\sigma_0^2} - z_{\alpha/2}\sqrt{\frac{\sigma_0^2}{1 + t\sigma_0^2}} \, , \; \frac{\theta_0 + b\sigma_0^2}{1 + t\sigma_0^2} + z_{\alpha/2}\sqrt{\frac{\sigma_0^2}{1 + t\sigma_0^2}} \right). \qquad (10.3)$$

A Bayesian might stop at an interim analysis if the credibility interval lies entirely to the right of a "worthwhile" threshold θ_W "which explicitly trades off benefit against possible side effects" (Spiegelhalter and Freedman, 1988 [SF88]); the greater the risk of side effects, the larger θ_W must be to justify using the treatment. Given that regulatory agencies approve or disapprove drugs on the basis of whether the null hypothesis $\theta = 0$ has been rejected in favor of $\theta > 0$, it might also be reasonable to choose $\theta_W = 0$. This was the approach taken in Freedman and Spiegelhalter (1989) [FS89], Grossman, et al. (1994) [GPS94], and Fayers, Ashby, and Parmar (1997) [FAP97]. The resulting stopping boundary for efficacy, obtained by requiring the lower limit of (10.3) to be greater than 0, is

$$\frac{(\theta_0 + b\sigma_0^2)/(1 + t\sigma_0^2)}{\sqrt{\sigma_0^2/(1 + t\sigma_0^2)}} > z_{\alpha/2}.$$

Expressing this boundary in terms of the B-value and z-score yields

$$B(t) > \frac{z_{\alpha/2}\sigma_0\sqrt{1 + t\sigma_0^2} - \theta_0}{\sigma_0^2} \qquad (10.4)$$

$$Z(t) > \frac{z_{\alpha/2}\sigma_0\sqrt{1 + t\sigma_0^2} - \theta_0}{\sigma_0^2\sqrt{t}}. \qquad (10.5)$$

The symmetric boundary for the flip-side of efficacy is obtained by requiring the upper limit of (10.3) to be less than 0, resulting in:

$$B(t) < \frac{-z_{\alpha/2}\sigma_0\sqrt{1 + t\sigma_0^2} - \theta_0}{\sigma_0^2}$$

$$Z(t) < \frac{-z_{\alpha/2}\sigma_0\sqrt{1 + t\sigma_0^2} - \theta_0}{\sigma_0^2\sqrt{t}}.$$

10.3 The Need for a Skeptical Prior

The stopping boundary at the end of the preceding section has a provocative interpretation. Let N be the sample size per arm if the trial is not stopped early. Suppose at an interim analysis we augment our clinical trial data with N/σ_0^2 "imaginary" observations per arm such that the difference between the treatment and control sample means of the imaginary observations is δ_0, where $\delta_0/(2\sigma^2/N)^{1/2} = \theta_0$. The frequentist drift parameter estimate using the actual plus imaginary observations would be (10.1). In the case of known σ^2, adding

N/σ_0^2 imaginary observations to each arm reduces the variance of the drift parameter estimate by a factor of $n/(n + N/\sigma_0^2) = t\sigma_0^2/(1 + t\sigma_0^2)$, where n is the sample size per arm at the interim analysis without including imaginary observations and $t = n/N$. Thus, the variance of the drift parameter estimate using actual plus imaginary observations is

$$\frac{t\sigma_0^2}{1 + t\sigma_0^2}\,\mathrm{var}(B(t)/t) = \frac{\sigma_0^2}{1 + t\sigma_0^2}.$$

The mean and variance of the frequentist drift parameter estimate using actual plus imaginary observations are identical to (10.1) and (10.2). In other words, a frequentist who simply added N/σ_0^2 imaginary observations, computed a z-score, and rejected the null hypothesis if it exceeded $z_{\alpha/2}$ would arrive at exactly the same conclusion as a Bayesian who uses a normal prior with mean θ_0 and variance σ_0^2.

The disturbing connection between Bayesian methodology using the conjugate prior and fabricating data suggests that Bayesian methods are potentially subject to abuse unless a skeptical value is selected for θ_0. An investigator who made up data that supported a treatment benefit would be fired, so trying to accomplish the same end using Bayesian machinery should be strongly discouraged. Selecting $\theta_0 = 0$ avoids this criticism. In effect, we are forcing the results of the clinical trial to overcome a handicap caused by saddling the actual data with imaginary data forced to follow the null hypothesis. Grossman, et al. (1994) [GPS94] point out that this rule is intuitively appealing even without regarding it formally as a Bayesian method. The smaller σ_0^2 is, the larger the handicap.

Choosing a skeptical prior distribution also counters the criticism that Bayesian methods might depend heavily on the prior distribution. We are more confident in our findings if results are promising even assuming a skeptical prior distribution.

When $\theta_0 = 0$, the posterior mean (10.1), credibility interval (10.3), B-value boundary (10.4), and z-score boundary (10.5) reduce to

$$\mathrm{E}(\theta \mid B(t) = b) = \left\{\frac{\sigma_0^2}{\sigma_0^2 + 1/t}\right\}(b/t), \tag{10.6}$$

$$\left(\frac{b\sigma_0^2}{1 + t\sigma_0^2} - z_{\alpha/2}\sqrt{\frac{\sigma_0^2}{1 + t\sigma_0^2}}, \ \frac{b\sigma_0^2}{1 + t\sigma_0^2} + z_{\alpha/2}\sqrt{\frac{\sigma_0^2}{1 + t\sigma_0^2}}\right), \tag{10.7}$$

$$B(t) > \frac{z_{\alpha/2}\sqrt{1 + t\sigma_0^2}}{\sigma_0}, \quad \text{and} \tag{10.8}$$

$$Z(t) > \frac{z_{\alpha/2}\sqrt{1 + t\sigma_0^2}}{\sigma_0\sqrt{t}}. \tag{10.9}$$

Estimator (10.6) shrinks the empirical estimate b/t toward the mean 0 of the prior distribution (Figure 10.1). The degree of shrinkage depends on the variance σ_0^2 of the prior distribution. As $\sigma_0^2 \to 0$, the posterior mean approaches

0 irrespective of the empirical estimate. This makes sense; we choose a very small value for σ_0^2 only if we are very confident that θ is near 0. In that case it takes overwhelming evidence (i.e., a very large value for the empirical estimate b/t) to convince us otherwise. As $\sigma_0^2 \to \infty$, the posterior mean approaches the empirical estimate b/t, and the stopping rule becomes equivalent to rejecting the null hypothesis at an interim analysis if the z-score exceeds $z_{\alpha/2}$. We have seen in Section 4.1 that such a rule causes substantial inflation of the type 1 error rate.

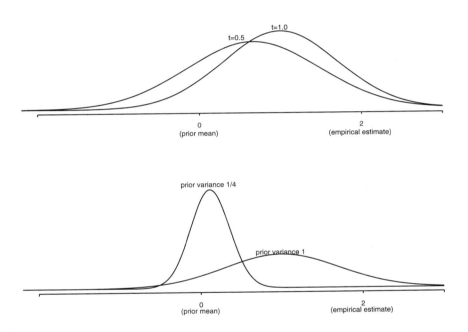

Fig. 10.1. Top panel: The posterior distribution of θ given $B(t)/t = 2$ for $t = 0.5$ and $t = 1$. The prior distribution is standard normal. The posterior mean shrinks the empirical estimate, $B(t)/t = 2$, toward the prior mean 0. The degree of shrinkage is greater earlier in the study ($t = 0.5$) when there is less empirical data to overrule the prior. At the end of the trial ($t = 1.0$) the posterior mean is closer to the empirical estimate and the posterior variance becomes smaller. Bottom panel: The posterior distribution of θ given $B(1)/1 = 2$ for a normal prior with mean 0 and variance $\sigma_0^2 = 1$ or $\sigma_0^2 = 1/4$. Again the posterior mean shrinks the empirical estimate toward the prior mean 0. The degree of shrinkage decreases and the posterior variance increases as the prior variance increases.

A closer look reveals the folly of choosing a huge value of σ_0^2. Though on the surface a diffuse prior seems desirable because it appears to reflect complete uncertainty, it in fact reflects certainty that the treatment effect is either very positive or very negative. That is, as $\sigma_0^2 \to \infty$, the prior probability that $|\theta| \leq B$ tends to 0 for *every* B. How often do we feel that the treatment effect is either extremely large and positive or extremely large and negative, but not moderate?

10.4 A Comparison of Bayesian and Frequentist Boundaries

The preceding section showed that injudicious choice of the prior variance can lead to monitoring boundaries with a very low or very high type 1 error rate. Like Goldilocks, we can select a value of σ_0^2 that is "just right," i.e., has type 1 error rate exactly equal to a desired level. The corresponding boundaries lie between those of Pocock and O'Brien-Fleming (Freedman and Spiegelhalter, 1989 [FS89]; Grossman et al. 1994 [GPS94]). For example, Grossman et al. (1994) [GPS94] express the z-score boundary (10.9) and its symmetric lower boundary in terms of $f = 1/\sigma_0^2$, which they call the *handicap*. The resulting two-tailed boundary is

$$|Z(t)| > z_{\alpha/2} \sqrt{\frac{f+t}{t}}, \tag{10.10}$$

where f is chosen to yield type 1 error rate 0.05 or 0.01 (Table 10.1).

Table 10.1. The handicap $f = 1/\sigma_0^2$ ensuring that the Bayesian two-tailed boundary for equally-spaced looks has type 1 error rate 0.01 or 0.05 (Grossman et al., 1994 [GPS94]).

	Handicap (f)	
k	$\alpha = 0.05$	$\alpha = 0.01$.
1	0	0
2	0.16	0.11
3	0.22	0.15
4	0.25	0.17
5	0.27	0.18
6	0.29	0.20
7	0.30	0.21
8	0.32	0.22
9	0.33	0.22
10	0.33	0.23

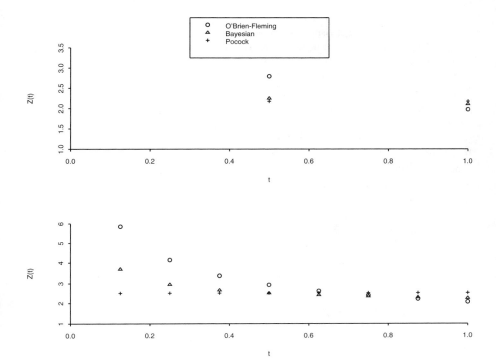

Fig. 10.2. A comparison of Bayesian and frequentist boundaries for a trial with two equally spaced looks (upper panel) and eight equally spaced looks (lower panel). The prior distribution is normal with mean 0 and variance chosen to yield type 1 error rate 0.05.

For example, in a trial with four looks equally spaced in terms of information, selecting $f = 0.25$ and applying boundary (10.10) produces an $\alpha = 0.05$ level procedure. Recall that a normal prior with mean 0 and variance σ_0^2 is like augmenting the trial data with $N/\sigma_0^2 = Nf$ observations such that $\bar{X}_T - \bar{X}_C = 0$. Thus, f may be interpreted as a proportion: $f = 0.25$ is like combining our trial with another trial, one fourth the final size of our trial, with sample mean difference 0.

Figure 10.2 compares Bayesian boundaries with those of O'Brien-Fleming and Pocock for two and eight equally spaced looks. With only two looks, the Bayesian boundary looks very similar to the Pocock boundary. As the number of looks increases, the Bayesian boundary becomes more intermediate between O'Brien-Fleming and Pocock boundaries. As the number of looks tends to infinity, the Bayesian boundary becomes more similar to the O'Brien-Fleming boundary. To see this, note that from (10.10), the boundary for $B(t)$ is $c_t = z_{\alpha/2}(f+t)^{1/2}$. The ratio of B-value boundaries at information fractions

t_1 and t_2 is $c_{t_1}/c_{t_2} = \{(f+t_1)/(f+t_2)\}^{1/2}$. As the number of looks tends to ∞, f tends to ∞ (albeit very slowly) and c_{t_1}/c_{t_2} tends to 1. In other words, the Bayesian boundary approaches a constant boundary for the B-value, which is the O'Brien-Fleming boundary. Still, the convergence is so slow that, from a practical standpoint, the most we can say is that the Bayesian boundary lies between the Pocock and O'Brien-Fleming boundaries, and is closer to the Pocock boundary when the number of looks is quite small.

Some Bayesians might scoff at the idea of choosing σ_0^2 to achieve a given type 1 error rate. After all, narrowly focusing on type 1 error rate is the reason we had to punish ourselves for peeking at data. Moreover, pure Bayesians feel that the prior distribution should reflect actual prior opinion, which has nothing to do with type 1 error rate. Nonetheless, there are advantages of adopting a middle ground between frequentist and Bayesian monitoring. One such middle ground might be to specify initially the number of equally spaced looks we plan to take and select σ_0^2 to yield type 1 error rate 0.05. If the looks turn out not to be equally spaced or we decide to take additional looks, we still use the Bayesian boundary obtained by seeing if the posterior credibility interval lies to the right of 0. This may slightly inflate the type 1 error rate, but this drawback is partially offset by the ease of estimation at the end of the trial; we simply use the posterior credibility interval.

We have thus far considered only the normal prior distribution. Greenhouse and Wasserman (1995) [GW95] investigated how sensitive Bayesian methods are to the prior distribution selected. They considered mixtures of the form $(1 - \epsilon)\pi_0 + \epsilon q$, where π_0 denotes the prior actually selected and q is an arbitrary distribution. They showed that in many cases the conclusions are rather insensitive to the prior.

10.5 Example

This example shows how a non-Bayesian who wishes to avoid the unpleasantries of frequentist inference can use Bayesian methodology to monitor a trial and still protect the type 1 error rate. We warn the reader that pure Bayesians might criticize our mixture of Bayesian and frequentist components (e.g., using a prior distribution to determine boundaries, but then computing conditional, rather than predictive, power).

Consider a trial comparing hormone replacement therapy to placebo with respect to change from baseline to 3 years in minimum lumen diameter of coronary arteries measured on an angiogram. The standard deviation of change is expected to be 0.35 mm, and we are trying to detect a treatment difference of 0.12 mm. Recruitment will occur over the first 3 years, so the first and last woman recruited will have their end of study angiograms 3 and 6 years after the trial begins, respectively. Looks at the primary endpoint are scheduled at the end of years 4, 5, and 6 (the final analysis). Because recruitment is expected to occur uniformly over the first 3 years, the fraction of women with outcome data at analysis i is expected to be $i/3$, $i = 1, 2, 3$.

To monitor using Bayesian boundaries while still paying attention to the type 1 error rate, we specify a normal prior with mean 0 and "handicap" (determined from Table 10.1) $f = 0.22$ (prior variance $\sigma_0^2 = 1/f = 4.55$). From (10.10), the boundaries at the three looks are expected to be $1.96\{(0.22 + 1/3)/(1/3)\}^{1/2} = 2.525$, $1.96\{(0.22+2/3)/(2/3)\}^{1/2} = 2.260$, and $1.96\{(0.22 + 1)/1\}^{1/2} = 2.165$, respectively.

Our first step is to use the software at www.medsch.wisc.edu/landemets/ to compute the required sample size assuming equally spaced looks. We specify that we want to compute the drift parameter, and we enter these boundaries after selecting "User Input" from the "**Power and Bounds Parameters, Determine Bounds**" box. Clicking on "Calculate," we find the drift parameter to be 3.381. Equating the drift parameter $\delta/(2\sigma^2/N)^{1/2}$ to 3.381 and solving yields $N = 2\sigma^2(3.381)^2/\delta^2 = 2(0.35)^2(3.381)^2/(0.12)^2 = 195$. We round up to 200 participants per arm.

Suppose the first analysis occurs after 71 and 68 women are evaluated in the treatment and control arms; i.e., the information fraction is $t = (1/71 + 1/68)^{-1}/(2/200)^{-1} = 0.347$. From (10.10), the boundary at the first look is $1.96\{(0.22 + 0.347)/(0.347)\}^{1/2} = 2.505$. Suppose that the actual z-score is -0.5. We proceed to the next look.

At the second look, with 122 and 120 women per arm, the information fraction is $(1/122 + 1/120)^{-1}/(2/200)^{-1} = 0.605$. From (10.10), the boundary is $1.96\{(0.22 + 0.605)/0.605\}^{1/2} = 2.289$. Suppose the actual z-score is -0.75. At this point it is clear that the expected benefit from hormone replacement therapy has not materialized. The conditional probability that $\theta > 0$ given the observed data can be computed as follows. The current B-value is $(0.605)^{1/2}(-0.75) = -0.583$, so from (10.1) and (10.2), the posterior distribution of θ given $B(0.605) = -0.583$ is normal with mean and variance

$$E\{\theta \mid B(0.605) = -0.583\} = \frac{0 - 0.583(4.55)}{1 + 0.605(4.55)} = -0.707, \tag{10.11}$$

$$\text{var}\{\theta \mid B(0.605) = -0.583\} = \frac{4.55}{1 + 0.605(4.55)} = 1.212. \tag{10.12}$$

The conditional probability that $\theta > 0$ given the observed data is only $1 - \Phi\{(0 + 0.707)/(1.212)^{1/2}\} = 0.26$. Thus, the probability that $\theta > 0$ has dropped from 0.50 at the outset of the trial (because the prior distribution had mean 0) to 0.26 now.

A closet frequentist might also compute conditional power under the original alternative hypothesis to help decide whether continuation is futile. The drift parameter under the original hypothesis is $\theta = 3.381$, and the boundary at the end of the trial will be $1.96\{(0.22 + 1)/1\}^{1/2} = 2.165$, so conditional power given $B(0.605) = -0.583$ is

$$CP_{3.381}(0.605) = 1 - \Phi \left\{ \frac{2.165 - (-0.583) - 3.381(1 - 0.605)}{\sqrt{1 - 0.605}} \right\} = 0.012.$$

Even assuming the original hypothesis, which appears quite optimistic in light of the data, conditional power is about 1 percent. After considering both the posterior probability that $\theta > 0$ and conditional power, the Data and Safety Monitoring Board recommends termination of the trial for futility.

The Bayesian has an easy time estimating the drift parameter following the trial. From (10.11), the posterior mean is -0.707. From (10.7), the credibility interval for $\theta = \delta/(2\sigma^2/200)^{1/2}$ is $(-0.707 - 2.158, -0.707 + 2.158) = (-2.865, 1.451)$. The final step is to express the drift parameter estimate and its credibility interval in terms of the natural parameter δ, the difference in mean baseline to end-of-study changes in the treatment and control arms. Substituting the current pooled estimate of the standard deviation of changes, $\hat{\sigma} = 0.15$, for σ and solving for δ gives

$$\hat{\delta} = (-0.707)\{2(0.15)^2/200\}^{1/2} = -0.011.$$

In other words, the minimum lumen diameter decreased by an estimated 0.011 mm more in the treatment arm than in the control arm. The credibility interval for δ becomes

$$(-2.865\{2(0.15)^2/200\}^{1/2}, 1.451\{2(0.15)^2/200\}^{1/2}) = (-0.043, 0.022).$$

10.6 Summary

Bayesian monitoring of clinical trials has advantages and disadvantages over classical monitoring. The boundaries depend only on the current data, not on how many looks have been taken or how the data arose. The Bayesian approach also provides a natural way to incorporate external data; point and interval estimation following the trial are easy and natural. By far the biggest disadvantage is the dependence of conclusions on the prior distribution selected. The Data and Safety Monitoring Board may choose a prior different from what most practicing physicians might chose, and therefore might stop the trial when the data would not convince most physicians. Choosing a prior distribution that puts high probability on the alternative hypothesis creates a self-fulfilling prophecy, i.e., one is likely to conclude there is a treatment effect even if there is none. That is why it is wise to choose a skeptical prior with mean 0.

An appealing option is to choose a normal prior with mean 0 and variance selected to yield an alpha level procedure if the originally planned number and spacings of the looks is maintained. This produces a boundary intermediate between the Pocock and O'Brien-Fleming boundaries. If the originally scheduled looks are altered, the procedure will have type 1 error rate close to the target level unless the number of looks is increased dramatically or the spacings are markedly different from those originally anticipated.

11

Adaptive Sample Size Methods

11.1 Introduction

Thus far we have focused on clinical trials with either a fixed number of patients or a fixed number of events at the end, but recent advances have spawned the development of methods for changing the sample size on the basis of accumulating data. These so-called *adaptive* methods allow greater flexibility than group-sequential monitoring with a fixed maximum sample size. The idea is simple: the parameters needed for calculating sample size are better estimated from a subset of the data from the current trial than from observational data or from other trials enrolling less similar patients.

Adaptive methods are of two very different types: those incorporating data about a nuisance parameter only (such as the variance in a continuous outcome setting or the control event probability or overall event probability in a dichotomous outcome setting) and those also incorporating data about the treatment effect. Accurate estimation of nuisance parameters is crucial lest the sample size be too large or too small. For example, if the true standard deviation is 20 percent larger than anticipated, the sample size for a two-tailed t-test with 90 percent power must be increased by 44 percent. Similarly, in a dichotomous outcome trial, overestimation of the control event rate in a trial powered to detect a fixed relative risk produces an underpowered trial. The role of the treatment effect in sample size calculations differs from that of the nuisance parameter; accurate *estimation* of the treatment effect is less important than appropriate *specification* of the treatment effect based partly on clinical relevance and partly on results from similar trials. For example, it may be that, unbeknownst to us, the true systolic blood pressure lowering effect of a drug is only 1 mm Hg, yet no one would power a drug trial to detect such a clinically insignificant blood pressure reduction. One might instead assume the smallest clinically relevant difference—perhaps 3 or 4 mm Hg—that would justify the use of medication. On the other hand, if other trials or other evidence led us to believe that the true effect was likely to be at least 10 mm Hg, we would probably not power the trial using the minimal clinically relevant difference because that would result in a sample size much larger than needed.

In this book we focus more on sample size modification based on a nuisance parameter rather than on the treatment effect for two primary reasons. First, we would ordinarily not undertake a clinical trial if we could not specify either a minimally relevant or an expected treatment difference. Second, adaptive methods based on the treatment effect are much more controversial than those based on a nuisance parameter. Criticisms have focused on both specific methodology and larger issues such as the necessity of unblinding and its potential bias, and the possibility of increasing the sample size to detect clinically meaningless differences. Nonetheless, in trials designed with only very limited information about the treatment effect, some allowance for sample size modification is desirable.

Before proceeding, we shall use a different notational convention than what we have followed thus far. In previous chapters, we have used $n_1, \ldots, n_k$ and $Z_1, \ldots, Z_k$ to denote cumulative sample sizes and z-scores. In this chapter, unless otherwise stated, these stand for stagewise quantities. Thus, n_i and Z_i are the sample size per arm and z-score corresponding to the data in stage i only. We use no subscript when we refer to a quantity computed over the entire trial. Thus, n and Z refer to the sample size per arm and z-score for all data in the trial.

11.2 Methods Using Nuisance Parameter Estimates: The Continuous Outcome Case

We closely follow the review paper of Proschan (2005) [Pr05].

The approximate sample size formula to achieve power $1 - \beta$ to detect a mean difference δ using a two-tailed t-test at level α was obtained in Chapter 3 by equating the expected z-score to $z_{\alpha/2} + z_\beta$ and solving for the per-arm sample size n:

$$n = \frac{2\sigma^2(z_{\alpha/2} + z_\beta)^2}{\delta^2}. \tag{11.1}$$

We now consider two-stage methods where we use the first stage to estimate σ^2, and apply that estimate to determine the total sample size.

A central question is whether the first stage variance estimate gives any information about the current or future treatment effect estimate. Intuition suggests that it does not because in a one-sample setting with normally distributed observations $X_1, \ldots, X_n$, the sample mean and variance are independent (Mood, Graybill, and Boes, 1974 [MGB74], page 243). Logically, a future sample mean should likewise be independent of the current sample variance. An indirect way to see this uses Basu's theorem; for normally distributed data $X_1, \ldots, X_{n+r}$ with known variance, $\bar{X}_{n+r}$ is complete and sufficient, while s_n^2 is ancillary with respect to μ, so $\bar{X}_{n+r}$ and s_n^2 are independent. A more direct proof uses the fact that $(\bar{X}_{n+r}, X_1 - \bar{X}_n, \ldots, X_n - \bar{X}_n)$ are jointly multivariate normal with $\mathrm{cov}(\bar{X}_{n+r}, X_i - \bar{X}_n) = 0$ for each i, so $\bar{X}_{n+r}$ is independent of $(X_1 - \bar{X}_n, \ldots, X_n - \bar{X}_n)$, and therefore of any function (e.g., the sample variance) of the latter set. In fact, a similar approach shows that the set of all past and present sample variances is independent of the set of all present and future treatment effect estimates. A similar result holds in the two-sample setting:

Result 11.1

a) In a one-sample setting, the set of past and present cumulative variances $(s_2^2, \ldots, s_n^2)$ is independent of the set of present and future cumulative sample means $(\bar{X}_n, \bar{X}_{n+1}, \ldots)$ and cumulative z-scores $(n^{1/2}\bar{X}_n/\sigma, (n+1)^{1/2}\bar{X}_{n+1}/\sigma, \ldots)$.

b) In a two-sample setting, the set of past and present cumulative pooled variances is independent of the set of present and future cumulative treatment effect estimates and cumulative z-scores.

Result 11.1 is comforting because it shows that peeking at sample variances gives no information about the current or future treatment effect. It suggests that we may be able to analyze the data at the end of an adaptive trial as if the sample size had been fixed in advance.

11.2.1 Stein's Method

Stein (1945) [S45] devised a two-stage procedure to construct a t-test in a one-sample setting with power at least a specified value irrespective of the true variance. We devote considerable attention to his method because the way he achieved this remarkable feat is instructive. We can apply his method in a two-sample clinical trial as follows. At the first stage with n_1 participants per arm, we calculate the pooled variance s_1^2 with $2(n_1 - 1)$ degrees of freedom. Wittes and Brittain (1990) [WB90] called the first stage of a two-stage design an *internal pilot study*. Let $t_{a,m}$ denote the upper ath quantile of a t-distribution with m degrees of freedom. For power $1 - \beta$, we determine the final sample size n per arm using Equation (11.1) but replace σ^2 by s_1^2 and the standard normal critical points by those of a t-distribution with $2(n_1 - 1)$ degrees of freedom. If the resulting sample size is smaller than n_1, we take no additional observations. Thus, the final sample size per arm is

$$n = \max\{n_1, 2s_1^2(t_{\alpha/2,2(n_1-1)} + t_{\beta,2(n_1-1)})^2/\delta^2\}. \tag{11.2}$$

After randomizing $n_2 = n - n_1$ additional patients per arm, we compute the Stein t-statistic t_S:

$$t_S = \frac{\bar{X}_T - \bar{X}_C}{\sqrt{2s_1^2/n}}, \tag{11.3}$$

where $\bar{X}_T$ and $\bar{X}_C$ are the sample means of all n patients per arm. (If the treatment and control internal pilot sample sizes n_{T1} and n_{C1} differ, replace

$2s_1^2/n$ in the denominator of (11.3) with $s_1^2(1/n_{T1} + 1/n_{C1})$, and use $n_{C1} + n_{T1} - 2$ degrees of freedom instead of $2(n_1 - 1)$ in (11.2). Notice that the pooled variance estimate s_1^2 in the denominator is that of the internal pilot study only. We shall soon see that this crucial difference between the Stein and usual t-statistics is what allows us to achieve any given power irrespective of the true variance σ^2.

We know that in a nonadaptive setting, the numerator and denominator of the t-statistic are independent; we now show that independence holds for T_S in the adaptive setting as well. For added clarity, we write $\bar{X}_{Tn}$ and $\bar{X}_{Cn}$ to emphasize the per-arm sample sizes upon which they are based.

$$
\begin{aligned}
\Pr\left(\frac{\bar{X}_{Tn} - \bar{X}_{Cn}}{\sqrt{2\sigma^2/n}} \le z, s_1^2 \le u\right) &= \sum_{r=n_1}^{\infty} \Pr\left(\frac{\bar{X}_{Tn} - \bar{X}_{Cn}}{\sqrt{2\sigma^2/n}} \le z, s_1^2 \le u, n = r\right) \\
&= \sum_{r=n_1}^{\infty} \Pr\left(\frac{\bar{X}_{Tr} - \bar{X}_{Cr}}{\sqrt{2\sigma^2/r}} \le z, s_1^2 \le u, n = r\right) \\
&= \sum_{r=n_1}^{\infty} \Pr\left(\frac{\bar{X}_{Tr} - \bar{X}_{Cr}}{\sqrt{2\sigma^2/r}} \le z\right)\Pr(s_1^2 \le u, n = r) \\
&= \Phi(z) \sum_{r=n_1}^{\infty} \Pr(s_1^2 \le u, n = r) \\
&= \Phi(z)\Pr(s_1^2 \le u).
\end{aligned}
$$

The third line follows from Result 11.1. Because the joint distribution of $(\bar{X}_{Tn} - \bar{X}_{Cn})/(2\sigma^2/n)^{1/2}$ and s_1^2 factors into the product of the marginal distributions, they are independent. Also, the null distributions of Z and $2(n_1 - 1)s_1^2/\sigma^2$ are standard normal and chi-squared with $2(n_1 - 1)$ degrees of freedom, respectively. Thus, the null distribution of t_S is t with $2(n_1 - 1)$ degrees of freedom.

To show that we can obtain power $1 - \beta$ irrespective of σ^2, we need to consider the distribution of t_S under the alternative hypothesis, $\mu_T - \mu_C = \delta$. Subtract μ_T and μ_C from the infinite pool of potential treatment and control observations, respectively, and apply Stein's t-test to the transformed data set $(\underline{X}_T', \underline{X}_C')$. Denote the t-statistic applied to the transformed data by t_S'. The numerator of t_S' is $\bar{X}_T - \bar{X}_C - \delta$, where $\bar{X}_T$ and $\bar{X}_C$ are the sample means of the untransformed data. The pooled variance of the transformed data is that of the untransformed data because the sample variance in each arm is unaffected by location shifts. Thus, $t_S' = (\bar{X}_T - \bar{X}_C - \delta)/(2s_1^2/n)^{1/2} = t_S - \delta/(2s_1^2/n)^{1/2}$. Because the transformed data have equal population means (both are 0) in the treatment and control arms, t_S' has a t-distribution with $2(n_1 - 1)$ degrees of freedom. Power is

$$
P_{\mu_C,\mu_T}(t_S > t_{\alpha/2,2(n_1-1)}) = P_{\mu_C,\mu_T}\left\{t_S - \frac{\delta}{\sqrt{2s_1^2/n}} > t_{\alpha/2,2(n_1-1)} - \frac{\delta}{\sqrt{2s_1^2/n}}\right\}
$$

$$= P_{\mu_C,\mu_T} \left\{ t'_S > t_{\alpha/2,2(n_1-1)} - \frac{\delta}{\sqrt{2s_1^2/n}} \right\}$$

$$\geq P_{\mu_C,\mu_T}(t'_S > -t_{\beta,2(n_1-1)})$$
$$= P_{0,0}(t_S > -t_{\beta,2(n_1-1)}) = 1 - \beta. \tag{11.4}$$

The inequality in the second to last line follows from the fact $\delta/(2s_1^2/n)^{1/2} \geq t_{\alpha/2,2(n_1-1)} + t_{\beta,2(n_1-1)}$ [see Equation (11.2)]. This remarkable result means that power is at least $1 - \beta$ irrespective of the true variance σ^2.

A slight modification of Stein's procedure allows one to obtain confidence intevals of a given length, again using the pivotal fact that after the first stage, s_1^2 is fixed. The above argument that t'_S has a t-distribution with $2(n_1 - 1)$ degrees of freedom is valid for any sample size rule $n(s_1^2)$ based on the variance, not just the one defined by (11.2). It follows that

$$\bar{X}_T - \bar{X}_C \pm t_{\alpha/2,2(n_1-1)} \sqrt{2s_1^2/n} \tag{11.5}$$

provides a $100(1 - \alpha)$ percent confidence interval for δ for any sample size function $n(s_1^2)$ based on the variance. We can therefore select n to make the half-width of the confidence interval (11.5) any desired value. We simply equate $t_{\alpha/2,2(n_1-1)}(2s_1^2/n)^{1/2}$ to a desired width w and solve for n, which yields $n = 2t_{\alpha/2,2(n_1-1)}^2 s_1^2/w^2$.

Example 11.1. Consider a trial comparing glucosamine to placebo for the relief of pain in patients with osteoarthritis of the knee. The primary outcome is the change from baseline to 6 months in a visual analog scale (VAS) reflecting pain; patients indicate their degree of pain on a scale from 0 (no pain) to 100 (worst possible pain). A t-test is used to compare the treatment arms. Suppose that prior to the trial, little is known about the standard deviation of such changes. The best guess is that it should be 15 or less. Investigators wish to detect a difference of 5 points between the treatment arms. The sample size for 80 percent power to detect a 5-point decrease in VAS score in the glucosamine arm compared to placebo is approximately $2(15)^2(1.96 + .84)^2/5^2 = 142$ per arm (rounding up). An internal pilot study is conducted at the planned halfway point, and the pooled variance of the 70 control and 72 glucosamine patients is $s_1^2 = 144$. The estimated standard deviation of $(144)^{1/2} = 12$ is smaller than the initial estimate of 15, giving us hope of decreasing the sample size. To use (11.2), we must compute the tail points $t_{0.025,140}$ and $t_{0.20,140}$ of the t-distribution with $70 + 72 - 2 = 140$ degrees of freedom; $t_{0.025,140} = 1.977$ and $t_{0.20,140} = 0.844$. The resulting calculated sample size per arm is $2(12)^2(1.977 + 0.844)^2/5^2 = 92$. Thus, we need 22 more control and 20 more glucosamine patients. Of course, it is often difficult to recruit precisely the number of participants required. Suppose in this case the final sample size turns out to be slightly larger, 95 and 94 patients in the placebo and glucosamine arms. The means and pooled variance at the end of the trial are $\bar{X}_T = -3$, $\bar{X}_C = +1$, and $s^2 = 174$, so the standard deviation estimate at the end of the trial is $(174)^{1/2} = 13.191$. The data from this trial are summarized in Table 11.1. Even though the pooled standard deviation of the 95 control and 94 glucosamine patients is 13.191, Stein's t-statistic uses the interim standard deviation estimate $s_1 = 12$:

$$t_S = \frac{-3 - 1}{\sqrt{12^2(1/95 + 1/94)}} = -2.291.$$

By referring -2.291 to a t-distribution with $70 + 72 - 2 = 140$ degrees of freedom corresponding to the interim variance, we calculate $p = 0.023$.

Table 11.1. Summary of data from the example.

	Control	Glucosamine
Interim	$n_{C1} = 70$	$n_{T1} = 72$
	$s_1 = 12$	
End	$n_C = 95$	$n_T = 94$
	$\bar{X}_C = +1$	$\bar{X}_T = -3$
	$s = 13.191$	

Suppose that at stage 1 we had selected n not on the basis of achieving a given power, but on the basis of obtaining a confidence interval with half width no larger than 3. The confidence interval at the end of the trial is given by equation (11.5) with $2(n_1 - 1)$ replaced by $72 + 70 - 2 = 140$:

$$\bar{X}_T - \bar{X}_C \pm 1.977\{2(144)/n\}^{1/2}. \tag{11.6}$$

Equating the half width $1.977\{2(144)/n\}^{1/2}$ to 3 and solving for n yields $(1.977)^2\{2(144)\}/3^2 = 126$. Thus, we would need 126 patients per arm. The final confidence interval would again use (11.6) (i.e., 1.977 standard errors corresponding to a t with 140 degrees of freedom) even though the total sample size is $2(126) = 252$.

Stein's method is seldom used in clinical trials for several reasons. First is the perceived inefficiency and undesirability of not using all of the data to estimate the variance. Second is the fact that the variance might actually change over the course of the trial. Patients may initially be plentiful and later sparse; patients may have to be recruited from different sources later in the trial, and they might have a different variance. In this setting, using the first stage variance can be anticonservative and increase the type 1 error rate (Proschan and Wittes, 2000 [PW00]). A third criticism is that Stein's method controls the type 1 error rate unconditionally, but not conditioned on the sample size actually selected (Zucker et al., 1999 [ZWS99]). The final sample size is independent of the treatment effect, so it is almost as if the sample size had been determined by a completely random mechanism such as a coin flip, in which case we would make inferences conditional on the sample size actually selected. But the conditional distribution of t_S given $N = n$ is no longer t with $2(n_1 - 1)$ degrees of freedom.

To elaborate on the conditional type 1 error rate of Stein's t-test, let $\sigma = 1$, and suppose that we are trying to detect a treatment effect of $\delta = 1$ with 80 percent power. Suppose also that the first-stage sample size is only 5 per arm; $t_{0.025,8} = 2.306$ and $t_{0.20,8} = 0.889$. If $2s_1^2(2.306 + 0.889)^2/1^2 \leq 5$, then (11.2) implies that we require no additional observations. Thus, if $s_1 \leq [5/\{2(3.195)^2\}]^{1/2} = 0.495$, we will not take any additional observations. The resulting Stein t-statistic has *unconditional* type 1 error rate 0.05, but the *conditional* type 1 error rate given that $n = 5$ is

$$\Pr\left(|\hat{\delta}_1| > 2.306\sqrt{\frac{2s_1^2}{5}} \;\middle|\; s_1 \leq .495\right) \geq \Pr\left(|\hat{\delta}_1| > 2.306\sqrt{\frac{2(.495)^2}{5}} \;\middle|\; s_1 \leq .495\right)$$

$$= \Pr\left(\frac{|\hat{\delta}_1|}{\sqrt{2/5}} > 2.306(0.495)\right)$$

$$= 2\{1 - \Phi(1.141)\} = 0.25.$$

It is of little consolation that the type 1 error rate averaged over all possible sample sizes is 0.05 if the type 1 error rate given the sample size actually selected is 0.25. The problem is ameliorated if we use restricted designs with sample size at least as large as originally planned (Wittes et al., 1999 [WSZ99]).

11.2.2 The Naive t-Test

A more natural procedure is to compute the usual pooled t-statistic and refer it to a t-distribution with $2n - 2$ degrees of freedom as if n had been determined before the trial. Thus, in Example 11.1, the final t-statistic would be $t = (-3-1)/\{(13.191)^2(1/95+1/94)\}^{1/2} = -2.084$, and we would refer this value to a t-distribution with $95 + 94 - 2 = 187$ degrees of freedom; the two-tailed p-value would be .039. Wittes and Brittain (1990) [WB90] proposed this "naive" t-statistic. Its advantage is that it uses all of the data for the variance estimate. Its disadvantage is that it uses all of the data for the variance estimate! That is, unlike with Stein's method, the final variance of the naive method cannot be predicted perfectly at the first stage, so there is no way to guarantee a given power level. Still, several papers have shown that this naive method controls type 1 and type 2 error rates near the desired levels. Wittes and Brittain (1990) [WB90] evaluated error rates by simulation in the context of an example. They considered *restricted designs* with final sample size at least as great as originally planned. Birkett and Day (1994) [BD94] extended this work by allowing an unrestricted design. Numerical integration confirms that error rates are close to target levels (Wittes et al., 1999 [WSZ99]).

A closer inspection of the naive method is revealing. It is not difficult to show that under the null hypothesis, $\hat{\delta}/\sqrt{2\sigma^2/n}$ has a standard normal distribution and is independent of the pooled variance s^2 of all $2n$ observations. Thus, if $(2n-2)s^2/\sigma^2$ had a chi-squared distribution with $2n-2$ degrees of freedom, the naive t-statistic would have a t-distribution with $2n-2$ degrees of freedom. But if $(2n-2)s^2/\sigma^2$ really were chi-squared with $2n-2$ degrees of freedom, then s^2 would be an unbiased estimate of σ^2. On the contrary, s^2 tends to underestimate σ^2. A rigorous proof may be found in Wittes et al. (1999) [WSZ99] or Proschan (2005) [Pr05]. Here we give the following heuristic argument. Consider a simpler adaptive sample size setting in which we choose from only two possible sample sizes, either $n = n_1$ per arm or $n = 2n_1$ per arm. Denote the pooled variance under these two scenarios by $\hat{\sigma}_1^2$ and $\hat{\sigma}_2^2$, respectively. Of course $\hat{\sigma}_1^2$ is the first-stage pooled variance. Both $\hat{\sigma}_1^2$ and $\hat{\sigma}_2^2$ are unbiased for σ^2, but $\hat{\sigma}_1^2$ is used to determine whether we choose $\hat{\sigma}_1^2$ or $\hat{\sigma}_2^2$; if $\hat{\sigma}_1^2$ is small, we choose it, but if $\hat{\sigma}_1^2$ is large, we dilute it with more observations, resulting in $\hat{\sigma}_2^2$. Clearly, this process will tend to underestimate σ^2. Nonetheless, Wittes et al. (1999) [WSZ99] showed that the bias is small and the type 1 error rate and power are quite close to the target values under both restricted and unrestricted designs. See Tables 11.2-11.4.

11.2.3 A Restricted t-Test

Proschan and Wittes (2000) [PW00] considered restricted designs requiring the final sample size per arm to be at least as large as initially planned, n_0. The idea is that, because the second stage will have at least $n_0 - n_1$ observations per arm, we could randomly select $n_0 - n_1$ second-stage observations per arm to include in the final variance estimate. That way, the final variance estimate will be unbiased and should be more accurate than s_1^2. Furthermore, the resulting t-statistic will have an exact t-distribution with $2n_0 - 2$ degrees of freedom under the null hypothesis. But of course different selections of the $n_0 - n_1$ second-stage observations per arm could result in different inferences. Proschan and Wittes (2000) [PW00] essentially averaged over all possible random selections of $n_0 - n_1$ observations per arm from the second stage, resulting in the variance estimate

$$\tilde{\sigma}^2 = \left(\frac{n_1 - 1}{n_0 - 1}\right) s_1^2 + \left(\frac{n_0 - n_1}{n_0 - 1}\right) \left\{\frac{(n-1)s^2 - (n_1 - 1)s_1^2}{n - n_1}\right\}.$$

They showed that referring their t-statistic to a t-distribution with $2n_0 - 2$ degrees of freedom is more robust than Stein's method to drifts over time in the population variance. They also proved that the type 1 error rate is no greater than α.

Had we used the restricted test in Example 11.1, we would have continued to 142 per arm instead of reducing the sample size. Suppose that with $n = 142/\text{arm}$, the pooled standard variance had been 169. We use the average first stage sample size $(70 + 72)/2 = 71$ for n_1 in the calculation of $\tilde{\sigma}^2$

Table 11.2. Type 1 error rate of the naive, nominal 0.05 level t-test for a restricted design with sample size recalculation after fraction π (n_1 observations per arm) of the originally planned sample size. The original sample size yields 90 percent power to detect an effect size of $e_0 = \delta/\sigma_0$, where δ is the treatment effect and σ_0 is the guessed value of the standard deviation σ (Wittes et al., 1999 [WSZ99]).

$1/e_0^2$	π	n_1	$\tau^2 = \sigma_0^2/\sigma^2$				
			.25	.50	1	2	4
1	.10	3	.0528	.0522	.0514	.0503	.0500
1	.25	6	.0518	.0528	.0515	.0501	.0500
1	.50	11	.0517	.0532	.0515	.0500	.0500
1	.75	17	.0516	.0533	.0514	.0500	.0500
1	.90	20	.0517	.0532	.0503	.0499	.0499
2	.10	5	.0497	.0512	.0508	.0501	.0500
2	.25	11	.0508	.0515	.0509	.0500	.0500
2	.50	22	.0507	.0515	.0509	.0500	.0500
2	.75	33	.0507	.0515	.0508	.0500	.0500
2	.90	39	.0504	.0519	.0513	.0493	.0502
5	.10	11	.0511	.0507	.0504	.0500	.0500
5	.25	27	.0504	.0506	.0504	.0500	.0500
5	.50	53	.0503	.0506	.0504	.0500	.0500
5	.75	80	.0503	.0506	.0504	.0500	.0500
5	.90	96	.0514	.0511	.0506	.0505	.0497
10	.10	22	.0516	.0505	.0502	.0500	.0496
10	.25	53	.0499	.0503	.0502	.0500	.0499
10	.50	106	.0502	.0503	.0502	.0500	.0500
10	.75	159	.0500	.0503	.0502	.0500	.0499
10	.90	190	.0512	.0504	.0497	.0504	.0492

$$\tilde{\sigma}^2 = \left(\frac{71-1}{142-1}\right)(12^2) + \left(\frac{142-71}{142-1}\right)\left\{\frac{(142-1)(13)^2 - (71-1)(12)^2}{142-71}\right\}$$
$$= 71.4894 + 97.5106 = 169 = s^2.$$

Not surprisingly, because the sample size did not change from the original plan, the restricted variance estimate is the usual pooled variance. Thus, the t-test at the end of the trial is identical to the fixed sample t-test with 142/arm. This would not have been the case had we increased the sample size.

11.2.4 Variance Shmariance?

Other variance estimates have also been proposed (Kieser and Friede, 2000 [KF00]), but does it really matter which variance is used? Results of Zucker

Table 11.3. Type 1 error rate of the naive, nominal 0.05 level t-test for an unrestricted design with sample size recalculation after fraction π (n_1 observations per arm) of the originally planned sample size. The original sample size yields 90 percent power to detect an effect size of $e_0 = \delta/\sigma_0$, where δ is the treatment effect and σ_0 is the guessed value of the standard deviation σ (Wittes et al., 1999 [WSZ99]).

$1/e_0^2$	π	n_1	$\tau^2 = \sigma_0^2/\sigma^2$				
			.25	.50	1	2	4
1	.10	3	.0551	.0604	.0714	.0790	.0690
1	.25	6	.0520	.0547	.0607	.0625	.0527
1	.50	11	.0517	.0537	.0572	.0523	.0500
1	.75	17	.0516	.0535	.0540	.0500	.0500
1	.90	20	.0517	.0533	.0520	.0495	.0505
2	.10	5	.0510	.0522	.0551	.0615	.0665
2	.25	11	.0508	.0517	.0537	.0567	.0523
2	.50	22	.0507	.0516	.0533	.0510	.0500
2	.75	33	.0507	.0515	.0524	.0500	.0500
2	.90	39	.0504	.0519	.0520	.0505	.0500
5	.10	11	.0503	.0506	.0513	.0528	.0565
5	.25	27	.0503	.0506	.0512	.0519	.0511
5	.50	53	.0503	.0506	.0512	.0496	.0500
5	.75	80	.0503	.0506	.0510	.0500	.0500
5	.90	96	.0514	.0511	.0503	.0505	.0501
10	.10	22	.0501	.0503	.0506	.0512	.0527
10	.25	53	.0501	.0503	.0506	.0511	.0506
10	.50	106	.0502	.0503	.0506	.0485	.0500
10	.75	159	.0500	.0503	.0505	.0500	.0500
10	.90	190	.0512	.0504	.0503	.0515	.0496

et al. (1999) [ZWS99] show that in terms of unconditional type 1 error rate and power, the original Stein procedure does at least as well as more contemporary variants. They compared the naive t-test to the following hypothetical procedure: at the end of the trial God reveals the population variance, σ^2, and we mortals use it to form the z-score $Z = (\bar{X}_T - \bar{X}_C)/(2\sigma^2/n)^{1/2}$. That z-score has a standard normal distribution under the null hypothesis. Stein's test outpowered the hypothetical z-test in most of the scenarios considered! In other words, it was better from a power standpoint to use the first-stage variance than the population variance. This confirms our earlier observation that a *dis*advantage of the naive test is that it uses more data than Stein's to estimate the variance; using more data makes the final variance less predictable. Even if the Stein variance estimate is inaccurate, it is 100 percent predictable after the first stage, ensuring the desired level of power or greater

Table 11.4. Power for the naive t-tests described in Tables 11.2 and 11.3 (Wittes et al., 1999 [WSZ99]).

Design	$1/e_0^2$	$\tau^2 = \sigma_0^2/\sigma^2$	π				
			.10	.25	050	.75	.90
Restricted	1	.25	.79	.84	.87	.88	.89
		.50	.83	.86	.88	.89	.89
		1	.93	.93	.93	.94	.94
		2	1	1	1	1	1
		4	1	1	1	1	1
Unrestricted	1	.25	.77	.84	.87	.88	.89
		.50	.78	.85	.88	.89	.89
		1	.80	.86	.89	.90	.91
		2	.81	.87	.92	.98	.99
		4	.85	.93	.99	1	1
Restricted	10	.25	.90	.89	.90	.90	.90
		.50	.89	.89	.90	.90	.90
		1	.92	.91	.91	.91	.91
		2	1	1	1	1	1
		4	.99	1	1	1	1
Unrestricted	10	.25	.88	.89	.90	.90	.90
		.50	.88	.89	.90	.90	.90
		1	.88	.89	.90	.90	.90
		2	.89	.90	.87	.98	.99
		4	.89	.91	1	1	1

by (11.4). Zucker et al. (1999) [ZWS99] show by simulation that the naive t-test lies between Stein's t and the hypothetical z-test, and often is closer to the hypothetical z-test.

The strongest argument against Stein's method is that the population standard deviation could change over the course of the trial because earlier patients might differ from later ones. The variance estimate of the naive t-test is more robust; if the second-stage variance estimate is larger than the first, the naive variance will essentially be a weighted average of the two variances, with weights proportional to the sample sizes of the two stages. Stein's t-test will use an anticonservative variance that results in inflation of the type 1 error rate (Proschan and Wittes, 2000 [PW00]).

11.2.5 Incorporating Monitoring

We next consider incorporating both sample size modification and monitoring. The simplest way is to monitor only after modifying the sample size. Suppose we reassess the sample size after $n_1 = n_0/2$ observations per arm, where n_0 is the originally planned, per-arm sample size. We determine a new sample size $n(s_1^2)$ based on the pooled variance. A simple modification of Stein's procedure is to use the internal pilot variance estimate s_1^2 in all future t-scores (Denne and Jennison 2000 [DJ00]). The t-score at the end of the trial is $Y/(s_1^2/\sigma^2)^{1/2}$, where $Y = (\bar{X}_T - \bar{X}_C)/(2\sigma^2/n)^{1/2}$ is the z-statistic using the population variance in the denominator. Similarly, we may write the t-statistics at looks $1, \ldots, k$ as $(Y_1, \ldots, Y_k)/(s_1^2/\sigma^2)^{1/2}$, where Y_i is the z-statistic on all data up to and including look i. By Result 11.1, the vector $(Y_1, \ldots, Y_k)$ is independent of s_1^2. Thus, the conditional distribution function of $(Y_1, \ldots, Y_k)$ given s_1^2 is its unconditional distribution function $F(y_1, \ldots, y_k)$, which is that of $B(t_1)/t_1^{1/2}, \ldots, B(t_k)/t_k^{1/2}$. That is, $F(y_1, \ldots, y_k)$ is multivariate normal with zero mean vector and correlation matrix $\mathrm{cov}(Y_i, Y_j) = (t_i/t_j)^{1/2}$. Also, $2(n_1-1)s_1^2/\sigma^2$ has a chi-square distribution $G_{2(n_1-1)}(x)$ with $2(n_1-1)$ degrees of freedom. The distribution of the cumulative t-statistics is therefore

$$\Pr\{(Y_1, \ldots, Y_k)/(s_1^2/\sigma^2)^{1/2} \leq (u_1, \ldots, u_k)\}$$

$$= \int_0^\infty F\left(u_1\sqrt{\frac{x}{2(n_1-1)}}, \ldots, u_k\sqrt{\frac{x}{2(n_1-1)}}\right) G_{2(n_1-1)}(x)dx.$$

We can compute boundaries using this joint distribution.

This generalization of Stein's method has the same drawback as Stein's method, namely the variance estimate does not use all of the observations. A more appealing method is to use, at each stage, the variance of all available observations. We describe a method that works well when the sample size is large. For small sample sizes, see the method of Denne and Jennison (2000) (DJ00). We first determine the per-arm sample size $n(s_1^2)$ based on the pooled variance s_1^2. Once n is fixed, we can convert group-sequential z-score boundaries to p-value boundaries as in Chapter 8, as shown in Example 11.2 below.

Example 11.2. A pilot study is undertaken to compare a structured diet and exercise program to advice only with respect to lowering hemoglobin A1c (HbA1c) among people with impaired glucose tolerance, a risk factor for development of diabetes. The primary outcome is the change in HbA1c from baseline to end of study. Suppose that the little information available about the variance σ^2 of such changes indicates that $\sigma^2 \approx 1$. We would like to detect an HbA1c difference between treatment arms of 0.4. We determine an initial sample size and use part of that sample to determine a new sample size $n(s_1^2)$ based on the internal pilot pooled variance s_1^2. We will then take interim looks after $(1/2)n$, $(3/4)n$, and n observations per arm using the O'Brien-Fleming spending function. Before the trial begins, we use the Lan-DeMets software to calculate the needed sample size taking monitoring into account. We choose "Drift" from the "Compute" menu, enter "3" for "Interim Analyses," choose "User Input" under "Information times," and enter $0.50, 0.75$, and

1 in the "Time" column of the matrix at the upper right of the screen. Making sure to select "Two-Sided Symmetric" under "Test Boundaries," "Spending Function" under "Determine Bounds," and "O'Brien-Fleming" from "Function," we set power and alpha at 0.90 and 0.05 and hit enter to find that the drift parameter θ, the expected value of the final z-score, is 3.2711. Because we expect a treatment difference of 0.4 and a variance of 1, it follows that $\theta = 0.4/(2/N)^{1/2}$. Equating θ to 3.2711 and solving for N yields $N = 2(3.2711)^2/(0.4)^2 = 134$ per arm. This produces our original calculated sample size. We plan to reassess the necessary sample size after 50 per arm.

Suppose that after 50 observations per arm, the pooled variance is 1.69. With a standard deviation of 1.3 instead of 1, the expected z-score with n observations per arm at the end is $0.4/\{2(1.3)^2/n\}^{1/2}$. Equating this to 3.2711 and solving for n yields $n = 2(1.3)^2(3.2711)^2/0.4^2 = 227$ per arm, or 454 total, a substantial increase from the originally planned 268 participants. Suppose cost and other factors lead us to to a sample size of 175 per arm, 350 total. If we take the efficacy looks after 87, 131, and 175 per arm, the z-score boundaries are 2.9626, 2.3590, and 2.0140, respectively. Converting these to p-value boundaries yields $2\{1 - \Phi(2.9626)\} = .003$, $2\{1 - \Phi(2.3590)\} = .018$, and $2\{1 - \Phi(2.0140)\} = .044$. After 87 participants per arm, we compute the nominal p-value using the t-distribution with $2(87 - 1) = 172$ degrees of freedom; if it is .003 or less, we stop the trial and reject the null hypothesis. If the p-value exceeds .003, we proceed to the next analysis with 131 per arm and compute the nominal p-value using the t-distribution with $2(131 - 1) = 260$ degrees of freedom. We will stop the trial and reject the null hypothesis if that p-value is .018 or less. If the p-value exceeds .018, we proceed to the final analysis with 175 per arm. We reject the null hypothesis at the end of the trial if the p-value using the t-distribution with $2(175 - 1) = 348$ degrees of freedom is .044 or less.

11.2.6 Blinded Sample Size Reassessment

Decisions about whether to stop a trial are often left to the unblinded DSMB, but sometimes the investigators themselves want to increase the sample size of a trial. Unblinding them can compromise the trial's integrity in many possible ways. Suppose, for example, that the investigator is aware of interim data from the trial indicating an apparently large treatment effect. An investigator who believes that a particular participant is on placebo may try to compensate by making exercise and dietary recommendations that might not be made if the patient is thought to be on the active drug. An investigator who believes, rightly or wrongly, that the answer is already in might recruit future patients less aggressively (investigators are often less likely than a DSMB to appreciate the fact that repeated looks at the data diminish the strength of evidence of a nominally significant treatment difference). For these and other reasons, investigators should remain blinded yet still be able to make an informed decision about whether to increase the sample size.

It may seem innocuous enough to reveal the pooled variance or even the variances in each arm to a blinded investigator. After all, variances are a far cry from treatment differences. Still, a clever investigator will be able to deduce the treatment effect as follows. First compute the "lumped" variance of the $2n_1$ observations in the internal pilot study:

$$s_{L1}^2 = \frac{1}{2n_1 - 1} \sum_{i=1}^{2n_1} (X_i - \bar{X}_1)^2,$$

where $\bar{X}_1$ is the mean of all $2n_1$ observations in stage 1. Even blinded investigators can compute this quantity if they have access to outcome data for individual participants. Note that

$(2n_1 - 1)s_{L1}^2$

$$= \sum_{i \in T} (X_i - \bar{X}_{T1} + \bar{X}_{T1} - \bar{X}_1)^2 + \sum_{i \in C} (X_i - \bar{X}_{C1} + \bar{X}_{C1} - \bar{X}_1)^2$$

$$= n_1 \{ (\bar{X}_{T1} - \bar{X}_1)^2 + (\bar{X}_{C1} - \bar{X}_1)^2 \} + \sum_{i \in T} (X_i - \bar{X}_{T1})^2 + \sum_{i \in C} (X_i - \bar{X}_{C1})^2$$

$$= n_1 (\bar{X}_{T1} - \bar{X}_{C1})^2 / 2 + \sum_{i \in T} (X_i - \bar{X}_{T1})^2 + \sum_{i \in C} (X_i - \bar{X}_{C1})^2$$

$$= n_1 \hat{\delta}_1^2 / 2 + 2(n_1 - 1)s_1^2. \tag{11.7}$$

The third line follows from the fact that $(\bar{X}_{T1} + \bar{X}_{C1})/2 = \bar{X}_1$. Equation (11.7) shows that we can write the first-stage treatment effect estimate $\hat{\delta}_1$ as a function of the lumped and pooled variances. Thus, a mathematically clever investigator can deduce the treatment effect from knowledge of these two variances.

Gould and Shih (1992) [GS92] and Gould (1995) [G95] proposed ways to adjust the sample size using only blinded data. One can avoid unblinding by making sample size decisions based on the lumped variance s_{L1}^2 and the originally hypothesized treatment effect δ_0. If the originally hypothesized treatment effect is accurate, we can estimate the pooled variance from the lumped variance using (11.7):

$$\hat{s}^2 = \frac{(2n_1 - 1)s_{L1}^2 - n_1 \delta_0^2 / 2}{2(n_1 - 1)}. \tag{11.8}$$

We could substitute (11.8) for σ^2 in the approximate sample size formula (11.1). If the assumed treatment effect is overly optimistic, the variance estimate (11.8) will be too small. One could instead substitute s_{L1}^2 for s_1^2 in (11.1). We use these variance estimates only to determine the final sample size; we use the usual fixed-sample t-statistic at the end of the trial.

The lumped variance seems overly conservative because if the treatment effect is much larger than expected, the lumped variance will also be large. From (11.7) and the fact that $\hat{\delta}_1$ will be close to δ as $n_1 \to \infty$, the lumped variance tends to ∞ as $\delta \to \infty$. Of course, in realistic settings the treatment effect is rarely huge. From (11.7), the ratio of lumped to pooled variances is

$$\frac{s_{L1}^2}{s_1^2} = \frac{n_1 \hat{e}_1^2}{2(2n_1 - 1)} + \frac{2(n_1 - 1)}{2n_1 - 1}$$
$$\approx 1 + \hat{e}_1^2/4, \tag{11.9}$$

where $\hat{e}_1 = \hat{\delta}_1/s_1$ is the estimated effect size. The effect size in a typical clinical trial might be on the order of one quarter or one third. Equation (11.9) shows that if $e = 1/3$, the lumped variance is less than 3 percent larger, on average, than the pooled variance; the lumped standard deviation is less than 1.5 percent larger than the pooled variance. Even if the effect size is one half, the lumped standard deviation is only 3 percent larger than the pooled standard deviation.

Gould and Shih (1992) [GS92] and Gould (1995) [G95] used the expectation maximization (EM) algorithm to obtain a more complicated variance estimator, but it does not appear to offer substantial improvement over the lumped variance. It has also been the source of some recent controversy (Friede and Kieser, 2002 [FK02]; Gould and Shih, 2005 [GS05]).

We emphasize that although the lumped variance is used to compute the sample size, the usual fixed-sample t-test is used at the end of the trial. The distribution of the fixed-sample t-test using adaptive sample size modification based on the lumped variance is not exactly t, just as the distribution of the naive t-test using sample size modification based on the pooled variance was not exactly t. Those who prefer an exact p-value can consult Kieser and Friede (2003) [KF03], who computed the exact distribution of the fixed sample t-test under adaptive sample size modification based on the lumped variance.

Govindarajulu (2003) [G03] considered a different final test statistic more akin to Stein's method. Just as Stein's method uses the first-stage pooled variance in the final t-statistic, Govindarajulu (2003) used the first-stage lumped variance in the final t-statistic, and proved that the procedure was asymptotically valid even for nonnormal data.

11.3 Methods Using Nuisance Parameter Estimates: The Binary Outcome Case

We can obtain an approximate sample size formula for trials with a dichotomous endpoint by using formula (11.1) with $\delta = p_C - p_T$. The variance σ^2 is $p(1 - p)$, where $p = (p_T + p_C)/2$ is the event probability among all patients in the trial. Because $p(1 - p)$ increases in p for $p \le 0.50$, it might seem that overestimation of p leads to overestimation of the variance when p is small, which ought to be conservative. This is true for a fixed value of $\delta = p_C - p_T$, but we often express treatment effects for a binary outcome trial in terms of a percentage reduction. For example, a 20 percent treatment reduction means that $p_T = 0.80p_C$; the size of the absolute treatment difference, $p_C - 0.80p_C$, increases as p_C increases. If we think the control rate will be 0.30 when in fact it is 0.20, the overestimate of the absolute treatment difference makes the trial underpowered even though $\sigma^2 = p(1-p)$ may be overestimated. We illustrate using the slightly more accurate and commonly used per-arm sample size formula

$$n = \frac{\left\{ z_{\alpha/2} \sqrt{2p(1-p)} + z_\beta \sqrt{p_C(1-p_C) + p_T(1-p_T)} \right\}^2}{(p_C - p_T)^2}, \qquad (11.10)$$

where again $p = (p_C + p_T)/2$ is the event probability among all patients in the trial. Suppose the control probability is expected to be 0.25. A 20 percent treatment reduction gives $p_C = 0.25$ and $p_T = (0.80)(0.25) = 0.20$. The sample size from (11.10) under this scenario is 1464 per arm. Sample size calculation is very sensitive to the control probability. For example, if the true control probability is 0.22 instead of 0.25, the sample size would be 1722 per arm; the total sample size increases by more than 500 even though the control event probability was overestimated by a fairly small amount. Overestimation of the control probability is common; it can result from different sources. Control event rates may be estimated from observational studies; patients volunteering for clinical trials are typically healthier than the general population. Patients in clinical trials may receive better background care than they would if they were not in the trial. Furthermore, data used to estimate the control event probability may be a few years or even a few decades old. Medical care is likely to have improved since then, resulting in lower event rates. Less commonly, the event probability is underestimated, resulting in a trial that is larger, and therefore more expensive, than necessary.

We might be able to avoid these problems by changing the sample size on the basis of an estimate of the control probability derived from an internal pilot study. For example, suppose that the control proportion after 500 patients turned out to be $105/500 = 0.21$. If we continued to assume a 20 percent reduction, then $p_T = (0.80)(0.21) = 0.168$, so the sample size using (11.10) would be 1824 per arm. Because we peeked only at the control event proportion, maintaining the originally hypothesized treatment effect, the situation seems analogous to the continuous outcome setting whereby the pooled variance gave us no information about the treatment effect. A closer examination reveals a potential problem. The first-stage control proportion $\hat{p}_{C1}$ and treatment effect estimate $\hat{\delta}_1 = \hat{p}_{C1} - \hat{p}_{T1}$ are correlated: $\text{cov}(\hat{p}_{C1}, \hat{p}_{C1} - \hat{p}_{T1}) = \text{var}(\hat{p}_{C1}) = p_C(1-p_C)/n_1$. For a fixed percentage treatment reduction, the final sample size decreases as the first-stage control proportion $\hat{p}_{C1}$ increases, and because $\hat{p}_{C1}$ is positively correlated with $\hat{\delta}_1 = \hat{p}_{C1} - \hat{p}_{T1}$, a larger than expected first-stage treatment effect estimate means a smaller than expected final sample size. In an extreme situation, a huge interim control proportion might require no additional observations. But a huge control event proportion probably also means a large treatment effect estimate (because of the positive correlation between $\hat{p}_{C1}$ and $\hat{p}_{C1} - \hat{p}_{T1}$), so the trial might stop precisely when the treatment effect is large. That suggests the possibility of inflating the type 1 error rate when the sample size is increased on the basis of the control event proportion.

Fortunately, simulation studies have not borne out the theoretical possibility of type 1 error rate inflation, and asymptotic arguments support the validity of modifying the sample size on the basis of the control event proportion.

11.3.1 Blinded Sample Size Reassessment

For binary outcome trials without an independent DSMB, maintaining the blind is highly desirable for the same reasons as in continuous outcome trials. Gould (1992) [G92] showed how to maintain the blind and still make an informed sample size choice (see also Gould, 1995 [G95]). He considered three different ways to express the treatment effect: a difference in proportions, a ratio of proportions, or an odds ratio. The approach is the same whichever way we express the treatment effect; instead of peeking at the control proportion, we look at the overall event proportion among all trial participants. From the overall event proportion and the originally assumed treatment effect we deduce the event probabilities in each arm, from which we compute the sample size. We illustrate using the ratio of proportions approach, which corresponds to a treatment effect expressed as a fixed percentage reduction.

Recall that in the example above we expected the control probability to be 0.25, so we originally anticipated a sample size of 1464 per arm. But suppose after 496 and 502 control and treatment participants have been evaluated, the overall event proportion is $320/998 = 0.321$. We use this as an estimate of $(p_C + p_T)/2$. We continue to assume the same treatment effect, namely $p_T/p_C = 0.80$. Simultaneously solving $(p_C + p_T)/2 =$ and $p_T/p_C = 0.80$ results in $p_C = 0.357$ and $p_T = 0.285$. Substituting these values into formula (11.10) results in a sample size of 882 per arm. More generally, if the first-stage overall event proportion is $\hat{p}_1 = (n_{C1}\hat{p}_{C1} + n_{T1}\hat{p}_{T1})/(n_{C1} + n_{T1})$ and the originally hypothesized relative treatment effect is R, we solve the simultaneous equations

$$p_T/p_C = R \text{ and } \frac{p_C + p_T}{2} = \hat{p}_1$$

to find

$$p_C = \frac{2\hat{p}_1}{1 + R} \text{ and } p_T = \frac{2R\hat{p}_1}{1 + R}.$$

We substitute these values into (11.10) to obtain the per-arm sample size.

Compare sample size recalculation based on the overall event proportion to that based on the control proportion. The overall proportion, $\hat{p}_1 = (n_{C1}\hat{p}_{C1} + n_{T1}\hat{p}_{T1})/(n_{C1} + n_{T1})$, is uncorrelated with the treatment effect estimate, $\hat{p}_{C1} - \hat{p}_{T1}$: $\text{cov}(\hat{p}_1, \hat{p}_{C1} - \hat{p}_{T1}) = (n_{C1} + n_{T1})^{-1}\{\text{cov}(n_{C1}\hat{p}_{C1}, \hat{p}_{C1}) + $

$0 + 0 - \text{cov}(n_{T1}\hat{p}_{T1}, \hat{p}_{T1})\} = (n_{C1} + n_{T1})^{-1}\{p_C(1 - p_C) - p_T(1 - p_T)\}$. Under the null hypothesis, $p_C = p_T$, so $\hat{p}_1$ is uncorrelated with the treatment effect estimate. This lack of correlation does not imply independence of $\hat{\delta}_1$ and $\hat{p}_{C1} - \hat{p}_{T1}$. Indeed, they cannot be independent, as the following simple argument shows: if $\hat{p}_1 = 0$ or $\hat{p}_1 = 1$, then $\hat{p}_{C1}$ and $\hat{p}_{T1}$ are both 0 or both 1, respectively. Thus, knowledge that $\hat{p}_1 = 0$ or $\hat{p}_1 = 1$ gives us complete knowledge of $\hat{p}_{C1}$ and $\hat{p}_{T1}$, and therefore of $\hat{\delta}_1$. Nonetheless, the fact that $\hat{p}_1$ and $\hat{p}_{C1} - \hat{p}_{T1}$ are asymptotically bivariate normal and uncorrelated means that they are asymptotically independent. By contrast, recall that the control event proportion was correlated with the treatment effect estimate. The following result is analogous to Result 11.1.

Result 11.2 *If the ratio of the treatment to control sample sizes remains constant throughout a trial, the set of current and past overall event proportions is uncorrelated with, and asymptotically independent of, the set of current and future treatment effect estimates.*

There is nothing to preclude folding in evidence from other sources in the sample size decision. Gould (1992) [G92] suggests a Bayesian strategy quantifying prior information using a beta prior density $f(p) = p^{a-1}(1 - p)^{b-1}/\{B(a, b)\}$ for the overall event probability p. One appealing way to do this is analogous to the method outlined in Chapter 10 for a normal prior distribution for the drift parameter in that it involves specification of a prior estimate and the number of observations that estimate is worth. Let X and p be the total number of events and the overall probability of event, respectively. Under the null hypothesis, the conditional distribution of X given p is binomial (n, p). The posterior distribution of p given $X = x$ is beta with parameters $x + a$ and $n - x + b$. It is as if the prior information were comparable to observing $a + b$ patients, a of whom had an event; when we put together this prior "pseudo data" with the actual data consisting of x patients with and $n - x$ patients without an event, we get $x + a$ patients with and $n - x + b$ patients without an event, hence the parameters of the posterior distribution. With this interpretation in mind, we choose $a + b$ on the basis of how many patients we feel our prior opinion is worth. We then equate $a/(a + b)$ to our estimate of the overall event probability. For example, if we expect the overall event probability to be 0.25, and we deem the prior information to be worth 50 patients, we set $a + b = 50$ and $a/(a + b) = 0.25$. This yields $a = 12.5$ and $b = 37.5$.

We saw that the variance estimator at the end of an adaptive continuous outcome trial is slightly too small. The nuisance parameter estimate at the end of a binary outcome trial is slightly too large. For example, consider sample size recalculation based on the interim control proportion. Conditioned on $\hat{p}_{C1}$, the expected value of the control event proportion at the end of the trial is

$$E(\hat{p}_C \,|\, \hat{p}_{C1}) = E\left\{(1/n)\left(n_1\hat{p}_{C1} + \sum_{i=n_1+1}^{n} X_i\right) \,\Big|\, \hat{p}_{C1}\right\}$$

$$= \frac{n_1\hat{p}_{C1} + (n - n_1)p_C}{n}$$

$$= p_C + \frac{n_1(\hat{p}_{C1} - p_C)}{n}$$

and therefore the unconditional expectation of $\hat{p}_C$ is

$$E(\hat{p}_C) = p_C + n_1 E\{(\hat{p}_{C1} - p_C)(1/n)\}$$
$$= p_C + n_1 \text{cov}(\hat{p}_{C1}, 1/n).$$

For a trial powered to detect a given percentage reduction, n decreases as $\hat{p}_{C1}$ increases. Thus, $1/n$ is an increasing function of $\hat{p}_{C1}$, so the above covariance is positive. Thus, $\hat{p}_C$ slightly overestimates p_C.

11.4 Adaptive Methods Based on the Treatment Effect

11.4.1 Methods

In our experience, most trials do not require adaptive methods to change the sample size on the basis of the treatment effect, but once in a while trials start with virtually no information about the treatment effect. This has led to the development of extremely flexible methods allowing changes in sample size, or even other features such as the primary endpoint, after seeing accumulating data. Flexibility is good, but it is not without cost. Indeed, monitoring itself was developed because of the need for flexibility; we would have more statistical power if we examined the data only at the end, but ethics and practicality demand interim monitoring.

Example 11.3. Consider a trial comparing the change in LDL cholesterol from baseline to end of study in a control and intervention diet. Before the trial begins, we expect the standard deviation of change to be 12 mg/dl, and we want to detect a difference of 6 mg/dl between the diets. The sample size for 90 percent power is about 84/arm. For simplicity, assume that we are very confident that the standard deviation is 12, so we will treat it as known. After 42/arm, the estimated treatment effect is smaller than expected. Is it valid to increase the sample size, from 84/arm to, say, 100/arm and analyze the results as if the sample size of 100/arm had been fixed in advance?

The final treatment effect estimate is $\hat{\delta} = (n_1\hat{\delta}_1 + n_2\hat{\delta}_2)/(n_1 + n_2) = w_1\hat{\delta}_1 + w_2\hat{\delta}_2$, where $w_i = n_i/(n_1 + n_2)$ and δ_i is the treatment effect estimate using only data from stage i, $i = 1, 2$. We have seen this scenario before (Section 7.5); $\hat{\delta}_1$ and $\hat{\delta}_2$ are both unbiased estimators, but the weight attached to each depends on the size of $\hat{\delta}_1$. In fact, if $\hat{\delta}_1$ is large enough, we will not even proceed to the second stage, so $\hat{\delta}_1$ will receive full weight. Similarly, the final z-score

$$Z = \frac{\sqrt{n_1}Z_1 + \sqrt{n_2}Z_2}{\sqrt{n_1 + n_2}}$$

is the weighted combination $w_1^{1/2}Z_1 + w_2^{1/2}Z_2$ of the stage-specific z-scores Z_1 and Z_2. It is as if we had data from two different studies, but hid the data from the second study if the first study's results showed a strong benefit. Clearly, this tack must yield an overly optimistic picture of the treatment's effectiveness. Proschan and Hunsberger (1995) [PH95] showed that for a one-tailed test at level α, the actual type 1 error rate can be as high as $\alpha + \exp(-z_\alpha^2/2)/4$. The actual type 1 error rate is more than doubled for a one-tailed test at level 0.05.

How can we solve this problem? One way is to weight the first- and second-stage z-scores as originally intended. We originally planned to have 84 observations per arm, so the originally planned first- and second-stage weights were $w_1 = w_2 = 1/2$. Suppose we agree to use the z-score

$$Z = \frac{Z_1 + Z_2}{\sqrt{2}} \tag{11.11}$$

irrespective of the actual second-stage sample size. We will show that even when the second-stage sample size is changed on the basis of the first-stage results, Z_1 and Z_2 are independent standard normals under the null hypothesis. To see this, consider the conditional distribution of Z_2 given Z_1. The only information Z_1 gives is the second-stage sample size $n_2 = n_2(Z_1)$; given n_2, Z_2 has a standard normal distribution under H_0. Because the null conditional distribution of Z_2 given Z_1 is standard normal irrespective of the value of Z_1, it follows that Z_1 and Z_2 are independent under H_0 (note: if we stop at stage 1, we could artificially generate Z_2 from a standard normal distribution; it would not be used anyway). Thus, the null distribution of $Z = (Z_1 + Z_2)/2^{1/2}$ is standard normal even if the second-stage sample size changes on the basis of Z_1. One adaptive two-stage procedure would examine the first-stage z-score Z_1, determine the second-stage sample size $n_2(Z_1)$, and then refer (11.11) to a standard normal distribution at the end of the trial. We will call this the equally weighted z-method because it weights the stage 1 and 2 z-scores equally regardless of the sample sizes.

Once again, we have good news and bad news. The good news is that we can refer (11.11) to a standard normal distribution irrespective of the second-stage sample size. The bad news is that we refer (11.11) to a standard normal distribution irrespective of the second-stage sample size! That is, we weight the two z-scores equally even if the second stage is much larger than the first, and herein lies the controversy over adaptive methods. If the second-stage sample size changes too drastically, the adaptive procedure has very poor operating characteristics. For example, if $Z_1 = 0$ and $Z_2 = 2.5$, then $(Z_1 + Z_2)/\sqrt{2} = 1.77 < 1.96$ is not statistically significant even if n_2 is astronomically large.

Worse yet, it is possible to reject the null hypothesis $H_0 : \mu = 0$ in favor of $H_1 : \mu > 0$ when the usual fixed-sample z-score is negative (Proschan and Hunsberger, 1995 [PH95]). Thus, adaptive methods perform poorly in extreme circumstances. We return to these controversies after we briefly review the history of adaptive methods based on the treatment effect.

For simplicity, we assumed that the variance is known, but we can avoid this by using the inverse normal method outlined in Chapter 8: we first compute the p-value p_i corresponding to the t-statistic applied only to the data of stage i, $i = 1, 2$, and then compute $Z_i = \Phi^{-1}(1 - p_i)$. We apply adaptive methods to the i.i.d. standard normals Z_1 and Z_2. This method was proposed for adaptive designs by Lehmacher and Wassmer (1999) [LW99], though its history in nonadaptive settings dates much further back (Hedges and Olkin, 1985 [HO85]).

One of the earliest papers on adaptive methods using the treatment effect, Bauer and Köhne (1994) [BK94], worked directly with the p-values p_1 and p_2 rather than transforming them to i.i.d. normals. They noted that p_1 and p_2 are i.i.d. uniforms under the null hypothesis even if the second-stage sample size is changed. The argument is essentially the same as above: given p_1, the second-stage sample size is fixed, and the conditional distribution of p_2 given p_1 is uniform. Because the conditional distribution of p_2 given p_1 is the same for all values of p_1, p_1 and p_2 are independent. Bauer and Köhne (1994) [BK94] proposed using Fisher's combination of p-values

$$-2 \ln(p_1 p_2),$$

whose null distribution is chi-squared with 4 degrees of freedom. The two-stage procedure uses the first-stage p-value to determine the second-stage sample size, and then rejects the null hypothesis at the end of the second stage if $-2 \ln(p_1 p_2) \geq \chi^2_{4,\alpha}$, where $\chi^2_{4,\alpha}$ is the $1 - \alpha$th percentile of a chi-squared distribution with 4 degrees of freedom. Note that if $-2 \ln(p_1) \geq \chi^2_{4,\alpha}$, then rejection at the end of the second stage is assured, so we can stop at the first stage. We will call Bauer and Köhne's procedure the equally weighted p-method because it equally weights the first- and second-stage p-values. This method is very flexible because it can accommodate more drastic design changes. For example, one could conceivably change the primary outcome halfway through the trial; under mild conditions, the p-values from the first and second stages are still independent uniforms under the null hypothesis. Of course, drastic adaptations may not be readily accepted by the clinical trial community.

Proschan and Hunsberger (1995) [PH95] looked at two-stage adaptive methods from a different perspective. They were interested in increasing the sample size to achieve a given conditional power. For example, for the equally weighted z-method, we can compute conditional power by fixing z_1 and determining the values of Z_2 leading to rejection of the null hypothesis. That is, we re-express the rejection region $(Z_1 + Z_2)/2^{1/2} > z_\alpha$ as $Z_2 > 2^{1/2} z_\alpha - z_1$ (Figure 11.1). Conditioned on $Z_1 = z_1$, it is as if we conducted a test on the second-stage data only, using the boundary $\sqrt{2}z_\alpha - z_1$. The type 1 error rate for a test using boundary $\sqrt{2}z_\alpha - z_1$ is

$$A(z_1) = P_0(Z_2 \geq \sqrt{2}z_\alpha - z_1)$$
$$= 1 - \Phi(\sqrt{2}z_\alpha - z_1).$$

Think of the "A" in $A(z_1)$ as signifying the "alpha" to use on the second-stage data. Proschan and Hunsberger called $A(z_1)$ a conditional error function because it dictates the amount of conditional type 1 error rate to use given z_1. Thus, the equally weighted z-method is fully equivalent to the following: determine, on the basis of the observed first-stage z-score z_1, the alpha level $A(z_1)$ to use for the second-stage z-score Z_2. Reject at the second stage if $Z_2 \geq z_A$, where z_A is the standard normal deviate exceeded with probability $A(z_1)$.

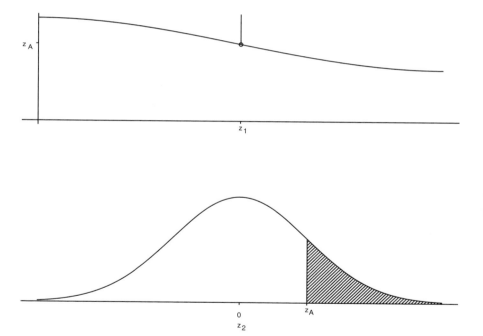

Fig. 11.1. The boundary of a rejection region in the plane (top panel). Having observed $Z_1 = z_1$, we can express the rejection region for Z_2 as $Z_2 \geq c_2(z_1)$; the associated (conditional) type 1 error rate is $A(z_1) = 1 - \Phi(c_2(z_1))$. Thus, we may also express $c_2(z_1)$ as z_A, the point on the standard normal curve whose area to the right is $A = A(z_1)$ (bottom panel).

This equivalent formulation makes it very easy to compute conditional power. With second-stage sample size n_2, Z_2 is $N(\delta/(2\sigma^2/n_2)^{1/2}, 1)$, and conditional power is

$$CP(n_2, \delta) = 1 - \Phi\left(z_A - \frac{\delta}{\sqrt{2\sigma^2/n_2}}\right). \qquad (11.12)$$

To achieve conditional power $1 - \beta$, we equate (11.12) to $1 - \beta$ and solve for n_2. The solution is

$$n_2 = 2\sigma^2(z_A + z_\beta)^2/\delta^2. \qquad (11.13)$$

Notice that formulas (11.12) and (11.13) are unconditional power and sample size formulas for a z-test conducted at alpha level $A(z_1)$.

Consider the common elements of the equally weighted z- and p-methods. Both use a rejection region in the (z_1, z_2)-plane. For the equally weighted z-method, the region is $(z_1 + z_2)/2^{1/2} \geq z_\alpha$; for the equally weighted p-method, the region can be expressed as $-2\ln[\{1 - \Phi(z_1)\}\{1 - \Phi(z_2)\}] \geq \chi^2_{4,\alpha}$. Both methods use the rejection region even if the second-stage sample size changes. In both cases, we can express the rejection region in the equivalent form $Z_2 \geq z_A$, where $A = A(z_1)$ is the conditional error function, a function satisfying

$$0 \leq A(z_1) \text{ and } \int A(z_1)\phi(z_1)dz_1 = \alpha.$$

Conditional power depends on the adaptive method selected only through z_A.

These common features hold for more general adaptive methods. The basic idea of most adaptive procedures is to apply an alpha-level rejection region in the plane even if the second-stage sample size changes. The properties of the procedure depend on z_A, where $A(z_1)$ is its induced conditional error function. Thus, a two-stage adaptive procedure can be described either by its rejection region in the plane or, equivalently, by the conditional error function it induces.

We now present heuristic reasoning behind the choice of rejection region $(z_1, z_2) \in R$. Notice that the mean of Z_1 is $n_1^{1/2}\delta/(2\sigma^2)^{1/2}$, and the conditional mean of Z_2 given n_2 is $n_2^{1/2}\delta/(2\sigma^2)^{1/2}$. We don't know n_2 in advance, so we don't know $\{E(Z_1), E(Z_2 \mid n_2)\}$ in advance. All we know is that $\{E(Z_1), E(Z_2 \mid n_2)\}$ should lie in the positive quadrant if the treatment is effective; as n_2 ranges from 0 to ∞, $\{E(Z_1), E(Z_2 \mid n_2)\}$ ranges over the positive quadrant under the hypothesis that $\delta > 0$. This property makes positive quadrant tests attractive (Proschan, 2004 [P04]). To protect ourself against possibly large departures of n_2 from its original target, we could consider the likelihood ratio test for alternatives in the positive quadrant, leading to the rejection region $Z_1^2 + Z_2^2 \geq k^2$. The boundary of this rejection region is a quarter circle; the associated conditional error function satisfying $z_1^2 + z_A^2 = k^2$ is called the "circular" conditional error function. If we took a more local view, we would protect ourselves against smaller increases or decreases of sample size. If $n_2 = n_1$ were fixed, the most powerful test would be $Z > z_\alpha$, where Z is the equally weighted z-score (11.11). Thus, we would expect the equally weighted z-method to behave well when n_2 does not change much from its original target. This is equivalent to using a "linear" conditional error function $A(z_1)$ such that $z_A = 2^{1/2} z_\alpha - z_1$. An important advantage of the equally weighted z-method is that we pay no penalty if we do not change the second-stage sample size. That is, when σ is known, the test at the end is identical to the fixed sample z-test if n_2 does not change. For these reasons, we focus on the equally weighted z-method.

Adaptive methods can also also incorporate stopping at stage 1 if Z_1 is quite small (stopping for futility). Lan and Trost (1997) [LT97] proposed the following rule for stopping early for futility. If conditional power a) drops below a lower limit l, stop for futility; b) if it exceeds an upper limit u, continue to the originally planned sample size; c) if it lies between l and u, extend the trial to achieve conditional power u. The authors showed that with the interim look at the planned halfway point, and $l = 0.1$, $u = 0.85$, and $\alpha = 0.025$, the type 1 error rate estimated from a million simulations was 0.022.

We could combine adaptive sample size methods with early stopping for benefit. For example, to extend the equally weighted z-method to incorporate early stopping, we could apply standard monitoring boundaries to the equally weighted z-scores irrespective of n_2. Lehmacher and Wassmer (1999) [LW99] and Cui, Hung, and Wang (1999) [CHW99] independently proposed the same k-stage analog incorporating monitoring. Suppose we plan k looks after equal increments of information, and we specify the monitoring boundaries $c_1, \ldots, c_k$. That is, we plan to reject the null hypothesis at stage i if

$$\frac{z_1 + \ldots + z_i}{\sqrt{i}} \geq c_i. \tag{11.14}$$

At a fixed interim analysis (at the planned halfway point, for example) we may decide to increase the sample size and therefore to change the future stage sizes. As long as we continue to weight the z-scores equally as in (11.14), the procedure maintains level α. Similarly, if the planned look times were not equally spaced, as long as we use the original weighted combination of z-scores, the procedure maintains its type 1 error rate. In fact, Fisher (1998) [F98] proved that as long as the weight attached to the z-score at the current stage depends only on previous z-scores, not the current one, these "self-designing" trials maintain the correct type 1 error rate (see also Shen and Fisher, 1999 [SF99]). We will restrict attention to methods maintaining the originally planned weights.

Example 11.4. Consider a trial with three planned looks, after 100, 150, and 200 observations per arm and using the O'Brien-Fleming-like spending function. The boundaries using the O'Brien-Fleming-like spending function and information fractions $1/2$, $3/4$, and 1 are 2.9626, 2.3590, and 2.0140. We use the first-stage z-score to reevaluate the second- and third-stage sample sizes. Even if we decide to change the second- and third-stage sample sizes, the weights attached to the stagewise z-scores are those corresponding to fixed sample sizes 100, 50, and 50. For example, suppose the first-stage z-score is smaller than expected, say $Z_1 = 0.20$. As a result, we decide to increase each of the second- and third-stage looks to 100 per arm. If the z-score for the second-stage data were $Z_2 = 0.55$, then the cumulative z-score at the second stage would be $\sqrt{100/150}\,Z_1 + \sqrt{50/150}\,Z_2 = (0.8165)(0.20) + (0.5774)(0.55) = 0.481$ (even though the second-stage sample size is the same as the first), just as it would be with fixed first- and second-stage sample sizes of 100 and 50. Because this cumulative z-score is less than the boundary value 2.3590, we proceed to the third look. The cumulative z-score at the third look will be $\sqrt{100/200}\,Z_1 + \sqrt{50/200}\,Z_2 + \sqrt{50/200}\,Z_3$, just as with fixed sample sizes of 100, 50, and 50. We compare this cumulative z-score to the boundary 2.0140.

11.4.2 Pros and Cons

Adaptive methods offer great flexibility in clinical trials. For example, consider two-stage methods. Having observed z_1, we may select the second-stage sample size based on conditional power under various assumptions about the treatment effect and other factors. We need not specify in advance a rule $n(z_1)$ dictating what we would do for every conceivable value of z_1; instead we consider only the value z_1 actually observed, making the mild assumption that the human mind behaves like a measurable function of z_1. With the equally weighted z-method, if we decide to maintain the original sample size, the analysis is the same as for a fixed sample size test.

Flexibility has a price; the downside of adaptive methods is that if the sample size is changed, the weights attached to the z-scores are suboptimal. Another way to express the problem is to say that that because inference is not based on the sufficient statistic, these methods lose efficiency (Jennison and Turnbull, 2003 [JT03]). In that regard, Tsiatis and Mehta (2003) [TM03] proved that a two-look adaptive method in which the final sample size could take one of K possible values is less efficient than a group-sequential method with looks at each of the possible sample sizes of the adaptive method. Thus, if the final sample size of the adaptive design could take on any of 200 different values, the group-sequential design would require 200 looks, which is generally not practical. The comparison also assumes a fixed maximum sample size, whereas the point of adaptive designs is that one need not prespecify a maximum sample size.

One can make adaptive designs look either bad or good depending on one's perspective. Given an adaptive design and a fixed maximum sample size, one can find a more powerful group-sequential design (with possibly an impractical number of look times). On the other hand, given *that* group-sequential design, one can make it more powerful by increasing the sample size and using the same boundaries, as in Example 11.4. This endless one-upsmanship is reminiscent of an exchange between the federal government and Frank Proschan (Michael Proschan's father), who was seeking employment (Hollander, 1995 [H95]). The government issued a craftily worded letter asking, "Would you accept, if offered, a position as statistician at a salary of..." Proschan recognized that it was not an offer, but rather an attempt to gain the upper hand by assessing his willingness to accept such an offer. Not to be outdone, he contemplated responding with, "Would you offer, if I were to accept, if offered, a position as statistician at a salary of ..." The specification of a maximum sample size might seem at first very practical. But is it reasonable to specify that one is entirely willing to entertain sample sizes up to and including 1, 000, but entirely unwilling to consider a sample size of 1, 001 under any circumstances? The debate over adaptive methods is likely to continue, and in the process, spawn improved methods.

In some situations there is no substitute for adaptive methods (Mehta, 2005 [M05]). For example, suppose a pharmaceutical company initially powers a trial to detect a 25 percent benefit, but is then bought by another company that would be satisfied to show a 20 percent reduction. Halfway through the trial, the company wants to consider increasing the sample size. But whether it should increase the sample size surely depends on whether interim results are promising. The new company would want to make sure that *conditional* power to detect a 20 percent benefit is high. Only adaptive methods allow an increase in sample size under such circumstances (Shih, 2005 [S05]). As Lan and Soo (2005) [LS05] point out, the sample size choice might be made on the basis of either conditional or unconditional power, depending on the goal and the interim results of the trial.

11.5 Summary

Adaptive methods recalculate sample size using data from an internal pilot study. The methods come in two flavors: those estimating nuisance parameters only, and those estimating both the treatment effect and nuisance parameters. The former, which are less controversial, are of two types: those breaking the blind and those maintaining the blind. In either case, one can usually analyze the final data as if the sample size had been fixed in advance. Table 11.5 summarizes adaptive methods based on a nuisance parameter. Coffey and Muller (1999) [CM99] show how to calculate exact test size and power under various scenarios.

Adaptive methods that estimate the treatment effect are very flexible but controversial. One concern is that they could be used to try to detect effects that are smaller than the minimally clinically relevant difference. Another is their lack of efficiency. If the sample size is changed greatly from what was originally planned, adaptive methods can be quite inefficient. Nonetheless, when used correctly, some adaptive methods based on the treatment effect (namely

Table 11.5. Comparison of sample size recalculation methods based on the nuisance parameter for trials with a continuous or dichotomous outcome.

	Continuous	Dichotomous
	\multicolumn{2}{c}{Unblinded Method}	
nuisance parameter	σ^2	p_C
nuisance par. estimator	pooled variance	control proportion
$(\hat{\delta}_1, n)$	independent	negatively correlated
method at end	Stein & variants, naive t	naive proportions test
asymptotically valid?	yes	yes
	\multicolumn{2}{c}{Blinded Method}	
nuisance parameter	σ^2	overall p
nuisance par. estimator	lumped variance	combined event proportion
method at end	naive t	naive proportions test
asymptotically valid?	yes	yes

the equally weighted z-method) allow small increases in sample size and power at no additional cost in the sense that if the sample size is not changed, the test at the end is the same as a fixed-sample t-test. Furthermore, in some situations it is important to have high conditional, rather than unconditional, power. In such cases there is no substitute for adaptive methods. Sample size methods based on the treatment effect are like antidepressants: it is best not to need them, but if you do, they work reasonably well.

12

Topics Not Covered

12.1 Introduction

Our goal in writing this book has been to present a unified approach to data monitoring. The methods we describe allow the statistician to create monitoring boundaries for efficacy, safety, and futility to provide a DSMB with a firm probabilistic structure as well as flexibility in its response to data. Moreover, we hope that the mathematical foundations developed in the previous chapters will give the reader enough tools to derive boundaries for situations not identical to the ones we have described.

The methods in this book are not, however, the only techniques available in the literature for use in clinical trials. This chapter introduces some other approaches one can take in establishing monitoring boundaries. We briefly describe in Sections 12.2 and 12.3 some of these other methods with comments on why they are not the methods we prefer. In our view, the strength of the methods described in earlier chapters is that they allow the boundaries to be guidelines without sacrificing statistical rigor.

Another subject we have not addressed is so-called reverse stochastic curtailing. Section 12.4 points to the literature on this topic.

Nearly all the examples in this book thus far have considered two-arm studies that aim to show that a new treatment is better than placebo or better than an active control already in use. Many trials, however, study more than two arms. We indicate in Section 12.5 how to adapt the methods of this book to such trials, but we warn that the more arms in a study, the more caution a DSMB should take before recommending a major change in the protocol, the dropping of a study arm, or the stopping of the entire study.

The problem of monitoring a trial that aims to show equivalence or non-inferiority of two therapies is another topic not yet addressed. In 12.6 we provide some tentative guidance to those who try to monitor such trials.

Although we have discussed confidence intervals computed after a group-sequential trial is stopped, we have not discussed repeated confidence intervals

(RCIs) computed throughout a trial. Section 12.7 touches on RCIs and explains why we did not cover them extensively.

For a comprehensive review of sequential methods and their application to medicine as well as other fields, see Lai (2001) [L01] and the discussions following the paper.

12.2 Continuous Sequential Boundaries

We have concentrated on group-sequential methods, that is, boundaries derived under the assumption that the DSMB will look at the data not one observation at a time, but rather at intervals. The looks may be defined by calendar time, by number of participants randomized, by information time, or according to some other preference of the DSMB. The first sequential methods developed, however, looked at data not in groups but as individual observations (Wald, 1947 [W47]) or as pairs (Armitage, 1975 [A75]) accrued.

Wald's (1947) [W47] sequential probability ratio test took one observation at a time, plotted the result against the prespecified boundaries, and if the trajectory did not cross a boundary, took another observation. The study ended when the trajectory crossed a boundary. The sequence could theoretically continue infinitely, although the probability of very large sample sizes under either the null or alternative hypotheses is very small. Armitage (1957) [A57] developed methods, called restricted designs, that fixed the maximum sample size. These methods are of great interest historically for clinical trials because they paved the way for the methods of sequential analysis we use today. They are still applicable in many fields, including in some specialized medical settings where recruitment is slow and the outcome determined quickly after randomization. We have not found these designs useful in the types of trials with which we have experience. Part of the reason is practical: data are often not available in the order in which patients have been accrued. For paired designs, the pairings artificially link two patients who happen to enter the study close in time but who otherwise may differ considerably from each other. Another practical concern is that few DSMBs like to be involved in a trial on a day-to-day basis in the way these methods require. A more statistical concern is that, as we amplify below, these boundaries indeed act as boundaries and not as guidelines; failure to stop a study when it crosses a boundary invalidates their probabilistic interpretation.

Since those early days, a considerable literature has developed regarding these methods. These modern continuous sequential boundaries have many variant designs whose names reflect the shape of the boundaries—e.g., triangular, wedge, and Christmas tree. Their mathematical foundation is the same as those of the methods of this book—they all rely on Brownian motion. In fact, the group-sequential methods are the discretized versions of continuous monitoring. As described by Whitehead (1997) [W97], many of these newer continuous designs no longer require determining the outcome of each observation prior to entering the next patient. Some trials, even large ones, have adopted these plans. See, for example, Moss et al., (1996) [MHC96], who describe early stopping of a trial with an implanted defibrillator. Some argue that they are superior to the types of boundaries we recommend in this book because they allow acceptance of the null hypothesis during the course of the trial. Again, we see this property not as an advantage, but a disadvantage, because of the constraints it puts on the DSMB to obey a crossing (see 12.3).

12.3 Other Types of Group-Sequential Boundaries

The methods of this book address upper bounds (efficacy) and lower bounds (futility and safety) separately, regarding the monitoring as two one-sided activities. This separation of the top and bottom boundaries reflect, we believe, the actual behavior of DSMBs—they think about efficacy, futility, and safety in different ways. An example is the Clopidogrel in Unstable Angina to Prevent Recurrent Events (CURE) Trial, a trial comparing clopidogrel to placebo in patients with unstable angina. The primary endpoint in CURE was a composite of cardiovascular death, nonfatal myocardial infarction, or nonfatal stroke [CLOP91]. At the last DSMB meeting before the trial was due to end, the data crossed the boundary that allowed declaration of efficacy of clopidogrel. Nonetheless, the DSMB did not recommend stopping the trial because the data were showing that patients on the treatment arm were experiencing a high incidence of serious bleeding. Because the mortality in the two arms was nearly equal with most of the endpoints being nonfatal myocardial infarction, the board believed that more complete data on serious bleeding would provide practicing clinicians with useful assessment of risks and benefits.

As we have seen in Chapter 3, the data from a trial may cross a futility boundary but the DSMB may decide not to recommend stopping because it views the potential additional information useful. Conversely, the data may fail to cross a safety boundary (see Chapter 9) but the DSMB may recommend stopping anyway because, in the face of the observed data, it judges its prespecified safety boundary too extreme for ethical comfort. Because the methods of the previous chapters separate the upper and lower boundary, failing to behave as the lower boundary would guide a DSMB does not affect the probability structure of the upper, or efficacy, boundary.

Many of the methods to which we now refer do not separate the upper and lower boundaries. Instead, they exploit the fact that a random walk could—albeit with low probability—first cross a lower boundary and then later an upper boundary. This allows lowering of the upper boundary, thus increasing the efficiency of the trial. For example, imagine a trial with a single interim analysis at $t = 1/4$ to stop for futility if $Z(1/4) < 0$; otherwise the trial proceeds to the end and uses upper boundary c. Its actual type 1 error rate is $\Pr[\{Z(1/4) \geq 0\} \cap \{Z(1) \geq c\}]$. Using $c = 1.96$ results in a one-tailed type

1 error rate of 0.0227. We can lower the final critical value to 1.916 for a one-tailed type 1 error rate of 0.025. We view this gain in efficiency a price too high to pay for the loss in flexibility, for it forces a DSMB to stop when the data cross the lower boundary.

12.4 Reverse Stochastic Curtailing

One criticism leveled against sequential analysis is that it provides no guarantee that a study with data that cross a boundary at an interim look would be statistically significant had the trial continued to its planned end. While such paths are unlikely, they can occur and standard methods do not explicitly limit such events. A criticism leveled against stochastic curtailing is that it is extremely conservative, especially in the beginning of a trial, for it relies on estimates of the drift parameter that may be highly unlikely given the data observed thus far. Reverse stochastic curtailing addresses both these issues (Tan, Xiong, and Kutner, 1998 [TXK98]).

Recall from Chapter 3 that the conditional power (CP), which forms the basis for stochastic curtailing, is the probability conditional on the data observed thus far of rejecting the null hypothesis given the drift parameter θ. In practice, we calculate conditional power for a range of values of θ and make a judgment regarding what action to recommend. Reverse conditional power, on the other hand, asks for the distribution of the data at time t conditional on being at the edge of the rejection region at the end of the trial. The advantage is that this conditional distribution does not depend on the drift parameter θ because the statistic at the end of the trial is sufficient for θ (recall that, by definition, the conditional distribution of the data given a sufficient statistic does not depend on the parameter). Thus, reverse conditional power does not require us to specify values of θ.

To construct monitoring boundaries based on reverse conditional power, one specifies not only the type 1 and type 2 error rates, but also the value ρ, the maximum conditional probability of a discordant result, that is, the probability of crossing a boundary at an interim analysis for a study that would not reject the null hypothesis if it were to continue to the planned end of the trial. Under these conditions, one can construct either continuous or group-sequential boundaries. Tan et al. (1998) [TXK98] present examples showing boundaries based on reverse conditional power with considerably lower probabilities of discordant results than either O'Brien-Fleming or Pocock boundaries.

This method can apply to studies that end for administrative reasons. For example, Thompson et al. (2001) [TLC01] describe a study of the neurocognitive effects of methylphenidate on learning-impaired survivors of childhood cancer. The study, which stopped early because of slow recruitment, found a statistically significant benefit of treatment. The authors calculated the reverse conditional probability "to estimate the probability of discordant findings if the trial had been completed as planned."

12.5 Monitoring Studies with More Than Two Arms

Some trials have more than two arms. They may, for instance, compare two different doses of a drug to placebo, they may compare more than one drug to an active control (e.g., ALLHAT [A02]) or to each other, or they may use a factorial design to evaluate the effect of two or more treatments. Monitoring such trials is more complex than monitoring a two-arm study. In the simplest approach, a DSMB might regard each arm separately, comparing each to the control with the boundary of its choice. More complicated methods are available under certain specific alternatives (e.g., Lin and Liu, 1992 [LL92]). In general, the more complicated the design, the more difficult it is to prespecify the possible outcomes of the trial; therefore, an experienced DSMB will place strong reliance in these cases on its judgment to augment the inference coming directly from the prespecified boundaries.

Suppose, for example, a trial has three arms: a placebo, a low-dose, and a high-dose group. The DSMB might opt for six looks at the data employing an O'Brien-Fleming-like spending function with a type 1 error rate of $\alpha/2$ for each active arm compared to placebo. This approach applies sequential boundaries to deal with the multiple looks and a Bonferroni correction to adjust for the two primary comparisons. In practice, monitoring a three-arm study is more complicated than monitoring two two-arm studies. Certain outcomes will cause a DSMB to pause in making a recommendation about changing the course of a trial. Stopping the low-dose arm of a study that is indicating futility of that arm is intuitively sensible, but it may risk unblinding the results. On the other hand, a trial for which the data cross the monitoring boundary for efficacy in the low-dose arm but not in the high-dose arm may lead a DSMB to question whether stopping the low-dose arm for efficacy is premature.

The situation becomes even more complicated with factorial studies, whose purpose may be not only to estimate the main effect of two treatments, but to evaluate the effect of the combination. Early stopping with a conclusion about the main effect of one treatment, or even both, may jeopardize the ability to make accurate inference about the combination.

In general, we recommend that a DSMB faced with monitoring a multi-arm study consider at the outset of the study the contrasts of most interest as well as outcomes that would appear potentially inconsistent and thus would caution against early stopping of an arm either for futility or efficacy, and, even, perhaps for safety. The methods of this book should allow the statistician to create a monitoring plan reasonably in harmony with these considerations, but all involved—the DSMB, the sponsor, and the investigators—should recognize that a responsible DSMB might well decide to make a recommendation that contradicts the monitoring plan.

12.6 Monitoring for Equivalence and Noninferiority

Over the last several years, partly in response to the reluctance of many to use placebo or standard of care controls, a number of trials have been designed to show equivalence or noninferiority of a new intervention to one already available. "Equivalence" here means "not very different from," while "noninferiority" means "not unacceptably worse than." These trials establish an equivalence or noninferiority margin δ with the view toward declaring success if the confidence limit for the estimated treatment effect falls within the interval $\pm\delta$ for equivalence or if the lower bound of the confidence interval falls above $-\delta$ for noninferiority.

The literature contains methods for sequential monitoring of such trials (e.g., Brannath et al. [BBM03]), but we find a DSMB's subjective judgment more important than statistical methods. For example, there is controversy over whether one can claim superiority of one treatment over the other if the trial was designed to show equivalence or noninferiority. Nonetheless, if one treatment appears clearly superior to the other, the DSMB has an ethical obligation to stop the trial and inform patients and clinicians of this finding. Less controversial is when the DSMB is contemplating early stopping because the treatments appear very similar. Still, only in rare settings would interim results be sufficiently compelling to demonstrate equivalence of two treatments because usually the interim sample size is too small to produce sufficiently tight confidence intervals. Given that there would be no ethical imperative to stop early in such a case—because the participant should be indifferent to the treatment received—it may be best to continue to the planned end.

12.7 Repeated Confidence Intervals

Another topic we have not discussed is repeated confidence intervals (RCIs). Repeated confidence intervals provide simultaneous coverage probability of confidence intervals computed throughout a trial. For example, suppose we use the Pocock two-tailed boundary $c_i = \pm 2.361$ with four equally spaced looks. If we simply compute 95 percent confidence intervals at each look, the probability that at least one interval will exclude the true parameter value is much higher than .05, just as the probability of at least one type 1 error using four level .05 tests is much higher than .05. To achieve simultaneous coverage probability .95, we would replace 1.96 in the formula $\bar{Y}_T - \bar{Y}_C \pm 1.96(2\sigma^2/n_i)^{1/2}$ at look i with the Pocock constant $c_i = 2.361$. This means that the confidence interval is wider than a nominal 95 percent confidence interval. The advantage of using this more conservative confidence interval is that we can be very confident that all of the intervals computed throughout the trial cover the true parameter value. Thus, we can use them as a monitoring tool to help aid the decision about whether to stop a trial. The problem is that stopping decisions are usually based on whether boundaries are crossed and other factors such as consistency of results across subgroups or similar endpoints, and not so much on confidence intervals. One important reason for this is that interim confidence intervals can be so wide as to be almost uninformative, even if no account of monitoring is taken. In a trial with no monitoring, the confidence interval at the end will have width $1.96\sigma_{\hat{\delta}_N}$, where $\sigma_{\hat{\delta}_N}$ is the standard error of the treatment effect estimate with N observations per arm. If the trial has 90 percent power to detect the treatment effect δ_0, then N was selected so that $\delta_0/\sigma_{\hat{\delta}_N} = 1.96 + 1.28 = 3.24$, and thus $\sigma_{\hat{\delta}_N} = \delta_0/3.24$. The lower limit of a 95 percent confidence interval is $\hat{\delta}_N - 1.96\delta_0/3.24$. Even if $\hat{\delta}_N$ exactly equals its expectation, δ_0, the lower limit of the confidence interval will be $1.28\delta_0/3.24 = 0.40\delta_0$. In other words, we would not be able to rule out a treatment effect less than half of what was originally expected. Now consider the confidence interval at an interim analysis after one fourth of the data are evaluated. Even if we make no adjustment for monitoring, the standard error of the treatment effect estimate and the width of the confidence interval are increased twofold. Further compound the problem by adjusting for monitoring using repeated confidence intervals. We must use 2.361 standard errors instead of 1.96 standard errors. The repeated confidence interval will be very wide. The problem is even worse with more conservative early boundaries such as those of O'Brien-Fleming. With O'Brien-Fleming, we would have to use 4.048 standard errors at the first of four equally spaced interim analyses.

Another potential problem with RCIs is that they do not match the confidence intervals of Chapter 7 computed when a group-sequential trial is terminated. In particular, the center of the RCI is the difference in sample means, which we saw in Chapter 7 is biased when the trial is stopped. Moreover, the RCI is usually wider than the confidence interval upon termination. We know we will want to compute a confidence interval when the trial ends, so using RCIs to aid the stopping decision may be confusing. It might be difficult to explain to a DSMB that now that they stopped the trial—in part because of the RCI—they must use a different confidence interval to report the final result. We believe it is more helpful to make the stopping decision on the basis of whether the boundary has been crossed. If it has, we stop the trial and compute the terminal confidence interval as in Chapter 7. If we are contemplating continuing the trial even though we crossed an efficacy boundary, again it seems preferable to use the terminal confidence interval computed as in Chapter 7 than an RCI to help decide whether to stop. After all, the crucial question is whether the confidence interval reported when the trial is stopped will be convincing to the medical community. If we are contemplating stopping a trial for futility, again we would not want to use a conservative interval such as an RCI. Instead we might look at an unadjusted confidence interval, arguing that even under the best possible circumstances (i.e., not adjusting for multiple looks), the trial has effectively no chance of demonstrating a treatment benefit.

13

Appendix I: The Logrank and Related Tests

We speak of "survival analysis" where the survival time refers to the period before the event of interest. In the most natural language, if we define "death" as the "failure" of interest, then a person who dies at time T has survived up to time T. When failure is an event other than death, "survival" is a handy misnomer. For an excellent introductory text, see Miller (1998) [M98].

To begin our discussion, assume that 1,000 participants enter a clinical trial simultaneously, and let T denote the survival time of a random patient. Table 13.1, called a *life table*, summarizes the observed survival data. During the first month, 50 of the 1,000 patients die, with an observed probability of dying equal to $q_1 = 50/1000 = 0.05$ for $\Pr(T \leq 1)$. The observed probability of surviving the first month is therefore $p_1 = 1 - q_1 = 0.95$. At the end of the first month, $\hat{S}_1 = 0.95$; that is, 95 percent of the patients survive. Assuming no loss to follow-up, 950 patients enter the second time interval. Suppose another 38 patients die during that interval. We estimate the conditional probability $\Pr(T \leq 2 \mid T > 1)$ by the observed $q_2 = 38/950 = 0.04$. Then $p_2 = 0.96$ estimates $\Pr(T > 2 \mid T > 1)$. At the end of month 2, $\hat{S}_2 = 0.95 \times 0.96 = 0.912$, or 91.2 percent of the patients survive. Of the 912 patients alive at the beginning of the third time interval, 30 die. The p, q, and $\hat{S}$ values of the third interval are evaluated in a similar manner. The p and q values are the observed conditional probabilities while $\hat{S}$ is the observed cumulative probability of survival. This type of presentation, called an actuarial life table, is common in demography and in actuarial mathematics.

In clinical trials, however, we rarely analyze data within fixed intervals of time; instead, we typically use intervals defined by the actual times of failure. We illustrate using an artificial example of a five-person trial studying death as the endpoint. If the times of death in years are 0.8, 1.3, 2.5, 3.0, and 3.7, then the estimated probability $\hat{S}(t)$ of surviving t years is 1 for $t < 0.8$, $(1)(4/5) = 4/5$ for $0.8 \leq t < 1.3$, $(1)(4/5)(3/4) = 3/5$ for $1.3 \leq t < 2.5$, etc. Denote the sample cumulative distribution function by $\hat{F}(t)$. Then, $\hat{S}(t) = 1 - \hat{F}(t)$.

Now suppose that the data point 2.5 represents not a death, but a *censored observation*, meaning that we only know that the time to event was

Table 13.1. A life table. Notes: t = the time, in months, at the beginning of the interval; N = the number alive at the beginning of the interval; d = the number of deaths in the interval $[t, t+1)$; $q = d/N$, the probability of dying in the interval conditional on being alive at the beginning of the interval; $p = 1 - q$, the conditional probability of surviving to the subsequent interval; $\hat{S}(t)$ = the estimated cumulative probability of surviving to t.

t	N	d	q	p	$\hat{S}$
0	1000	50	0.05	0.95	0.95
1	950	38	0.04	0.96	0.912
2	912	30	0.0329	0.9671	0.882
3	882	...	...	...	...
⋮					

at least 2.5 years. For example, suppose the patient moved away and was not heard from again after 2.5 years. The estimated survival probabilities at $t = 0.8$ and $t = 1.3$ remain unchanged; however, the probability of surviving 2.5 years is estimated by Pr(survive 1.3 years) Pr(survive 2.5 years | survive 1.3 years). Because all three people who survived 1.3 years survived at least 2.5 years (including the person with the censored observation), the estimated probability of surviving 2.5 years is $(3/5)(3/3) = 3/5$. On the other hand, because we know nothing about what happened after 2.5 years to the person with the censored observation, that person cannot enter into future calculations of conditional probabilities. Therefore, we estimate the probability of surviving 3.0 years by Pr(survive 2.5 years) Pr(survive 3.0 years | survive 2.5 years) $= (3/5)(1/2) = 3/10$. Here we used $1/2$ for the conditional probability of surviving 3 years given survival of 2.5 years because, of the two people who survived 2.5 years and had known vital status at 3 years, one survived. The estimated survival probability at 3.7 years is $(3/10)(0/1) = 0$.

The resulting survival plot, called a *Kaplan-Meier curve*, is shown in the top panel of Figure 13.1. The curve is clearly discontinuous, for it drops each time a death occurs. The bottom panel shows a Kaplan-Meier curve for a clinical trial with many more participants and many more deaths. In this case, the size of each drop is so small that the curve looks almost continuous.

13.1 Hazard Functions

As described above, a life table provides a discrete summary of survival times, whereas in clinical trials we usually assume that the survival time T is a continuous variable with distribution function $F(t)$, density function $f(t)$, and survival function $S(t) = 1 - F(t)$. The $\hat{S}$ column in the life table estimates the survival function at times $t = 1, 2, \ldots$. The q column of the life table on the

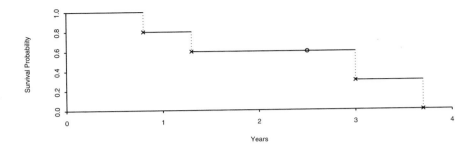

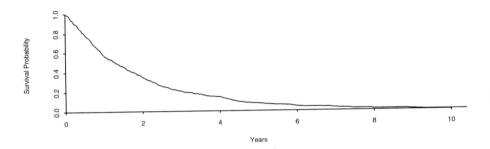

Fig. 13.1. Top panel: Kaplan-Meier survival plot for a small study with only five people, four of whom died (Xs) and one was censored at 2.5 years (circle). Bottom panel: Kaplan-Meier survival plot for a study with 500 people, all of whom died.

$(t+1)$st interval estimates the conditional probability $\Pr(t < T \le t+1 \,|\, T > t)$, which can be considered the discrete hazard rate during the time interval from t to $t + 1$. The continuous version of this concept is expressed as $\lambda(t)\Delta t \approx \Pr(t < T \le t + \Delta t \,|\, T > t)$, where the hazard function $\lambda(t)$ is defined as

$$\lambda(t) = \lim_{\Delta t \to 0} \frac{\Pr(t < T \le t + \Delta t \,|\, T > t)}{\Delta t}. \tag{13.1}$$

A useful alternative expression for the hazard function is obtained by rewriting (13.1) as

$$\left\{ \lim_{\Delta t \to 0} \frac{\Pr(t < T \le t + \Delta t)}{\Delta t} \right\} \Big/ \Pr(T > t) = f(t)/S(t).$$

This expression leads to:

$$\lambda(t) = \frac{f(t)}{S(t)} = \frac{dF(t)/dt}{S(t)} = -\frac{dS(t)/dt}{S(t)} = -\frac{d[\ln\{S(t)\}]}{dt}.$$

Thus, because $S(0) = 1$, it follows that $\ln\{S(0)\} = 0$, $\ln\{S(t)\} = -\int_0^t \lambda(u)du$, and $S(t) = \exp\{-\Gamma(t)\}$, where

$$\Gamma(t) = \int_0^t \lambda(u)du$$

is called the cumulative hazard function.

An interesting special case occurs when $\lambda(t) = \lambda$, a positive constant over time. In this case, the survival time T follows an exponential distribution with parameter λ. Symbolically, $T \sim \text{Exp}(\lambda)$. The distribution and density functions are $F(t) = 1 - \exp(-\lambda t)$ and $f(t) = \lambda \exp(-\lambda t)$, respectively, and the mean time to death is $1/\lambda$. An important feature of the exponential distribution is its "memoryless" property:

Result 13.1 *If $T \sim \text{Exp}(\lambda)$, then conditioned on $T > t$, the residual life $T - t$ also has an exponential distribution with parameter λ.*

While the exponential distribution is strictly valid for very few actual settings, it plays a role in survival analysis similar to the role played by the assumption of linearity in many areas of both physics and mathematics. The mathematical simplicity of the exponential distribution and the elegance of its memoryless property means that whenever we can appeal to it, we do so. Usually, it provides a good enough approximation to reality, at least for short intervals of time, just as the assumption of linearity plays a good enough approximation to many curves, at least for a narrow enough interval on the x-axis. Moreover, as we shall see below, in many cases a simple transformation of the true distribution can yield an exponential.

Consider a clinical trial comparing a new experimental treatment to the standard, or control, treatment. The new treatment is expected to reduce mortality. The phrase "reduce mortality" lacks a unique interpretation. One possible meaning is that the new treatment reduces the hazard function from $\lambda_C(t)$ to $\lambda_E(t)$, where $\lambda_E(t) \leq \lambda_C(t)$ for all $t \geq 0$. Unfortunately, there is no uniformly most efficient test statistic under this general assumption of hazard reduction. Instead, we often assume that reducing mortality means that the hazard is reduced by a constant proportion over time, so $\lambda_E(t)/\lambda_C(t) = R$ for all $t \geq 0$. This common assumption leads to the *proportional hazards model (PHM)*. The constant R is less than 1 when the treatment is beneficial, and is greater than 1 if the treatment is harmful. If the survival times T_E and T_C for the experimental and control treatment patients both follow exponential distributions, then the PHM is satisfied. Conversely, if $\lambda_E(t) = R\lambda_C(t)$ for all $t \geq 0$, we are going to show that after a monotone transformation of time from t to t^*, the survival times are exponentially distributed.

Let $U \sim U(0, 1)$ denote that the random variable U is distributed uniformly on the unit interval, or equivalently, that the density function for U is $f(u) = 1$, $0 < u < 1$. We exploit the following useful result several times in this book.

Result 13.2 *If X is a continuous random variable with distribution function G, then $G(X) \sim U(0,1)$. Conversely, if $U \sim U(0,1)$ then $G^{-1}(U) \sim X$. (Even if G is not invertible, the result is true if we define $G^{-1}(u)$ to be $\inf\{x : G(x) \geq u\}$.)*

Suppose the survival times follow the distributions $T_C \sim F_C$ and $T_E \sim F_E$. Under the PHM, $\lambda_E(t)/\lambda_C(t) = R$, $S_E(t) = \exp\{-\Gamma_E(t)\} = \exp\{-R\Gamma_C(t)\} = \{S_C(t)\}^R$.

Let $G_\lambda(t) = 1 - \exp(-\lambda t)$ be the distribution function for an exponential variable with parameter λ. Note that the inverse function $G_\lambda^{-1}(w) = -\ln(1-w)/\lambda$.

To transform T_C to an exponential random variable, we first transform it to a uniform, $U = F_C(T)$, and then transform U to an exponential with parameter 1 by $G_1^{-1}(U)$. Thus, the transformation is $G_1^{-1}(F_C)$. Now apply the analogous transformation to T_E:

$$G_1^{-1}\{F_C(T_E)\} = -\ln\{S_C(T_E)\} = -\ln[\{S_E(T_E)\}^{1/R}]$$

$$= -\ln\{S_E(T_E)\}/R = G_R^{-1}\{F_E(T_E)\}$$

which is exponential with parameter R because $F_E(T_E)$ is uniformly distributed. In other words, after the monotone transformation $G_1^{-1}\{F_C\}$, T_C and T_E follow exponential distributions with parameters 1 and R, respectively. This result is important because many statistics commonly used in survival analysis depend only on the order of the deaths, that is, on their *ranks*, not on the actual times of death.

The following sections discuss three different nonparametric approaches to survival analysis: linear rank statistics, U-statistics, and Mantel-Haenszel statistics. In the context of clinical trials, Mantel-Haenszel statistics are usually called logrank statistics. We first introduce these methods for complete observations, and then modify them for censored data.

13.2 Linear Rank Statistics

To introduce linear rank statistics, we appeal to an artificial setting—a video game for teenagers—as a didactive device, which we then apply to survival analysis in clinical trials. The purpose of thinking in terms of the game is to elucidate the relationship between scores and payments, which should help clarify the welter of statistical tests available in the survival setting. In particular, the example allows an easy metaphor for disentangling time to events from censoring. Lan and Wittes (1985) [LW85] use the video game example to introduce linear rank tests. Their paper includes citations giving the historical references to the various names of tests and scoring schemes described in this chapter. A thorough advanced mathematical treatment of rank statistics was given in Hajek and Sidak (1967) [HS67]. An intermediate version of the subject may be found in Randles and Wolfe (1979) [RW79], which we highly recommend for interested readers.

13.2.1 Complete Survival Times: Which Group Is Better?

Consider first the special class of two-sample rank statistics. Imagine two teams of teenagers, two boys and three girls, competing in a $5 = 2 + 3$ round video game contest where the players operate as airplane pilots in front of their video monitors. Missiles are fired randomly. Each player uses a joystick to control the plane and dodge the missiles. Skill is evaluated by the amount of time the player survives the game. Each player pays one dollar to enter the game. The game is fair in that all five dollars will be distributed to the players by the end of the fifth round.

The five players start the first round simultaneously. The first player whose plane is shot down is declared the first loser and is disqualified from further play. The game continues to the second and subsequent rounds, continuing until the missiles have shot down all five planes. Table 13.2 shows the observed survival times of these five players in seconds.

Table 13.2. Survival times in seconds of players in the video game.

Player	Pam	Gordon	Becky	Bill	Mary
Survival Time	67	121	254	517	795

These survival times clearly show that Pam performed the worst, Gordon the second worst,..., and Mary the best. But which team, the girls' (Pam, Becky, and Mary) or the boys' (Gordon and Bill) did better? The answer depends on how we define "better." Suppose that before the game started, we had specified the winning prizes for the players as indicated in Table 13.3: the second row, from left to right, shows the prizes for the first to the fifth loser. The last row of Table 13.3 is the net gain of the five players.

Table 13.3. Prizes, entry fees, and net gains of players in the video game.

Player	Pam	Gordon	Becky	Bill	Mary
Prize (score)	0.00	0.45	0.80	1.25	2.50
Entry fee	1.00	1.00	1.00	1.00	1.00
Net gain (centered score)	−1.00	−0.55	−0.20	0.25	1.50

Under the described scheme for prizes and fees, the girl's team has a total net gain of $-1.00 - 0.20 + 1.50 = 0.30$, which, because the game is fair, is the same as the loss of the boys' team. Therefore, we conclude that the girls' team played better. Of course, a different set of prizes could have led to a different conclusion.

More generally, to determine which team did better, we start with a set of scores and use the statistic $S = \sum$(centered scores of the girls) to determine the winning team. When $S > 0$, the girls' team wins. To complicate matters somewhat, even if the two teams have equal skill, a team may win just by chance. Therefore, we use a test statistic $Z = S/V^{1/2}$, where V is the variance or estimated variance of S, to determine whether one team performs "significantly" better than the other. Note that multiplying one set of scores by a nonzero constant changes S accordingly, but Z remains the same. The statistic S is called a *linear rank* statistic. It is *linear* because it is a sum of scores; it is a *rank* statistic because it is based not on the actual times of failures but on their orders, or ranks.

13.2.2 Ratings, Score Functions, and Payments

We now apply the notions just introduced to more general linear rank statistics. First, we shall rate each player in the game, or each participant in a clinical trial, on a scale from 0 to 1. We then apply a *score* to each rating. This score allows us to compare two or more teams in the video game example or two or more treatments (one of which may be a control) in the context of a clinical trial. For simplicity, the example continues with two groups.

We now show how to define payments and their association with scores. This device, while natural in the setting of games, is unusual for clinical trials. Nonetheless, we demonstrate that thinking in terms of *payments*, rather than in terms of *scores*, allows a natural bridge to censoring.

First, let $U_1, \ldots, U_N$ be i.i.d. uniform random variables and denote the ordered observations by $U[N, 1] < U[N, 2] < \ldots < U[N, N]$. We need double indices because, for samples of sizes m and n, the kth order statistics $U[m, k]$ and $U[n, k]$ follow different distributions. Similarly, let $T[N, i]$ denote the order statistics from an exponential distribution with parameter 1.

Result 13.3 *The expected values of $U[N, i]$ and $T[N, i]$ are:*
  a) $E\{U[N, i]\} = i/(N + 1)$ *and*
  b) $E\{T[N, i]\} = 1/N + 1/(N - 1) + \ldots + 1/(N - i + 1), \; i = 1, \ldots, N.$

We give a heuristic argument for this well-known result. For part (a), the uniform order statistics $U[N, 1], \ldots, U[N, N]$ partition the unit interval into $N + 1$ comparable spacings, $(0, U[N, 1]), (U[N, 1], U[N, 2]), \ldots, (U[N, N], 1)$, each of which has expectation $1/(N + 1)$. Thus, $E(U[N, i]) = E\{U[N, 1] - 0\} + \ldots + E\{U[N, i] - U[N, i - 1]\} = i/(N + 1)$.

For part (b), note that the smallest order statistic has an exponential distribution with parameter N because

$$\Pr(\min(T_1, \ldots, T_N) > t) = \Pr(T_1 > t) \ldots \Pr(T_N > t) = \exp(-Nt).$$

Therefore, $E\{T[N, 1]\} = 1/N$.

Given $T[N, 1] = t_1$, we may think of the time $T[N, 2] - t_1$ to the next order statistic as the minimum of the remaining $N - 1$ lifetimes. The memoryless property of the exponential distribution (Result 13.2) implies that each remaining person has survival time distribution $\text{Exp}(1)$. Thus, $T[N, 2] - t_1$, being the minimum of $N-1$ $\text{Exp}(1)$s, is $\text{Exp}(N-1)$. The expected value of the second order statistic is therefore $E\{T[N, 1]\} + E\{T[N, 2] - T[N, 1]\} = 1/N + 1/(N-1)$. Continuing in this fashion yields part (b). $\|$

Part (a) of this result gives a natural way to rate i.i.d. observations on a scale from 0 to 1. Assume $T_1, \ldots, T_N$ are i.i.d. random variables with distribution function F. The order statistics are $T[N, 1] < T[N, 2] < \ldots < T[N, N]$. The *rating* of $T[N, i]$, defined to be $i/(N + 1)$, is expressed as $\hat{F}(T \mid N, i) = i/(N + 1)$. $\hat{F}$ may be viewed as the empirical distribution function. This function differs slightly from the one introduced in almost all textbooks in statistics which typically use i/N rather than $i/(N + 1)$.

A score function ϕ is a monotone continuous function on $(0, 1)$ usually assumed to be square integrable. Associated with a given score function ϕ is a simple way to assign scores to the ordered statistics through the ratings: assign the observation $T[N, i]$ a score of $b[N, i] = \phi\{i/(N + 1)\}$, $i = 1, \ldots, N$. These scores can be rewritten as

$$b[N, i] = \phi\{i/(N + 1)\} = \phi\{E(U[N, i])\}, \ i = 1, 2, \ldots, N.$$

Alternatively, we could define scores through ϕ by reversing the order of ϕ and E and giving $T[N, i]$ a score of

$$a[N, i] = E\{\phi(U[N, i])\}.$$

In linear rank statistics, for a given score function ϕ, the quantities $\{a[N, i], \ i = 1, \ldots, N\}$ and $\{b[N, i], \ i = 1, \ldots, N\}$ are called the *exact* and *approximate* scores, respectively. The centered scores are obtained by subtracting the average of all the scores. The score function provides a useful tool to define a test statistic for comparing two distributions.

For two random variables $X \sim F$ and $Y \sim G$, we often want to know whether $H_0 : X \sim Y$ or $H_a : Y$ is "larger" than X. This question arises in many situations, not only in the setting of survival. Consider some possible ways to define the concept of "larger":

Definition 1. A random variable $Y \sim G$ is *stochastically larger* than $X \sim F$ if $\Pr(Y > t) \geq \Pr(X > t)$ for all t.

While this is probably the most intuitively natural candidate to define "larger," it is unfortunately impossible to find an optimal test under such a broad alternative space. One common strategy to deal with this difficulty is to consider a more limited alternative space.

Definition 2. A random variable Y is *larger* than X in the *shift sense* if Y has the same distribution as $X + a$ for some positive constant a.

This alternative definition is called a *location shift*. Optimal linear rank statistics can be derived for some specific parametric forms of F. This definition, while commonly used for normal distributions, is not usually applicable to survival settings because $Y > 0$.

Definition 3. A random variable Y is *larger* than X in the *Lehmann sense* if, for all t, $1 - G(t) = \{1 - F(t)\}^R$ for some $0 < R < 1$. These Lehmann alternatives correspond to the proportional hazards model for survival times X and Y.

Note that if Y is larger than X under definitions 2 or 3, Y is stochastically larger than X.

To test whether $Y \sim G$ is larger than $X \sim F$, we take m i.i.d. observations $X_1, \ldots, X_m$ from F and n i.i.d. observations $Y_1, \ldots, Y_n$ from G. We pool the two samples and rewrite the $N = m + n$ observations as $T_1, \ldots, T_m, \ldots, T_N$, and the order statistics as $T[N, 1], T[N, 2], \ldots, T[N, N]$. Under $H_0 : F = G$, the Ts are i.i.d.

Let $c[N, 1], \ldots, c[N, N]$ be a set of constants summing to 0. A statistic of the form

$$\sum c[N, i] I(T[N, i] \text{ is a } Y),$$

where $I\{\cdot\}$ denotes the indicator function, is called a *linear rank statistic*. The scores $\{c[N, i]\}$ are usually taken to be the approximate or exact scores derived from a score function ϕ, centered so that they sum to 0. When chosen appropriately, a linear rank statistic based on the exact scores will provide an optimal test (locally most powerful rank test) for two-sample comparisons under specific alternatives, and is asymptotically equivalent to the test based on the approximate scores. See Chapter 9 of Randles and Wolfe (1979) [RW79] for a nice description of optimal score functions.

We consider two important choices of score function ϕ.

Location: $\phi(w) = w$ is optimal for location shifts of a logistic distribution. The exact scores $a[N, i]$ equal the approximate scores $b[N, i] = i/(N + 1)$. These two sets of scores are proportional to the rank score $c[N, i] = i$. The corresponding linear rank test is the Wilcoxon test.

Scale: $\phi(w) = -\ln(1 - w)$ is optimal for Lehmann alternatives. This function gives rise to several sets of scores.

(a) Note that $-\ln(1 - w)$ is the inverse function of $w = 1 - \exp(-t)$, so if U is uniform, $-\ln(1 - U)$ is $\text{Exp}(1)$. The exact scores, which are known as the *Savage scores*, are the expected order statistics from an $\text{Exp}(1)$ distribution:

$$a[N, i] = 1/N + 1/(N - 1) + \ldots + 1/(N - i + 1) i = 1, \ldots, N.$$

(b) The *centered Savage scores* are $a^*[N, i] = 1/N + 1/(N - 1) + \ldots + 1/(N - i + 1) - 1$, $i = 1, \ldots, N$.

(c) The approximate scores $b[N, i] = -\ln\{1 - i/(N + 1)\}$, $i = 1, \ldots, N$ are called the *logrank scores*.

The Savage and logrank scores produce asymptotically equivalent tests. We consider only the Savage scores for the rest of this chapter because they are easier to handle mathematically than are the logrank scores.

We now present these two statistics, the Wilcoxon and the logrank, in terms of the video game and introduce the concept of payments by the losers as a way to determine the winning team. In linear rank statistics the payments and the scores have a natural connection which we shall exploit in connection with censoring.

Payment plan 1) The Savage payment: The ith loser pays $P_i = 1$ dollar to be divided equally among all players still competing at the end of the ith round. For instance, the first loser pays 1 dollar and each player, including the first loser, receives $1/N$ dollar. Therefore, the net gain of the first loser is $c[N, 1] = 1/N - 1$. In general, the ith loser receives $1/N$ from the first loser, $1/(N-1)$ from the second loser, ..., and $1/(N-i+1)$ from the ith loser; the ith loser's net gain is $c[N, i] = 1/N + 1/(N-1) + \ldots + 1/(N-i+1) - 1$, $i = 1, \ldots, N$. From above, these are the centered Savage scores; the corresponding statistic $S = \sum(\text{centered scores of the girls})$ is the Savage statistic. The censored version of the Savage statistic is commonly known as the *logrank statistic*.

Payment plan 2) The Wilcoxon payment: The ith loser pays $P_1 = 1$ dollar to each player competing at the end of the ith round. Thus, the first player pays N dollars, and each player, including the first loser, receives 1 dollar. Therefore, the net gain of the first loser is $1 - N$. In general, the ith loser receives 1 dollar from the first loser, 1 dollar from the second loser, ..., 1 dollar from the ith loser, and pays $N - i + 1$ dollars. Therefore, the ith loser's net gain is

$$c[N, i] = i - (N - i + 1) = 2i - (N + 1) = 2\{i - (N + 1)/2\}, \quad i = 1, \ldots, N.$$

These are twice the centered Wilcoxon scores.

Table 13.4 summarizes the survival times, scores, and payments for the centered Savage and Wilcoxon payment plans.

Table 13.4. Survival times, scores, and payments of players in the video game.

Player	Time	Rating	Savage Score (Prize)	Payment	Wilcoxon Score (Prize)	Payment
Pam	67	1/6	1/5	−1	1	−5
Gordon	121	1/5	1/5 + 1/4	−1	2	−4
Becky	254	1/4	1/5 + 1/4 + 1/3	−1	3	−3
Bill	517	1/3	1/5 + 1/4 + 1/3 + 1/2	−1	4	−2
Mary	795	1/2	1/5 + 1/4 + 1/3 + 1/2 + 1/1	−1	5	−1

Under the Savage payment plan, the net gain of the boys' team is $(1/5 + 1/4 - 1) + (1/5 + 1/4 + 1/3 + 1/2 - 1) = -0.27$, and the net gain of the girl's team is $+0.27$; i.e., the Savage statistic is 0.27.

Under the Wilcoxon payment plan, the net gain of the girls' team is $(1 - 5) + (3 - 3) + (5 - 1) = 0$, so the Wilcoxon statistic is 0.

In summary, the Savage statistic declares the girls' team the winner, whereas the Wilcoxon statistic declares the teams tied.

13.3 Payment Functions and Score Functions

Before moving to clinical trials, we explore the relationship between score functions and payment functions assuming no censoring. Once more we refer to the video game example to give us a natural way to think about payments. Prentice (1978) [P78] conjectured and Cuzick(1985) [C85] confirmed the equivalence of the score function and Mantel-Haenszel formulations of a test. A heuristic exploration of the two formulations was given in Lan and Wittes (1990) [LW90].

Because $F(T)$ is uniformly distributed for any survival time T with distribution function F, we may replace T by $F(T)$ and consider survival times only in the unit interval. Under this setting, the survival time T reflects the skill of a player in the population on a scale from 0 to 1. Imagine a video game with N players. At time t, $0 < t < 1$, each remaining player has the same amount of money, namely the average of all future scores. Thus, each player has, in dollars,

$$(1/N_t) \sum_{i=1}^{N} \phi(T_{(i)}) I\{T_{(i)} > t\}, \tag{13.2}$$

where N_t denotes the number of players still alive at time t. Rewrite (13.2) as

$$(N_t/N)^{-1}(1/N) \sum_{i=1}^{N} \phi(T_{(i)}) I\{T_{(i)} > t\} \to \{1 - F(t)\}^{-1} E\{\phi(T) I(T > t)\}$$

$$= E\{\phi(T) \mid T > t\} = \frac{1}{1-t} \int_t^1 \phi(u) du.$$

A player whose plane is shot down at time t and pays $p(t)$ has a net gain of

$$\phi(t) = \frac{1}{1-t} \int_t^1 \phi(u) du - p(t).$$

Equivalently, the payment function is

$$p(t) = \frac{1}{1-t} \int_t^1 \phi(u) du - \phi(t). \tag{13.3}$$

It is also possible to derive the score function for an arbitrary payment plan. For a given payment function $p(t)$, each surviving player at time t has received $N^{-1}p(t_1)$ dollars from the first loser at time $T_{(1)} = t_1$, $(N-1)^{-1}p(t_2)$ dollars from the second loser at time $T_{(2)} = t_2$, etc. The amount received from loser i is $(N - i + 1)^{-1}p(t_i)$, which can be written as

$$(1/N)\{(N - i + 1)/N\}^{-1}p(t_i) = (1/N)\{\hat{S}(t_i)\}^{-1}p(t_i),$$

where $\hat{S}(t_i)$ is the estimated survival function at time t_i. Because $\hat{S}(t_i)$ will be very close to the true survival function $1 - t_i$ when N is large, the amount received from loser i is very close to $(1/N)(1 - t_i)^{-1}p(t_i)$. The total amount received from all losers by time t is therefore very close to

$$\sum_{t_i \leq t} \frac{p(t_i)}{1 - t_i}(1/N) \approx \int_0^t \frac{P(u)}{1 - u}du.$$

This amount must equal $\Phi(t) = p(t) + \phi(t)$, so

$$\phi(t) = \int_0^t \frac{P(u)du}{1 - u} - p(t). \tag{13.4}$$

We can apply equations (13.3) and (13.4) to obtain the Savage and Wilcoxon statistics. For the Savage statistic, take score function $\phi(w) = -\ln(1 - w) - 1$ (we subtract 1 to make the expectation 0). From (13.3), the payment function is

$$p(t) = \frac{1}{1 - t}\int_t^1 \{-\ln(1 - u)du - 1\} - \{-\ln(1 - t) - 1\}$$
$$= \ln(1 - t) + \frac{1}{1 - t}\left\{(1 - u)\ln(1 - u) - (1 - u)\Big|_t^1\right\}$$
$$= 1.$$

Thus, in the setting of the video game, each loser would pay 1 dollar to be divided equally among the survivors.

Conversely, if the payment function is 1, equation (13.4) yields a score function of $\int_0^t (1 - u)^{-1}du - 1 = -\ln(1 - t) - 1$.

To obtain the Wilcoxon statistic, take $\phi(u) = 2N(u - 1/2)$. From (13.3), the payment function is

$$p(t) = \frac{1}{1 - t}\int_t^1 \{2N(u - 1/2)\}du - 2N(t - 1/2) = N(1 - t).$$

Because the number of surviving players at time t is approximately $N(1 - t)$, a loser pays each survivor 1 dollar.

Conversely, if the payment function is $N(1 - t)$, equation (13.4) yields a score function of

$$\phi(t) = \int_0^t N\,du - N(1-t) = 2N(t - 1/2).$$

In a clinical trial, of course, the participants do not actually pay to enroll, but the relationships articulated in this section hold there as well.

13.4 Censored Survival Data

In many clinical trials, the time to event for some participants is unknown at the end of the trial because their data are censored. Some people may have moved before the end of the trial and their clinical status is unknown at the time they move. Frequently, the trial ends before all participants have experienced the event of interest. Again, the future time when these participants will experience the event, if ever, is unknown. This type of censoring is called *noninformative* because the failure to know the time of event is unrelated to the probability of the event (unless, of course, the person moves in response to becoming healthier or sicker). To allow censoring in our video game example, we add a twist to the game. Suppose Becky's mother called at $t = 254$ and demanded that she come home immediately. At the time of the call, Becky's plane was still operative. How can we modify the rules of the game to adjust for this type of censoring? Assume that the occurrence of the phone call had nothing to do with what was happening in the video game. In other words, her mother did not know whether Becky's plane was still aloft. Thus, her time of being shot down would be noninformatively censored. We denote Becky's survival time as 254+ to reflect that her plane would have survived at least 254 seconds. Then we must modify the centered scores (net gains) for the players. Because the censoring does not affect either Pam's or Gordon's ranks, their centered scores should remain the same and their loss under the Savage payment plan remains $(1 - 1/5) + (1 - 1/5 - 1/4) = 1.35$. Becky deserves to receive one third of this amount (because she is one of three remaining players), and that is her net gain (centered score). It is not immediately clear how the remaining two players, Bill and Mary, should share the remaining two thirds of 1.35, but Mary certainly deserves to receive more than Bill.

Obviously, the analogous situation is much more complicated in a clinical trial where there may be hundreds or thousands of participants and dozens or even many hundreds of censored survival times. We can simplify this messy situation if, instead of thinking of scores, we think in terms of payments. Players need not pay a fee in advance to participate in the contest. Instead, they pay when their planes are shot down. When Pam's plane is shot down, she pays 1 (dollar), shared by all the competing players at $t = 67$. At that time, everyone, including Pam, receives $1/5$. At $t = 121$, Gordon's plane is shot down and he pays 1; everyone competing at that moment receives $1/4$. When her mother calls, Becky leaves with $1/5 + 1/4$, the amount she received from Pam and Gordon; however, she does not pay 1 (dollar) because her survival time is censored and she deserves to have the same amount of money as Bill and Mary have at that time. Finally, Bill pays 1, which he and Mary share, and Mary pays herself 1. The centered scores (net gains) of the players are summarized in Table 13.5.

Table 13.5. Survival times, scores, and payments of players in a video game with censoring.

Player	Time	Rating	Savage Score (Prize)	Payment	Wilcoxon Score (Prize)	Payment
Pam	67	1/6	1/5	−1	1	−5
Gordon	121	1/5	1/5 + 1/4	−1	2	−4
Becky	254+	1/4	1/5 + 1/4 + 1/3	0	3	0
Bill	517	1/3	1/5 + 1/4 + 1/3 + 1/2	−1	4	−2
Mary	795	1/2	1/5 + 1/4 + 1/3 + 1/2 + 1/1	−1	5	−1

Under the Savage scores, the net gain of the girls' team is $(1/5 - 1) + (1/5 + 1/4 - 0) + (1/5 + 1/4 + 1/2 + 1/1 - 1) = 0.60$. As we shall soon see, this is the logrank statistic with censoring.

Under the Wilcoxon payments applied to the same censored survival times, the net gain of the girls' team becomes $S_G = (1 - 5) + (2 - 0) + (4 - 1) = 1$. This censored version of the Wilcoxon statistic is called the Gehan statistic (Gehan, 1965 [Ge65]), discussed in the next section.

It is not surprising that the change of Becky's survival time from 254 to 254+ favors the girls' team. For the Savage payment plan, it increases their net gain from 0.27 to 0.60; for the Wilcoxon payment plan, it breaks the tie and makes the girls' team the winner.

Note that the under the Gehan payment plan, the adjustment for censored data depends heavily on the censoring times. A losing player pays each remaining player 1; if Becky's mother had called at time 120 instead of 254, Gordon would have had to pay only 2 instead of 3 dollars. With the Savage payment plan, Gordon would have paid 1 dollar irrespective of when Becky's mother called. In clinical trials, it is undesirable for inference to depend heavily on censoring times because we are interested in comparing survival functions, not censoring distributions.

13.5 The U-Statistic Approach to the Wilcoxon Statistic

After Wilcoxon (1945) [W45] introduced rank scores and the Wilcoxon statistic, Mann and Whitney (1947) [MW47] proposed an equivalent statistic which they called the U-statistic. They used a very natural approach to compare whether one variable is stochastically larger than the other. Again assume m Xs and n Ys, all continuous with no ties. Mann and Whitney (1947) considered the statistic $U(X < Y) =$ the number of (X, Y) pairs such that $X < Y$. (Earlier in the chapter we used U to denote the uniform distribution; this section uses U for the Mann-Whitney statistic.) Assume the variables are continuous and no tie occurs. Because there are mn pairs, the mean of U is $mn/2$ under H_0. We define

$$U = U(X, Y) - mn/2$$

which has mean 0. If we define $U(X > Y)$ to be the number of (X, Y) pairs such that $X > Y$, then $U(X < Y) + U(X > Y) = mn$ and

$$2U = U(X < Y) - U(X > Y).$$

This result led Gehan to suggest ignoring the (X, Y) pairs when censoring causes uncertainty in the ordering of X and Y; this generalization of the Mann-Whitney U statistic is called the Gehan statistic G [Ge65]. When we employ the Wilcoxon payments in the video game, the net gain of the girls' team is the amount of money the boys pay the girls minus the amount of money the girls pay the boys, which is $U(X < Y) - U(X > Y) = 2U$. In other words, the Wilcoxon payment plan produces a statistic equal to 2U. With censoring, there will be no payment between a boy and a girl when the order of the survival times X and Y cannot be determined; this scheme results in the Gehan statistic G. Although this generalization of the Wilcoxon statistic for censored data seems very natural, it has a crucial pitfall alluded to earlier and elaborated on in the next section.

13.6 The Logrank and Weighted Mantel-Haenszel Statistics

The original Mantel-Haenszel (1959) [MH59] procedure dealt with the problem of pooling 2×2 tables to evaluate the association of exposure and disease after adjusting the effects of covariates. Mantel (1966) [M66] suggested applying the procedure to survival analysis. Previous sections of this chapter describe the relationship between Savage scores and the logrank statistic. Here we briefly summarize Mantel's development of the logrank statistic, again referring at times to the video game for insight. For now, we consider only the numerator of the various statistics. Later we will see how to standardize them to obtain test statistics that are asymptotically standard normal.

Assume $N = m + n$ survival times, m Xs and n Ys. Denote the combined sample by $T_1, \ldots, T_m, \ldots, T_N$ and the order statistics by $T[N, 1], \ldots, T[N, N]$. With censored observations, some survival times will not be observable. Let $T_{(i)}$ denote the time of the ith observed event, and assume no tied observations

Table 13.6. A 2×2 table at the time of the ith death.

	D	A	
X	$O_i = I(T_{(i)}$ is an $X)$		m_i
Y			n_i
	1	$N_i - 1$	$m_i + n_i = N_i$

occur. Just before $T(i)$, suppose m_i Xs and n_i Ys are still alive (Table 13.6). The Mantel-Haenszel statistic at time t is

$$S_{\text{MH}}(t) = \sum_{T_{(i)} \le t} (O_i - E_i),$$

where $E_i = m_i/N_i$.

In the context of our video game example, X denotes a boy; under the Savage payment plan, at time $T_{(i)}$ the boys' team pays a total of O_i and receives $E_i = m_i/N_i$ from the loser. Therefore, $O_i - E_i$ is the net gain of the girls' team at $T_{(i)}$. Summing over time, $S_{\text{MH}}(\infty)$ is the logrank statistic presented earlier.

More generally, if the payment is p_i at time $T_{(i)}$, the boys' team pays a total of p_iO_i and receives $(p_i/N_i)m_i = p_iE_i$ from the loser. Thus, the net gain of the girls' team is

$$S = \sum_{T_{(i)}} p_i(O_i - E_i). \tag{13.5}$$

S is called a weighted Mantel-Haenszel statistic with weights p_i. The Wilcoxon and Gehan statistics described earlier are examples of weighted Mantel-Haenszel statistics; the Wilcoxon applies to trials without censoring while the Gehan statistic is used when there is censoring.

When there is no censoring, we can divide the Wilcoxon payment $N-i+1$ at time $T_{(i)}$ by $N+1$ to produce the Wilcoxon weights $p_{Wi} = (N - i + 1)/(N+1)$, which estimate the survival function $1 - F$ at $T_{(i)}$. When there is censoring, the Gehan payment reduces by 1 not only at each event, but also at each censoring. This Gehan adjusted payment estimates the survival function of $M = \min\{T, C\}$ at $T_{(i)}$, where C is the censoring variable. Therefore, the Gehan statistic does not follow the spirit of the original Wilcoxon statistic, even though it reduces to the Wilcoxon statistic when there is no censoring.

A natural remedy for the Gehan statistic is to replace the Gehan payment by the Kaplan-Meier estimate. This new adjustment results in the Peto-Prentice statistic.

We can standardize weighted Mantel-Haenszel statistics by dividing by their estimated standard error, $\{\sum_{T_{(i)}} p_i^2 E_i(1 - E_i)\}^{1/2}$. This results in

$$Z = \frac{\sum_{T_{(i)}} p_i(O_i - E_i)}{\sqrt{p_i^2 E_i(1 - E_i)}}, \tag{13.6}$$

where p_i is

$$\text{Logrank} : p_i = 1$$
$$\text{Wilcoxon (no censoring)} : p_i = N - i + 1$$
$$\text{Gehan} : p_i = N_i$$
$$\text{Peto} - \text{Prentice} : p_i = \hat{S}(T_{(i)}), \tag{13.7}$$

where $\hat{S}(T_{(i)})$ denotes the Kaplan-Meier estimate of the probability of surviving time $T_{(i)}$. For further discussion see Lan and Wittes (1985) [LW85] and the references therein. Throughout the book, when we speak of these survival statistics, we mean the standardized form given by (13.6).

13.7 Monitoring Survival Trials

For clinical trials comparing survival distributions, the most commonly used statistical approaches come from the family of weighted Maentel-Haenszel tests described in Section 13.6. The test most commonly used is the logrank test, but other weightings are sometimes employed. For example, the Women's Health Initiative [WHI02] used weighted logrank tests downweighting events that occurred early after randomization because of the investigators' hypothesis that the effect of hormone therapy would not become fully manifest immediately after initiation of therapy.

In selecting weights, one should be careful to choose a scheme that disentangles the survival and censoring distributions, with the former providing the basis of inference regarding the effect of treatment. Provided one follows this advice (e.g., uses the logrank or Peto-Prentice statistic), one can use Brownian motion to monitor the trial. One cannot use Brownian motion if the weighting scheme does not disentangle the censoring and survival distributions (e.g., the Gehan statistic).

14

Appendix II: Group-Sequential Software

14.1 Introduction

At least four commercial packages are available for calculating monitoring boundaries—East (Cytel Software Corporation), PEST (University of Reading, England), S+SeqTrial (Insightful Corporation), and PASS (Number Cruncher Statistical Systems; Ogden, Utah). The first two are fully stand-alone packages; the third integrates with S+, and the last is primarily a program to calculate sample size, but it has modules that calculate various sequential boundaries.

Free Windows or DOS software for computing boundaries, cumulative boundary crossing probabilities, drift parameters, and confidence intervals in a group-sequential trial can be downloaded from

www.medsch.wisc.edu/landemets/.

We use version 2.1 of this program in this book. (The developers of this software have generously agreed to include version 2.1 on their website even if they develop a newer version.) We illustrate features of the Windows version of the program in the context of a trial comparing two diets with respect to cholesterol change from baseline to end of study using a two-tailed test at level 0.05. We plan to monitor at four equally spaced looks using the linear spending function.

When we open the program, a title page explaining the program's features appears. Simply click on it to make it disappear. We are now ready to use the program. The following sections provide detailed information about the use of this program.

14.2 Before the Trial Begins: Power and Sample Size

Before the trial starts, we compute the sample size required to achieve 90 percent power, taking monitoring into account. To do so, we compute the drift parameter required for 90 percent power and then transform to the sample size. The drift parameter for a continuous outcome trial trial using the t-test is

$$\theta = \frac{\delta}{\sqrt{2\sigma^2/N}}, \tag{14.1}$$

where δ is the difference, $\mu_T - \mu_C$, in mean cholesterol level between treatment and control, σ^2 is the variance of the outcome measure, and N is the per-arm sample size at the end of the trial.

To calculate the required sample size, we go to the "Compute" menu at the upper left, which presents the options "Bounds," "Drift," "Probability," and "Confidence." We select "Drift," and hit enter (in this program we must remember to hit enter, otherwise our actions are not registered). Under the "Interim Analyses" box of "**Analysis Parameters**," we type 4. The default is to use equally spaced looks, which is what we want, so when we hit enter, we see 0.25, 0.50, 0.75, and 1.00 under the "Time" column of the data matrix at the upper right of the screen. The default value for "Test Boundaries" is Two-Sided Symmetric, which is also what we want. We next move to "**Power and Bounds Parameters**." The default for "Determine bounds" is "Spending Function" and the default power is 0.90, which again are what we want. We move to "**Spending Function**." The default value for "Overall Alpha" is 0.05, so we move to the "Function" box. The program allows several different types of spending functions for a two-tailed test at level α:

1. The O'Brien-Fleming-like spending function $\alpha_*(t) = 4\{1 - \Phi(z_{\alpha/4}/t^{1/2})\}$.
2. The Pocock-like spending function $\alpha_*(t) = \alpha \ln\{1 + (e - 1)t\}$.
3. The power family $\alpha_*(t) = \alpha t^\phi$ (Phi of 1 gives the linear spending function).
4. The Hwang, Shi, DeCani family $\alpha_*(t) = \alpha\{1 - \exp(-\phi t)\}/\{1 - \exp(-\phi)\}$.

We select "Power Family" and type 1 in the "Phi" box to get the linear spending function.

When we click on "Calculate," we see several things, the most important of which is 3.4376 under "**Drift**" just above the graph. This means that to achieve 90 percent power, we need a drift parameter of 3.4376 instead of $1.96 + 1.28 = 3.24$ for a trial with no monitoring. The ratio of the sample size to achieve 90 percent power when monitoring with the linear spending function and that with no monitoring is $(3.4376/3.24)^2 = 1.126$. That means the sample size must be 12.6 percent larger than a trial with no monitoring.

The table at the upper right of the screen gives other output. The lower and upper boundaries ± 2.4977, ± 2.4071, ± 2.3208, and ± 2.2448 are given for four equally spaced looks. Of course, when we begin monitoring we will use the actual information fractions and the boundaries will change somewhat. Also shown are the nominal upper alpha and cumulative exit probabilities at the different looks. For example, the nominal upper alpha at the third look is the null probability that $Z(0.75) > 2.3208$, which is 0.01015. The cumulative exit probability by the third look is $P_{3.4376}(|Z(0.25)| > 2.4977 \cup |Z(0.50)| > 2.4071 \cup |Z(0.75)| \geq 2.3208) = 0.76854$. In other words, the probability of rejecting by the third look, assuming a drift parameter of 3.4376, is about 77 percent. We see that the cumulative exit probability by the last look is 0.90, as it should be.

14.3 During the Trial: Computation of Boundaries

As mentioned above, once the trial begins, we use the actual information fractions to compute boundaries. For example, suppose that the first of the four planned interim looks occurs at information fraction 0.18 instead of 0.25. We can easily use the normal distribution function to calculate the first boundary of a trial, but we can also use the program to compute it. Because the current boundary does not depend on the number or timing of future looks, we could, without loss of generality, assume that future looks will occur as originally scheduled, namely at $t = 0.50$, $t = 0.75$, and $t = 1$.

Open the "Compute" menu and choose "Bounds." Then go to "**Analysis Parameters**" and type 4 in the "Interim analyses" box, remembering to hit enter. The default is to make the analyses equally spaced, so to make the first analysis at information fraction 0.18, go to the "Information times" box and select "User input." Then go to the "Time" column of the matrix at the upper right and type 0.18, 0.50, 0.75, and 1, remembering to hit enter after each. Then select "Power Family" from the "**Spending Function**," "Function" box and type 1 followed by enter for the "Phi" parameter. Click on "Calculate" to obtain the first boundary 2.6121. Thus, we reject at the first analysis if the z-score is less than or equal to -2.6121 or greater than or equal to 2.6121. (To see that the current boundary does not depend on future plans, try repeating the steps above but specify only two looks, one at $t = 0.18$ and the other at $t = 1$. The boundary at $t = 0.18$ remains 2.6121.)

Because the first look is not too far from its scheduled time, the effect on power of taking the first look at time 0.18 instead of 0.25 is likely to be minimal. To check that, compute the cumulative exit probability under drift 3.4376. Go to the "Compute" menu and choose "Probability." Again type 4 under the "Interim Analyses" box and choose "User Input" under "Information times." Type the information times 0.18, 0.50, 0.75, and 1 in the "Time" column of the matrix at the upper right. From "**Spending Function**" again choose "Power Family" and type 1 for "Phi." Go to "**Probability Parameters**" and type 3.4376 followed by enter in the "Drift" box. Click on "Calculate" to see that the cumulative exit probability by the last look is 0.90; taking the first look at $t = 0.18$ instead of $t = 0.25$ gives only a trivial change in power.

Suppose the second look actually takes place at $t = 0.60$. Repeat the bound computation process with the only difference being that the second look is at $t = 0.60$ instead of 0.50. After clicking on "Calculate," we find that the boundary at the second look is 2.2746. Thus, we reject at the second look if $|Z(0.60)| > 2.2746$.

The program also displays a graph of the boundaries. Go to "**Z-score**," "Observed Z," and choose "Yes." An "Observed Z" column is created in the table at the top right of the screen. Then type in the observed z-scores at the first two looks, hit enter, and click on "Calculate." The z-scores and boundaries are plotted.

Repeat the "Compute Bounds" steps for the third look, which takes place at $t = 0.80$. The boundary at the third look is 2.3110 (of course the first two boundaries, which are in the past, remain unchanged).

14.3.1 A Note on Upper and Lower Boundaries

If we request "Two-Sided Symmetric" boundaries, the program takes the lower boundary into account when constructing the upper boundary. On the other hand, if we request "Two-Sided Asymmetric" boundaries from the "**Analysis Parameters** Test Boundaries" box, the program computes autonomous upper and lower boundaries. The reader will not notice any difference for conventional alpha levels, but try computing "Two-Sided Symmetric" boundaries at level $\alpha = 0.40$ versus "Two-Sided Asymmetric" boundaries using $\alpha = 0.20$ for the lower boundary and $\alpha = 0.20$ for the upper boundary. For four equally spaced looks and the linear spending function, the "Two-Sided Symmetric" boundaries at level 0.40 versus the "Two-Sided Asymmetric" boundaries with $\alpha = 0.20$ for the lower and upper boundaries are (1.6449, 1.4368, 1.2533, 1.0875) and (1.6449, 1.4368, 1.2540, 1.0906), respectively. The "Two-Sided Symmetric" boundaries are slightly smaller because the program accounts for the lower boundary when constructing the upper boundary. See Section 5.2 for further discussion.

14.4 After the Trial: p-Value, Parameter Estimate, and Confidence Interval

Suppose that the above trial is stopped at the third look because $Z(0.80) = 2.66 > 2.3110$. Now that the trial is over, we want to compute a p-value. For the stagewise ordering, the two-tailed p-value with symmetric boundaries is

$$\Pr(|Z(0.18)| \geq 2.4376 \cup |Z(0.60)| \geq 2.2746| \cup |Z(0.80)| \geq 2.66),$$

which is computed under the null hypothesis. To compute the p-value, choose "Probability" from the "Compute" menu. Type 4 for "Interim Analyses" and choose "User Input" for "Information times." Then enter the times 0.18, 0.60, 0.80, and 1 under the "Time" column of the data at the upper right of the screen. For "Determine Bounds" in the "**Probability Parameters**" area select "User Input" to change the third boundary to 2.66. Type the bounds 2.4376, 2.2746, 2.66, and then any value for the last bound, e.g., 1. Click on "Calculate." The cumulative exit probability by the third look is .03719. Thus, the two-tailed p-value is approximately .037. No matter what value we use for the boundary at $t = 1$, the cumulative exit probability at the third look remains .03719.

We also would like a monitoring-adjusted estimate of the parameter. First we get a monitoring-adjusted estimate of the unitless drift parameter θ, which we then translate to the more natural parameter $\delta = (\mu_T - \mu_C)$ mg/dl. The naive drift parameter estimate $B(0.80)/0.80 = Z(0.80)/(0.80)^{1/2} = 2.66/(0.80)^{1/2} = 2.974$ is biased. As suggested by Kim (1989) [K89], one simple way to correct for bias is to determine the drift parameter value θ such that the one-tailed probability of results at least as extreme as those observed is 0.50. Under the stagewise ordering, outcomes at least as extreme as those observed are $E = \{Z(0.18) \geq 2.4376\} \cup \{\tau = 0.60 \cap Z(0.60) > 2.2746\} \cup \{\tau = 0.80 \cap Z > 2.66\}$. Note that $P_\theta(E) \approx P_\theta(A)$, where $A = \{Z(0.18) \geq 2.4376\} \cup \{Z(0.60) \geq 2.2746\} \cup \{Z(0.80) \geq 2.66\}$, because the event $A \cap E^C$ implies that both the lower and upper boundaries were crossed by time 0.80, an event with vanishingly low probability. Thus, we will determine θ such that

$$P_\theta\{Z(0.18) > 2.4376 \cup Z(0.60) > 2.2746 \cup Z(0.80) \geq 2.66\} = 0.50. \quad (14.2)$$

Select "Drift" from the "Compute" menu and enter 4 for the number of looks (even though we stopped after only three looks). After hitting enter, choose "User Input" from "Information times," and enter the times 0.18, 0.60, 0.80, and 1 under the "Time" column of the matrix at the upper right of the screen. Choose "One-Sided" from the "Test Boundaries" box of "**Analysis Parameters.**" For "**Power and Bounds Parameters,**" "Determine Bounds," select "User Input." Enter the upper bounds 2.4376, 2.2746, 2.66 for the first three looks. For the last look, simply enter a huge bound such as 25. Then go to the "Power" box of "**Power and Bounds Parameters**" and enter 0.50. Click on "Calculate." The program will determine the value θ such that

$$P_\theta(Z(0.18) \geq 2.4376 \cup Z(0.60) \geq 2.2746 \cup Z(0.80) \geq 2.66 \cup Z(1) \geq 25) = 0.50. \quad (14.3)$$

It is now apparent why we chose such a large final boundary: there is essentially no chance that $Z(1) \geq 25$, so the probability on the left side of (14.3) is virtually identical to that of (14.2). The drift parameter value printed at the lower left of the screen is 2.6655. Note that this estimate is smaller than the naive estimate $B(0.80)/0.80 = 2.974$.

Having obtained the drift parameter estimate, convert it to an estimate for the natural parameter $\delta = \mu_T - \mu_C$ using (14.1). This yields

$$\hat{\delta} = \hat{\theta}\sqrt{2\sigma^2/N},$$

where N is the originally planned sample size per arm. Substitute the pooled sample variance for σ^2. For example, if the planned sample size at the end of the trial is $N = 100$ per arm and the pooled variance at the time the trial is stopped is $(10.54 \text{ mg/dl})^2$, the estimated treatment effect is $2.6655\{2(10.54)^2/100\}^{1/2} = 3.97$ mg/dl. Thus, the estimated cholesterol difference between the two diets is about 4 mg/dl. Had we used the naive drift parameter estimate 2.974, the estimated difference would have been about 4.4 mg/dl.

To compute a confidence interval for the drift parameter at the time the trial was stopped, go to the "Compute" menu and select "Confidence." Go to "**Analysis Parameters**" and this time type 3 under "Interim Analyses" because the trial was stopped at the third look. This is the only time we must enter the number of looks that actually occurred rather than the number planned. Go to "Information times," select "User Input," move to the matrix at the upper right, and enter the information fractions 0.18, 0.60, and 0.80 under "Time." Choose "Power Family" from "Spending Function," and enter 1 for the power parameter "Phi." Under "**Confidence Interval Parameters**" enter 2.66 followed by enter under the "Standardized Statistic" box. It was crucial to enter 3 instead of 4 for "Interim Analyses," because the value in the "Standardized Statistic" box is applied to the last look. The default level for the confidence interval is 95 percent. If that is what we want, click on "Calculate" and see the confidence interval $(0.2432, 4.9763)$.

We must now translate this interval into an interval for the natural parameter, $\delta = \mu_T - \mu_C$, as we did for the parameter estimate. Because the planned sample size at the end of the trial is $N = 100$ participants per arm and the sample standard deviation is 10.54, the confidence interval for δ is $(0.2432\{2(10.54)^2/100\}^{1/2}, 4.9763\{2(10.54)^2/100\}^{1/2}) = (0.36, 7.42)$. Thus, we can be 95 percent confident that the cholesterol difference between the two diets is between 0.36 mg/dl and 7.42 mg/dl.

Note that the confidence interval for the *drift parameter* did not depend on the sample size. Sample size played a role only in transforming from the drift parameter to the natural parameter. For example, if the sample size per arm had been 200 instead of 100, the confidence interval for δ would have been $(0.2432\{2(10.54)^2/200\}^{1/2}, 4.9763\{2(10.54)^2/200\}^{1/2}) = (0.26, 5.25)$ instead of $(0.36, 7.42)$ when $N = 100$.

14.5 Other Features of the Program

One feature of the program we have not yet discussed is truncation of very large boundaries. For example, consider the O'Brien-Fleming-like spending function with five equally spaced looks. When we select "Bounds" from the

"Compute" menu, enter 5 for "Interim Analyses," use the default "Equally Spaced" for "Information times," select the O'Brien-Fleming spending function, and click on "Calculate," we get the boundaries 4.8769, 3.3569, 2.6803, 2.2898, and 2.0310. If we do not feel comfortable with the very large first two boundaries, we can elect to truncate them at, say, 3.

We can truncate boundaries by moving to the "Truncate bounds" box of "**Spending Functions**" and choosing "Yes." Then specify 3 under "Truncation Pt" and hit enter. Clicking on "Calculate," we find the truncated boundaries ±3.0000, ±3.0000, ±2.8968, ±2.3156, and ±2.0399. To maintain an overall alpha of 0.05, the program had to increase the third, fourth, and fifth boundaries to compensate for the decrease in the first two boundaries. In fact, as can be seen from the cumulative alpha portion of the output, the last three boundaries were modified to make the cumulative type 1 error rates by those times the same as with untruncated boundaries, 0.00762, 0.02442, and 0.05000.

Output from the program, including the graph, can be exported to a Word file by choosing "Send to Word" from the "File" menu.

A DOS version of the program is also available. The options are largely the same, though the DOS version allows the use of two time scales, one to determine how much alpha to spend and the other to calculate covariances of the test statistics and boundaries.

For example, suppose we monitor using the linear spending function applied to calendar time, and we monitor the trial every year for 4 years. That is, we have four equally spaced looks in terms of calendar time. At the first look, $t = 1/4 = 0.25$, but suppose only about 16 percent of expected events have occurred.

The program begins with the question:

Is this an interactive session (1=yes, 0=no).

When we type 1 and hit enter, the program responds:

interactive=1

Enter number for your option:

1. **Compute bounds using a spending function.**
2. **Compute drift given power and bounds.**
3. **Compute probabilities given bounds and drift.**
4. **Compute confidence interval.**

When we type 1 and hit enter, the program responds:

Option 1. You will be prompted for a spending function.

Number of interim analyses?

When we type 4 and hit enter, the program responds:

4 interim analyses.

Equally spaced times between 0 and 1? (1=yes, 0=no).

We type 1 and hit enter. The response is

Analysis times: 0.250, 0.500, 0.750, 1.000

Do you wish to specify a second time/information scale? (e.g. the inverse of parameter variance or number of events, as in Lan & DeMets 89?) (1=yes, 0=no)
We type 1 and hit enter. The program responds:
First time scale will be used in the spending function. Second time scale will estimate covariances. Information:
We type in 0.16 for the first information fraction and then specify arbitrary numbers for the future information fractions (except that the last number is 1). For example, we might enter 0.16, 0.44, 0.66, and 1. The program responds with
Information: 0.160 0.440, 0.660, 1.000.
Overall significance level? (> 0 and $<= 1$).
When we type 0.05 and hit enter, we see
alpha=0.050
One(1), two(2)-sided symmetric, or asymmetric(3) bounds?
We type 2 and hit enter, at which time the same spending function options are presented. We choose 1 and hit enter. The program responds with
Use function alpha-star 1
Do you want to truncate the standardized bounds (1 =yes, 0 =no).

We select 0 and hit enter. The program shows the first time scale (the one used to spend alpha, e.g., calendar time), the second (e.g., information) time scale, the lower and upper bounds, the incremental alpha, and the cumulative alpha. Note that the incremental alpha is not the same as the "nominal upper alpha" presented with the Windows version of the program. The incremental alpha is the probability of remaining within the boundary at previous looks but exceeding the boundary at the current look (i.e., it is a first exit probability), whereas the nominal upper alpha is simply $1 - \Phi(c)$, where c is the current boundary.

References

[A02]   The ALLHAT Officers and Coordinators for the ALLHAT Collaborative
          Research Group: Major outcomes in high-risk hypertensive patients ran-
          domized to angiotensin-converting enzyme inhibitor or calcium channel
          blocker vs diuretic: The Antihypertensive and Lipid-Lowering Treat-
          ment to Prevent Heart Attack Trial (ALLHAT). Journal of the Ameri-
          can Medical Association **288**, 2981–2997 (2002)

[ABG93]   Andersen, P.K., Borgan, O., Gill, R.D., Keiding, N. Statistical Models
          Based on Counting Processes. Springer-Verlag, New York (1993)

[A57]   Armitage, P.: Restricted sequential procedures. Biometrika **44**, 9–26
          (1957)

[A75]   Armitage, P.: Sequential Medical Trials. Wiley, New York (1975)

[AMR69]   Armitage, P., McPherson, C.K., Rowe, B.C.: Repeated significance tests
          on accumulating data. Journal of the Royal Statistical Society A. **132**,
          235–244 (1969)

[A81]   Arnold, S.F.: The Theory of Linear Models and Multivariate Analysis.
          Wiley, New York (1981)

[B55]   Basu, D.: On statistics independent of a complete sufficient statistic.
          Sankhya **15**, 377–380 (1955)

[BK94]   Bauer, P., Köhne, K.: Evaluations of experiments with adaptive interim
          analyses. Biometrics **50**, 1029–1041 (1994)

[BB88]   Berger, J.O., Berry, D.A.: Statistical analysis and the illusion of objec-
          tivity. American Scientist **76**, 159–165 (1988)

[B68]   Billingsley, P. Convergence of Probability Measures. Wiley, New York
          (1968)

[BD94]   Birkett, M.A., Day, S.J.: Internal pilot studies for estimating sample
          size. Statistics in Medicine **13**, 2455–2463 (1994)

[BBM03]   Brannath, W., Bauer, P., Maurer W., Posch, M.: Sequential tests for
          noninferiority and superiority. Biometrics **59**, 106–14 (2003)

[B05]   Bresalier, R.S., Sandler, R.S., Quan, H., et al.: Cardiovascular events
          associated with rofecoxib in a colorectal adenoma chemoprevention trial.
          The New England Journal of Medicine **352**, 1092–1102 (2005)

[B04]   Brown, E.G.: Using MedDRA. Implications for risk management. Drug
          Safety **27**, 591–602 (2004)

[BLF99]   Buxton, A.E., Lee, K.L., Fisher, J.D., Josephson, M.E., Prystowsky, Hafley, G. for the Multicenter Unsustained Tachycardia Trial Investigators: A randomized study of the prevention of sudden death in patients with coronary artery disease. The New England Journal of Medicine **341**, 1882–1890 (1999)

[CAST89]   Cardiac Arrhythmia Suppression Trial Investigators: Preliminary report: Effect of encainide and flecainide on mortality in a randomized trial of arrhythmia suppression after myocardial infarction. The New England Journal of Medicine **321**, 406–412 (1989)

[CAST92]   Cardiac Arrhythmia Suppression Trial II Investigators: Effect of the antiarrhythmic agent moricizine on survival after myocardial infarction. The New England Journal of Medicine **327**, 227–233 (1992)

[C89]   Chang, M.N.: Confidence intervals for a normal mean following a group sequential test. Biometrics **45**, 247–254 (1989)

[CTM95]   Charache, S., Terrin, M.L., Moore, R. et al.: Effect of hydroxyurea on the frequency of painful cises in sickle cell anemia. The New England Journal of Medicine **332**, 1317–1322 (1995)

[CLOP91]   The Clopidogrel in Unstable Angina to Prevent Recurrent Events Trial Investigators: Effects of clopidogrel in addition to aspirin in patients with acute coronary syndromes without ST-segment elevation. The New England Journal of Medicine **345**, 494–502 (2001)

[CM99]   Coffey, C.S., Muller, K.E.: Exact test size and power of a Gaussian error linear model for an internal pilot study. Statistics in Medicine **18**, 1199–1214 (1999)

[C46]   Cramér, H.: Mathematical Methods of Statistics. Princeton University Press, Princeton, New Jersey (1946)

[CHW99]   Cui, L., Hung, H.M., Wang, S.J.: Modification of sample size in group sequential clinical trials. Biometrics **55**, 853–857 (1999)

[C85]   Cuzick, J.: Asymptotic properties of censored linear rank tests. The Annals of Statistics **13**, 133–141 (1985)

[D81]   DeLong, D.M.: Crossing probabilities for a square root boundary by a Bessel process. Communications in Statistics—Theory and Methods **A10**, 2197–2213 (1981)

[DJ00]   Denne, J.S., Jennison, C.: A group sequential t-test with updating of sample size. Biometrika **87**, 125–134 (2000)

[D83]   Dupont, W.D.: Sequential stopping rules and sequentially adjusted p-values: Does one require the other? Controlled Clinical Trials 4, 3–10 (1983)

[EF90]   Emerson, S.S., Fleming, T.R.: Parameter estimation following sequential hypothesis testing. Biometrika, **77**, 875–892 (1990)

[FAP97]   Fayers, P.M., Ashby, D., Parmar, M.K.B.: Tutorial in biostatistics: Bayesian data monitoring in clinical trials. Statistics in Medicine **16**, 1413–1430 (1997)

[F98]   Fisher, L.: Self-designing clinical trials. Statistics in Medicine **17**, 1551–1562 (1998)

[F82]   Freedman, L.S.: Tables of the number of patients required in clinical trials using the log-rank test. Statistics in Medicine **1**, 121–129 (1982)

[FAK96]   Freedman, L., Anderson, G., Kipnis, V., et al.: Approaches to monitoring the results of long-term disease prevention trials: examples from the Women's Health Initiative. Controlled Clinical Trials **17**, 509–525 (1996)

[FS89]   Freedman, L.S., Spiegelhalter, D.J.: Comparison of Bayesian with group sequential methods for monitoring clinical trials. Controlled Clinical Trials **10**, 357–367 (1989)

[FK02]   Friede, T., Kieser, T.: On the inappropriateness of an EM-algorithm based procedure for blinded variance estimation. Statistics in Medicine **21**, 165–176 (2002)

[FBH93]   Friedman, L.M., Bristow, J.D., Hallstrom, A., et al.: Data monitoring in the Cardiac Arrhythmia Suppression Trial. The Online Journal of Current Clinical Trials **1993** (1993)

[Ge65]   Gehan, E.A.: A generalized Wilcoxon test for comparing arbitrarily singly-censored samples. Biometrika **52**, 203–223 (1965)

[GD74]   George, S.L., Desu, M.M.: Planning the size and duration of a clinical trial studying the time to some critical event. Journal of Chronic Diseases **27**, 15–24 (1974)

[Go65]   Good, I. The Estimation of Probabilities: An Essay on Modern Bayesian Methods. MIT Press, Cambridge, MA. (1965)

[G92]   Gould, A.: Interim analyses for monitoring clinical trials that do not materially affect the type I error rate. Statistics in Medicine **11**, 55–66 (1992)

[G95]   Gould, A.L.: Planning and revising the sample size in a trial. Statistics in Medicine **14**, 1039–1051 (1995)

[GS92]   Gould, A.L., Shih, W.J. Sample size re-estimation without unblinding for normally distributed outcomes with unknown variance. Communications in Statistics (A) **21**, 2833–2853 (1992)

[GS05]   Gould, A.L., Shih, W.J.: Letter to the editor. Statistics in Medicine **24**, 147–156 (2005)

[G03]   Govindarajulu, Z.: Robustness of sample size re-estimation procedure in clinical trials (arbitrary populations). Statistics in Medicine **22**, 1819–1828 (2003)

[GW95]   Greenhouse, J.B., Wasserman, L.: Robust Bayesian methods for monitoring clinical trials. Statistics in Medicine **14**, 1379–1391.

[GPS94]   Grossman, J., Parmar, M.K.B., Spiegelhalter, D.J., and Freedman, L.S.: A unified method for monitoring and analysing controlled trials. Statistics in Medicine **13**, 1815–1826 (1994)

[HS67]   Hajek, J., Sidak, Z.: Theory of Rank Tests. Academic Press, New York (1967)

[H71]   Haybittle, J.L.: Repeated assessment of results in clinical trials of cancer treatment. British Journal of Radiology, **44**, 793–797 (1971)

[HO85]   Hedges, L.V., Olkin, I.: Statistical Methods for Meta-Analysis. Academic Press, San Diego (1985)

[H82]   Helland, I.S.: Central limit theorems for martingales with discrete or continuous time. Scandinavian Journal of Statistics, **9**, 79–94 (1982)

[HT87]   Hochberg, Y., Tamhane, A.C.: Multiple Comparison Procedures. Wiley, New York (1987)

[H95]   Hollander, M.: A conversation with Frank Proschan. Statistical Science **10**, 118–133 (1995)

[HFN04]   Hurwitz, H., Fehrenbacher, L., Novotny, W., et al.: Bevacizumab plus irinotecan, fluorouracil, and leucovorin for metastatic colon cancer. The New England Journal of Medicine **350**, 2335–2342 (2004)

[HSD90]   Hwang, I.K., Shih, W.J., DeCani, J.S.: Group sequential designs using a family of type I error probability spending functions. Statistics in Medicine **9**, 1439–1445 (1990)

[JB97]   Jankovic, J., Beach, J.: Long-term effects of tetrabenazine in hyperkinetic movement disorders. Neurology **48**, 358–362 (1997)

[JT91]   Jennison, C., Turnbull, B.W.: Exact calculations for sequential t, χ^2, and F tests. Biometrika, **78**, 133–141 (1991)

[JT97]   Jennison, C., Turnbull, B.W.: Group-sequential analysis incorporating covariate information. Journal of the American Statistical Association **92**, 1330–1341 (1997)

[JT00]   Jennison, C., Turnbull, B.W.: Group Sequential Methods with Applications to Clinical Trials. Chapman and Hall/CRC, Boca Raton, FL (2000)

[JT03]   Jennison, C., Turnbull, B.W.: Mid-course sample size modification in clinical trials based on observed treatment effect. Statistics in Medicine **22**, 971–993 (2003)

[KF00]   Kieser, M., Friede, T.: Re-calculating the sample size in internal pilot study designs with control of the type I error rate. Statistics in Medicine **19**, 901–911 (2000)

[KF03]   Kieser, M., Friede, T.: Simple procedures for blinded sample size adjustment that do not affect the type I error rate. Statistics in Medicine **22**, 3571–3581 (2003)

[K89]   Kim, K.: Point estimation following group sequential tests. Biometrics, **45**, 613–617 (1989)

[KBP94]   Knatterud, G.,L. Bourassa, M.G., Pepine, C.J., et al. for the ACIP Investigators: Effects of treatment strategies to suppress ischemia in patients with coronary artery disease: 12-week results of the Asymptomatic Cardiac Ischemia Pilot (ACIP) study. Journal of the American College of Cardiology, **24**, 11–20 (1994)

[LW05]   Lachenbruch, P.A., Wittes, J.: Sentinel event methods for monitoring unanticipated adverse events. In press (2006)

[L01]   Lai, T.L.: Sequential analysis: some practical problems and new challenges. Statistica Sinica **11**, 303–408 (2001)

[L88]   Lakatos, E.: Sample size based on the logrank statistic in complex clinical trials. Biometrics **44**, 229–241 (1988)

[LD83]   Lan, K., DeMets, D.: Discrete sequential boundaries for clinical trials. Biometrika, **70**, 659–63 (1983)

[LD89a]   Lan, K.K., DeMets, D.L.: Group sequential procedures: Calendar versus information time. Statistics in Medicine, **8**, 1191–1198 (1989a).

[LD89b]   Lan, K.K., DeMets, D.L.: Changing frequency of interim analysis in sequential monitoring. Biometrics **45**, 1017–1020 (1989b)

[LSH82]   Lan, K.K., Simon, R., Halperin, M.: Stochastically curtailed tests in long-term clinical trials. Commun. Statist.-Sequential Analysis **1**, 207–19 (1982)

[LS05]   Lan, K.K., Soo, Y: Optimality and flexibility in sample size re-estimation. International Chinese Statistical Association Bulletin **July**, 45–47 (2005)

[LT97]   Lan, K.K., Trost, D.C.: Estimation of parameters and sample size re-estimation. American Statistical Association Proceedings of the Bio-pharmaceutical Section (1997)

[LW85]   Lan, K.K., Wittes, J.: Rank tests for survival analysis: A comparison by analogy with games 1063–1069 (1985)

[LW88]   Lan, K.K., Wittes, J.: The B-value: A tool for monitoring data. Biometrics, **44**, 579–85 (1988)

[LW90]   Lan, K.K., Wittes, J.: Linear rank tests for survival data: Equivalence of two formulations. The American Statistician **44**, 23–26 (1990)

[LZ93]   Lan, K.K., Zucker, D.M.: Sequential monitoring of clinical trials: The role of information and Brownian motion. Statistics in Medicine, **12**, 753–765 (1993)

[LW99]   Lehmacher, W., Wassmer, G.: Adaptive sample size calculations in group sequential trials. Biometrics, **55**, 1286–1290 (1999)

[LL92]   Lin, D.Y., and Liu, P.Y.: Nonparametric sequential tests against or-dered alternatives in multi-armed clinical trials. Biometrika **79**, 420–425 (1992)

[LAP04]   Liu, Q., Anderson, K.M., Pledger, G.W.: Benefit-risk evaluation of multi-stage adaptive designs. Sequential Analysis **23**, 317–331 (2004)

[LH99]   Liu, A., Hall, W.J.: Unbiased estimation following a group sequential test. Biometrika **86**, 71–78 (1999)

[LRO00]   Luepker, R.V., Raczynski, J.M., Osganian, S., et al. for the REACT study group: Effect of a community intervention on patient delay and emergency medical service use in acute coronary heart disease: The Rapid Early Action for Coronary Treatment (REACT) trial. Journal of the American Medical Association, **284**, 60–67 (2000)

[MW47]   Mann, H.B., Whitney, D.R.: On a test of whether one of two random variables is stochastically larger than the other. Annals of Mathematical Statistics **18**, 50–60 (1947)

[M66]   Mantel, N. Evaluation of survival data and two new rank order statistics arising in its consideration. Cancer Chemotherapy Reports, **50**, 163–170 (1966)

[MH59]   Mantel, N., Haenszel, W.: Statistical aspects of the analysis of data from retrospective studies of disease. Journal of the National Cancer Institute 22, 719–748 (1959)

[MWG97]   McMahon, R.P., Waclawiw, M.A., Geller, N.L., et al.: An extension of stochastic curtailment for incompletely reported and classified recurrent events: The Multicenter Study of Hydroxyurea in Sickle Cell Anemia (MSH). Controlled Clinical Trials **18**, 420–430 (1997)

[MH4]   Mehrota, D.V. and Heyse, J.F.: Use of the false discovery rate for eval-uating clinical safety data. Statistical Methods in Medical Research **13**, 227–238 (2004)

[M05]   Mehta, C. ENAR 2005 talk paper.

[M75]   Meier, P.: Statistics and medical experimentation. Biometrics **31**, 511–529 (1975)

[M98]   Miller, R.G. Jr.: Survival Analysis. Wiley, New York (1998)

[MDA05]   Montori, V.M., Devereaux, P.J., Adhikari, N.K. et al. Randomized trials stopped early for benefit. A systematic review. Journal of the American Medical Association **294**, 2203–2209 (2005)

[MGB74]   Mood, A.M., Graybill, F.A., Boes, D.C.: Introduction to the Theory of Statistics. McGraw-Hill, New York (1974)

[M95]   Moore, T.J.: Deadly Medicine: Why Tens of Thousands of Heart Patients Died in America's Worst Drug Disaster. Simon & Shuster, New York (1995)

[MHC96]   Moss, A.J., Hall, W.J., Cannom, D.S., et al.: Improved survival with an implanted defibrillator in patients with coronary disease at high risk for ventricular arrhythmia. The New England Journal of Medicine **335**, 1933–40 (1996)

[MB54]   Mosteller, F., Bush, R.R.: Selected Quantitative Techniques, in Handbook of Social Psychology (G. Lindzey, Ed.). Addison-Wesley, Cambridge, MA. (1954)

[OF79]   O'Brien, P.C., Fleming, T.R.: A multiple testing procedure for clinical trials. Biometrics **35**, 549–556 (1979)

[O45]   Orwell, G. Animal Farm. Harcourt Brace, New York (1945)

[PH90]   Pawitan, Y. and Hallstrom, A.: Statistical interim monitoring of the Cardiac Arrhythmia Suppression Trial. Statistics in Medicine **9**, 1081–1090 (1990)

[PP72]   Peto, R., Peto, J.: Asymptotically efficient rank invariant test procedures. Journal of the Royal Statistical Society A **135**, 185–198 (1972)

[PRZ03]   Pitt, B., Remme, W., Zannad, F., et al.: Eplerenone, a selective aldosterone blocker, in patients with left ventricular dysfunction after myocardial infarction. The New England Journal of Medicine **348**, 1309–21 (2003)

[PZW99]   Pitt, B., Zannad, F., Remme, W.J., et al. for the Randomized Aldactone Evaluation Study Investigators: The effect of spironolactone on morbidity and mortality in patients with severe heart failure. The New England Journal of Medicine **341**, 709–717 (1999)

[P77]   Pocock, S.J.: Group sequential methods in the design and analysis of clinical trials. Biometrika **64**, 191–199 (1977)

[Po05]   Pocock, S.J.: When (not) to stop a clinical trial for benefit. Journal of the American Medical Association **294**, 2228–2230 (2005)

[P78]   Prentice, R.L.: Linear rank tests with right censored data. Biometrika **65**, 167–179 (1978)

[Pr05]   Proschan, M.A.: Two-stage adaptive methods based on a nuisance parameter: A review. Journal of Biopharmaceutical Statistics **4**, 559–574 (2005)

[P99]   Proschan, M.A.: Properties of spending function boundaries. Biometrika **86**, 466–473 (1999)

[P04]   Proschan, M.A.: The geometry of two-stage tests. Statistica Sinica **13**, 163–177 (2004)

[PFW92]   Proschan, M.A., Follmann, D.A., Waclawiw, M.A.: Effects of assumption violations on type I error rate in group sequential monitoring. Biometrics **48**, 1131–1143 (1992)

[PH95]   Proschan M.A., Hunsberger, S.A.: Designed extension of studies based on conditional power. Biometrics **51**, 1315–1324 (1995)

[PMS01]   Proschan, M., McMahon, R., Shih, J., et al.: Sensitivity analysis using an imputation method for missing binary data in clinical trials. Journal of Statistical Planning and Inference **96**, 155–165 (2001)

[PW00]   Proschan, M.A., Wittes, J.: An improved double sampling procedure based on the variance. Biometrics **56**, 1183–1187 (2000)

[RW79]   Randles, R.H., Wolfe, D.A.: Introduction to the Theory of Nonparametric Statistics. Wiley, New York (1979)

[RT88]   Rosner, G.L., Tsiatis, A.A.: Exact confidence intervals following a group sequential trial: A comparison of methods. Biometrika **75**, 723–729 (1988)

[S56]   Savage, I.R.: Contributions to the theory of rank order statistics—the two sample case. Annals of Mathematical Statistics **27**, 590–615 (1956)

[S81]   Schoenfeld, D.: The asymptotic properties of nonparametric tests for comparing survival distributions. Biometrika **68**, 316–319 (1981)

[S80]   Serfling, R.J.: Approximation Theorems of Mathematical Statistics. Wiley, New York (1980)

[SF99]   Shen, Y., Fisher, L.: Statistical inference for self-designing clinical trials with a one-sided hypothesis. Biometrics **55**, 190–197 (1999)

[S05]   Shih, W.J.: Group sequential, sample size re-estimation and two-stage adaptive designs in clinical trials: a comparison. Statistics in Medicine **25**, 933–941 (2006)

[S04]   Singh, D.: Merck withdraws arthritis drug worldwide. British Medical Journal **329**, 816 (2004)

[SMP05]   Solomon, S.D., McMurray, J.J.V., Pfeffer, M.A., et al. for the Adenoma Prevention with Celecoxib (APC) study investigators: Cardiovascular risk associated with celecoxib in a clinical trial for colorectal ademoma prevention. The New England Journal of Medicine **352**, 1071–1080 (2005)

[SF88]   Spiegelhalter, D.J., Freedman, L.S.: Bayesian approaches to clinical trials. Bayesian Statistics **3**, 453–477 (1988)

[SFB86]   Spiegelhalter, D.J., Freedman, L.S., Blackburn, P.R.: Monitoring clinical trials: Conditional or predictive power? Controlled Clinical Trials **7**, 8–17 (1986)

[S45]   Stein, C.: A two-sample test for a linear hypothesis whose power is independent of the variance. Annals of Mathematical Statistics **16**, 243–258 (1945)

[SSD49]   Stouffer, S.A., Suchman, E.A., DeVinney, L.C., Star, S.A., Williams, R.M.: The American Soldier, Volume 1. Adjustment During Army Life. Princeton University Press, Princeton (1949)

[TXK98]   Tan, M., Xiong, X., Kutner, M. H.: Clinical trial designs based on sequential conditional probability ratio tests and reverse stochastic curtailing. Biometrics **54**, 682–695 (1998)

[TLC01]   Thompson, S.J., Leight, L., Christensen, R.: Immediate neurocognitive effects of methylphenidate on learning-impaired survivors of childhood cancer. Journal of Clinical Oncology **19**, 1802–1808 (2001)

[T82]   Tsiatis, A.A.: Repeated significance testing for a general class of statistics used in censored survival analysis. Journal of the American Statistical Association **77**, 855–861 (1982)

[TM03]   Tsiatis, A.A., Mehta, C.: On the inefficiency of the adaptive design for monitoring clinical trials. Biometrika **90**, 367–378 (2003)

[W47]   Wald, A.: Sequential Analysis. Wiley, New York (1947)

[W97]   Whitehead, J.: The Design and Analysis of Sequential Clinical Trials, 2nd ed. Wiley, New York (1997)

[W45]   Wilcoxon, F.: Individual comparisons by ranking methods. Biometrics **1**, 80–83 (1945)

[W96]   Wittes, J.: A statistical perspective on adverse event reporting in clinical trials. Biopharmaceutical Report, 5–10 (Fall 1996)

[WB90]   Wittes, J., Brittain, E.: The role of internal pilot studies in increasing the efficiency of clinical trials. Statistics in Medicine **9**, 65–72 (1990)

[WSZ99]   Wittes, J., Schabenberger, O., Zucker, D., et al.: Internal pilot studies I: Type I error rate of the naive t-test. Statistics in Medicine **18**, 3481–3491 (1999)

[WHI02]   Writing Group for the Women's Health Initiative Investigators: Risks and benefits of estrogen plus progestin in healthy postmenopausal women. Journal of the American Medical Association, **288**, 321–333 (2002)

[YPL85]   Yusuf, S., Peto, R., Lewis, J., et al.: Beta blockade during and after myocardial infarction: An overview of the randomized trials. Progress in Cardiovascular Diseases, **XXVII**, 335–371 (1985)

[ZWS99]   Zucker, D.M., Wittes, J.T., Schabenberger, O., Brittain, E.: Internal Pilot Studies II: Comparison of various procedures. Statistics in Medicine **18**, 3493–3509 (1999)

Index

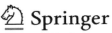
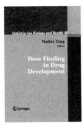

Dose Finding in Drug Development

Naitee Ting (Editor)

This book introduces the drug development process, the design and analysis of clinical trials. Many of the discussions are based on applications of statistical methods in the design and analysis of dose response studies. Although the book is prepared mainly for statisticians/biostatisticians, it also serves as a useful reference to a variety of professionals working for the pharmaceutical industry. The potential readers include pharmacokienticists, clinical scientists, clinical pharmacologists, pharmacists, project managers, pharmaceutical scientists, clinicians, programmers, data managers, regulatory specialists, and study report writers. This book is also a good reference for professionals working in a drug regulatory environment, for example, the FDA. Scientists and/or reviewers from both U.S. and foreign drug regulatory agencies can benefit greatly from this book. In addition, statistical and medical professionals in academia may find this book helpful in understanding the drug development process and practical concerns in selecting doses for a new drug.

2006. 255 p. (Statistics for Biology and Health) Hardcover ISBN 0-387-29074-5

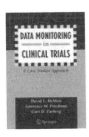

Data Monitoring in Clinical Trials: A Case Study Approach

David DeMets, Curt Furberg, and Lawrence Friedman (Editors)

Randomized clinical trials are the gold standard for establishing many clinical practice guidelines and are central to evidence based medicine. Obtaining the best evidence through clinical trials must be done within the boundaries of rigorous science and ethical principles. One fundamental principle is that trials should not continue longer than necessary to reach their objectives. Therefore, trials must be monitored for recruitment progress, quality of data, adherence to patient care or prevention standards, and early evidence of benefit or harm. Frequently, a group of external experts, independent from the investigators and trial sponsor, is charged with this monitoring responsibility, especially for safety and early benefit. This group is referred to by various names, such as a data monitoring committee or a data and safety monitoring board. This book, through a series of case studies presented by many distinguished clinical trial experts, illustrates the complexity of this monitoring process. The editors provide an overview of the process and a summary of a multitude of the lessons learned from the cases presented.

2005. 288 p. Softcover ISBN 0-387-20330-3

Printed in the United States of America.